In Vivo Atlas of Deep Brain Structures

Springer-Verlag Berlin Heidelberg GmbH

S. Lucerna  F. M. Salpietro
C. Alafaci  F. Tomasello

# In Vivo Atlas
# of Deep Brain Structures

## With 3D Reconstructions

With 54 Plates and 40 Figures
in 265 Separate Illustrations, Mostly in Color

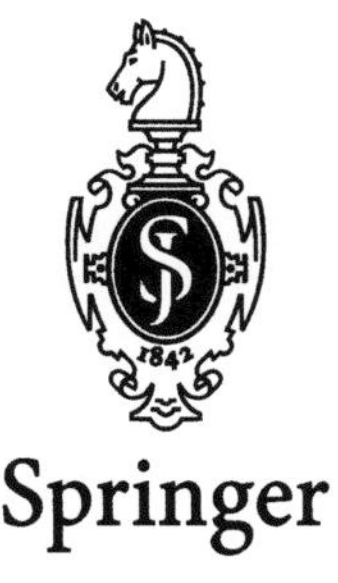

Springer

Dr. Sebastiano Lucerna
Prof. Dr. Francesco M. Salpietro
Prof. Concetta Alafaci
Prof. Francesco Tomasello

University of Messina
University Polyclinic "G.Martino", Department of Neurosurgery
Via Consolare Valeria 1, 98122, Messina, Italy

ISBN 978-3-642-62710-1

Library of Congress Cataloging-in-Publication Data
In vivo atlas of deep brain structures : with 3D reconstructions / S. Lucerna ... [et al.].
p. ; cm. Includes bibliographical references.
ISBN 978-3-642-62710-1      ISBN 978-3-642-56381-2 (eBook)
DOI 10.1007/978-3-642-56381-2
1. Brain - Anatomy - Atlases. 2. Brain - Imaging - Atlases. 3. Magnetic resonance imaging - Atlases.
I. Lucerna, S. (Sebastiano), 1957-.
[DNLM: 1. Brain - anatomy & histology - Atlases. 2. Magnetic Resonance Imaging - Atlases.
WL 17 I36 2002]   RC473.B7 I5 2002   611'.81'0222-dc21   2001049700



http://www.springer.de

© Springer-Verlag Berlin Heidelberg 2002
Originally published by Springer-Verlag Berlin Heidelberg New York in 2002
Softcover reprint of the hardcover 1st edition 2002



Cover design: Erich Kirchner, Heidelberg
Typesetting and reproduction of the figures: AM-productions GmbH, Wiesloch

Printed on acid-free paper          21/3111/op    5 4 3 2 1

# Preface

In the first half of the twentieth century, the study of neuroanatomy was essentially based on the observations made by scientists on brain cadavers fixed with standard techniques. These studies have produced well-known tools such as the stereotactic atlas, which have proven to be extremely useful and irreplaceable for neurosurgeons, neuroradiologists, neurologists and neuroanatomists. In particular, the Talairach and Schaltenbrandt atlases are considered the most prestigious and up-to-date work available today. The recent introduction of neuroimaging, especially nuclear magnetic resonance, together with the exciting and tremendous progress made in computer graphics, has allowed us to approach neuroanatomy directly in living patients with more accuracy and a high degree of detail.

This work, after a short introduction which explains the methodology used, is divided into four types of sections: three types of sections obtained from the same brain and orientated in the standard axial, sagittal, and coronal spatial planes and one type of section of three-dimensional pictures obtained from the computerized processing of the previous pictures.

The organization and the life-size tables obtained by magnetic resonance make this work similar to a classic stereotactic atlas, although the authors do not claim to reach the high level of precision which such atlases usually provide. The abbreviations used are based on Latin nomenclature, in order to be understood and recognized worldwide, and are supported by a system of color codes useful for the identification of brain structures.

By using the above techniques, the present atlas aims to make a contribution to the field of neuroanatomy. It emphasizes the importance of deep brain structures, as they are of great interest to neurosurgeons and neuroscientists, especially in light of the recent progress which has been made in the surgical treatment of Parkinson disease and other extrapyramidal disorders.

Messina, November 2001      The Authors

# Acknowledgements

The authors wish to express their gratitude to Professor M. Longo, Head of the Section of Neuroradiology at the University Polyclinic of Messina, for his invaluable help with the MRI documents. Special mention should also be made of Dr. G. Ricciardi, assistant to Prof. Longo, for his technical skill in performing MR imaging. Finally, we extend our most sincere thanks to Springer and especially to Ms. D. Mennecke-Bühler, Ms. I. Oppelt and Ms. A. Cerri (Springer Italia) for their kind cooperation during the preparation of this book.

Messina, November 2001                                          The Authors

# Contents

# The Reference System: The ca-cp Plane

Talairach (1955) and Schaltenbrandt (1977) suggested that the anterior and posterior commissure might be considered to have a constant relationship with the deep cerebral structures and proposed using a line between these two structures as the basic reference line. Talairach found only a negligible difference between the intercommissural distance in 26 brains (from 23 mm to 28.5 mm) and took the average of this distance as 25.5 mm in his proportional atlases (Talairach 1957, 1988, 1993).

The reference system used in our atlas is taken as the intercommissural plane passing through the center of the anterior and posterior commissures (Fig. 1). On such a plane, a system of Cartesian axes has been defined which originates in the center of the anterior commissure, with coordinates expressed in millimeters with a positive sign superiorly (axial plane), anteriorly (coronal plane), and laterally (sagittal plane) with respect to the origin. In this way each structure can be identified in the three-dimensional (3D) space from a triplet of coordinates (axial, coronal, sagittal) on the corresponding magnetic resonance imaging (MRI) slice on a 1:0.87* scale and on the relevant magnified plate. We have found it useful not to normalize such a system with a proportional scale, because the interindividual variability in the deep cerebral structures can be effectively compensated for through a simple proportion between the standard intercommissural distance of the present atlas, which is about 28 mm, and the corresponding measurement on the patient's MRI. Such a system of reference is also useful for the 3D reconstruction image tables. All plans constitute a kind of parallelepiped (Fig. 2) 48 mm high, 66 mm long, and 76 mm wide. The anatomical structures of our atlas are represented in this manner.

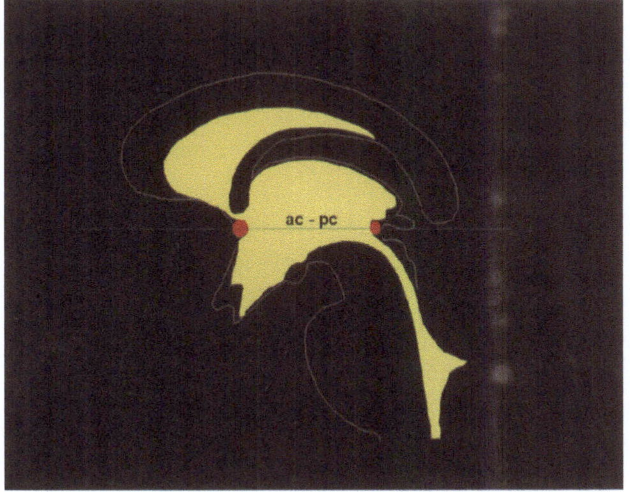


**Fig. 1.** The intercommissural plane

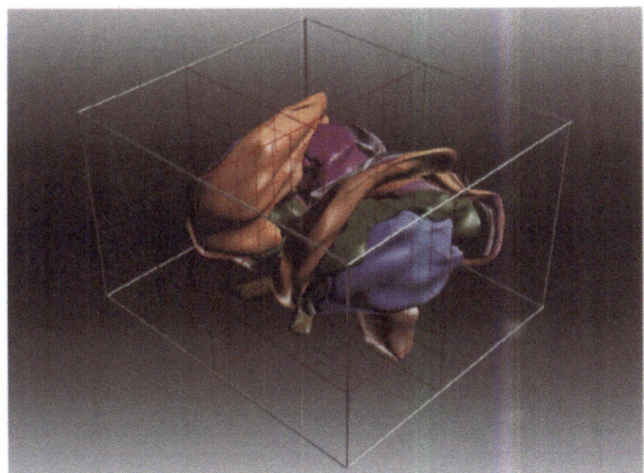

**Fig. 2.** Three-dimensional spatial limits

---

* Unfortunately, 1:1 scale could not be used for reasons of technical production.

# MRI Technique

The study of basal ganglia and other deep brain structures is one of the most remarkable examples of the utility of morphological MR studies not only for diagnostic purposes, but also for the preparation and accurate guidance of neurosurgery and stereotactic radiotherapy.

However, this is only true if high filed MR imagers with a homogeneous magnetic field and homogenous gradients are used. T1-weighted MR studies are the most suitable for morphological study of the basal ganglia, both because of their high fidelity in anatomical structure depiction and their high intrinsic gray matter to white matter (GM/WM) contrast.

The sequences most suitable for obtaining T1-w images with these characteristics are conventional spin echo (SE), volumetric gradient echo (GE-3D), and inversion recovery (IR) sequences. All three have complementary advantages and disadvantages, so that one or the other must be selected according to the type of information required.

Conventional SE is the least sensitive to motion artifacts and an intermediate number of sections can be obtained in an average time (15 with a TR of 750 ms). On the other hand, they are the least efficient as regards signal/noise ratio (S/N) and contrast/noise ratio (C/N).

The employment of turbo factors is significantly limited since the number of sections per acquisition and image contrast are greatly reduced.

Magnetization prepared rapid 3D-GE (MP-RAGE), also known as volumetric spoiled gradient echo (3D-SPGR), are globally the most efficient of the three groups of sequences. They demonstrate very good S/N and C/N ratios: a very high number of sections (>120) can be acquired which are so thin (1-1.5 mm) that it is possible to obtain nearly isotropic voxels and, as a consequence, produce high-quality multi-planar reconstructions. In addition, they are the least sensitive to distortion artifacts, commonly present when imaging structures situated near air-bone parenchyma interfaces.

However, these sequences also present significant drawbacks, such as a high sensitivity to motion artifacts and reconstruction artifacts as a result of processing algorithms and voxel anisotropy. In fact, the latter is a serious disadvantage because, due to 3D-Fourier transform (3D-FFT), this sequence produces significant aliasing artifacts in the head-to-feet direction, when obtained on the axial plane.

IR represents the last class of sequences which provide high-quality images of the brain. These utilize additional RF pulses (inversion pulses) to increase or modify the contrast between different structures. In particular, they better visualize the cerebral gray matter (cortex and deep nuclei) thanks to an inversion time (TI) of 250-400 ms, with which the signal from white matter is minimized and the GM/WM contrast optimized.

The sequence which can be attained by combining an IR showing these characteristics with the advantages of fast SE is commonly known as FIRMS (fast inversion recovery for myelin suppression).

This IR was optimized at the end of the 1990s at the radiology department of the New Jersey Medical School (USA).

The use of intermediary turbo factors (echo train length = ETL 5-9) does not alter the features of this sequence and enables optimal anatomical images to be achieved even in thin slices (2-3 mm), with high S/N and C/N ratios in short times (1 min 15 s per acquisition).

A 250-ms IT gives the best S/N and C/N ratios, while 16 kHz is the ideal bandwidth and 19-30 ms the optimal TE.

It has been shown that images obtained by means of FIRMS optimized with the above parameters show better performance in terms of signal and GM/WM contrast than other conventional SE and GE (2D or 3D) sequences.

In order to reduce acquisition time to a minimum and to enhance GM/WM contrast, FIRMS can be performed using a signal reconstruction technique based on the longitudinal magnetization magnitude

(magnitude reconstruction technique), rather than on its absolute value. The only drawback of this technique is cerebrospinal fluid (CSF) hyperintensity, which renders the images more like T2-weighted than T1-weighted ones.

The greatest disadvantages of FIRMS sequence are:

1. The notable deterioration of image quality when the slice thickness is reduced to below 3 mm
2. The presence of ghost artifacts due to pulsation of the main intracranial vessels and of CSF within cisterns and ventricles

A Magnetom Vision scanner (1.5 T, Siemens, Erlangen, Germany) was used for this atlas. Studies were always performed within 3 days from the last quality control of the main magnetic field and gradient homogeneity.

The FIRMS sequence which could be achieved with the above scanner had the following parameters: field of view (FOV) 220 · 165, matrix 168 · 256, slice thickness 3 mm, interslice gap 3 mm, ETL 7, TI 250 ms, TE 30, no. of acquisitions 3, TA 6 min – 7 min 20 s, no. of sections 7-12.

TR was the only parameter modified among the different acquisitions (value between 3,500 ms for seven sections and 5,600 for 12 sections), in order to obtain a sufficient number of sections to cover all the structures of interest in the shortest possible time.

To avoid any interference among contiguous sections, which is often responsible for disturbing artifacts mainly due to CSF flux, slices had a 3-mm thickness and were placed with an interslice gap of 3 mm (gap ratio =1).

Two images were acquired in each plane, offsetting the slices of the two studies by 3 mm in order to cover the whole region of interest and thus filling previously unacquired gaps.

We considered it useful to trigger all FIRMS sequences by heart cycles; in order to do this a rough ECG was obtained by applying three electrodes to the volunteer's back.

This technique prolonged the acquisition time by between 30% and 50% (on average from 6 min 30 s to 9 min 05 s), but resulted in almost complete elimination of ghost artifacts which, as already stated, are one of the major disadvantages of this sequence. Each study began with a careful positioning of the volunteer within the dedicated volumetric coil. Two laser beams intersecting at right angles were used as markers to place the head so that the basal ganglia region was as close as possible to the coil center and

to maintain a perfect symmetry between facial structures. Both the patients and the sections were always positioned by an expert radiographer (L.B.) under the author's supervision.

The first sequence to be acquired was a T1-weighted, rapid GE, lasting 16 s, with a wide FOV and one section for each of the three fundamental planes (scout). The resulting images were used to position a T1 SE (TR 300, TA 2 min) oriented on the sagittal plane and parallel to the interhemispheric fissure.

To avoid distortion effects caused by excessive use of slice selection gradients, when shift corrections of the sections at an angle to the magnetic field's longitudinal axis of greater than 2° were needed, the volunteer was repositioned.

The sagittal image passing through the interhemispheric fissure obtained with this sequence was used to localize the anterior and posterior white commissures. Only then was the study with FIRMS sequences started, in which a series of nine axial sections perpendicular to the median sagittal scan and parallel to the intercommissural plane were acquired. The anterior and posterior commissures were included in the central section.

The second group of axial sections was oriented in exactly the same way as the first, but shifted 3 mm cranially in order that the two groups could subsequently be perfectly interleaved. In this way a slab of brain covering the region between 28.5 mm cranially and 22.5 mm caudally to the intercommissural plane was studied, so that the entire basal ganglia region was included.

Subsequently, 12 coronal sections were positioned perpendicularly both to previously acquired axial scans and to the interhemispheric fissure. The center of the group was placed in order to correspond with the anterior commissure, so that the region between the more frontal part of the head of caudate nucleus anteriorly and the collicular plate posteriorly would be covered.

Twelve more coronal sections were acquired with the same orientation, but shifted 3 mm posteriorly in order to cover structures not included in the first group of images.

Finally, nine sagittal scans which were also perpendicular to the axial scans but parallel to the interhemispheric fissure were obtained. The most medial section was placed to run along the whole interhemispheric fissure and, therefore, included the anterior and posterior commissures, while the remaining sections covered the left hemisphere up to the internal part of the lobus insularis. In this case, the study was also completed by acquiring the nine sections shifted 3 mm to the left.

The entire procedure, including head positioning, scout performing, and acquisition of FIRMS images on the three planes, took on average 1 h. For the study to be valid, the volunteer's head should not have moved more than 2 mm from its original position. In order to verify this, the T1-weighted rapid GE on the three axis was repeated and superimposed, by means of a digital image addition, to the scout obtained at the beginning of the whole procedure. A mismatch greater than 2 mm in one of the three axes invalidated the study.

The gray scale of all the images obtained with FIRMS sequence was then inverted, so that a contrast between structures more similar to that of conventional T1-weighted IR sequences could be displayed.

Images of the whole study were finally transferred to a PC in a DICOM III format, by means of a service class provider (SCP) program.

# Magnified 2D Plate Reconstructions

## Spatial Limits and Magnification Factors

In the atlas, the spatial limits of 2D area reconstructions are given, taking into account the extension of the principal deep brain nuclei and their relationships with the ventricular system:

1. Anteriorly in the more frontal part of the head of caudate nucleus, about 27 mm from the anterior commissure
2. Posteriorly tangential to the collicular plate, about 39 mm from the anterior commissure
3. Superiorly in the more cranial part of the body of caudate nucleus, about 27 mm above the intercommissural plane
4. Inferiorly tangential to the lower part of the pituitary gland, about 21 mm below the intercommissural plane
5. Laterally tangential to the internal part of the lobus insularis, about 39 mm from the intercommissural plane
6. Medially on the midline

The magnification factor is 3x for axial and coronal reconstructions and 2x for sagittal reconstructions.

## Drawing Technique

The major advantages of an "in vivo brain" MRI atlas mainly consist in the absence of "post mortem" structural changes and artifacts induced by the techniques of prelevation, fixation, and histological sectioning. These changes may induce as a principal "side effect" a linear shrinkage of the brain which can be calculated from 5% (with a freezing technique) to more than 20% (celloidin or paraffin embedding). On the other hand, MRI slices have a limited spatial resolution and tissue characterization and a relatively large section thickness and may be affected by some distortion, particularly at the image margin.

These factors are the cause of the main problems of the drawing technique, which are correct outlining of the limits of the given structures in MRI slices and the overlapping of different structures in the same slice, the last being due to the 3-mm MRI slice thickness.

Concerning the first problem, the currently available graphic software offers several utilities to modify the contrast of the images, gray scales, and magnification, which, as a result of fine single pixel manipulation, offer better visualization of the transition zones between two different areas of the same image.

The second problem is very difficult to solve because many structures, such the nuclei of the thalamus, nucleus accumbens, the hypothalamic nuclei, and many others, are less than 3 mm in their maximum dimension and show the same signal in MRI images. For these reasons we believe that the 2D and 3D plates should be considered as "high probabilistic areas and volumes". We have not included in 2D and 3D reconstructions those structures which are not clearly documented on MRI or which show a high margin of reconstruction-induced error.

Although it is impossible to achieve a perfect result in terms of precision, reconstructions verified in stereotactic atlases (Schaltebrand, Talairach, Mai) have shown only minor differences, which are essentially due to interindividual anatomical variations.

The computerized post-MRI elaboration method of imaging utilized in the present atlas is described as follows:

1. Interpolated enhancement of resolution from 256x256 pixels in DICOM 3 format images to 1900x1900 pixels with conversion to TIFF (Tagged Image File Format) format, without modifying contrast or brightness (Figs. 3-5)
2. Correction of rotational errors greater than 0.2°

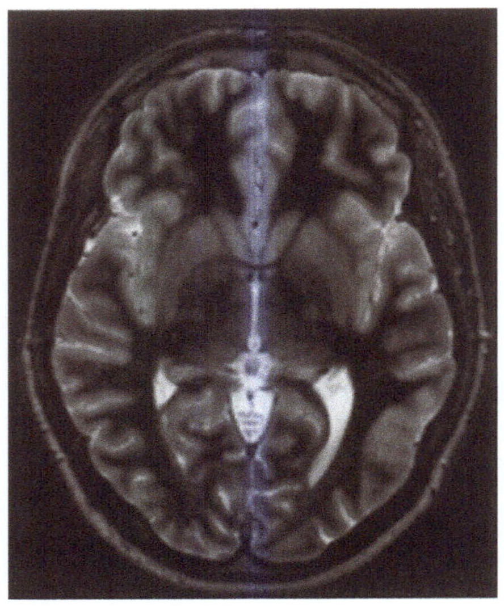

Fig. 3. MRI FIRMS original image

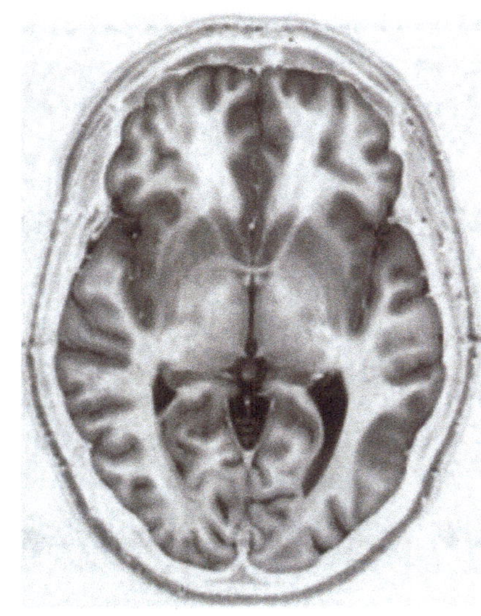

Fig. 4. MRI FIRMS inverted image

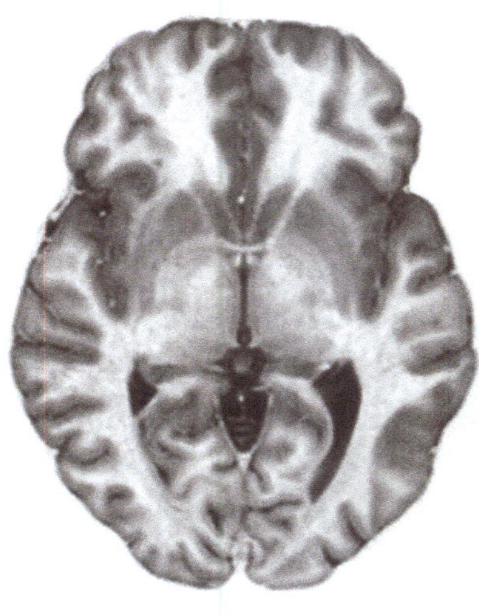

Fig. 5. MRI FIRMS image after computerized elaboration

3. Image marking with the reference system and the millimetric grid
4. Cropping of extracerebral structures (bone, muscles, and skin)
5. Outlining the structures of interest with a Bezier's curves drawing method (Fig. 6)
6. Image magnification and coloration according to a color code system
7. Image master printing with a high-resolution photographic printer

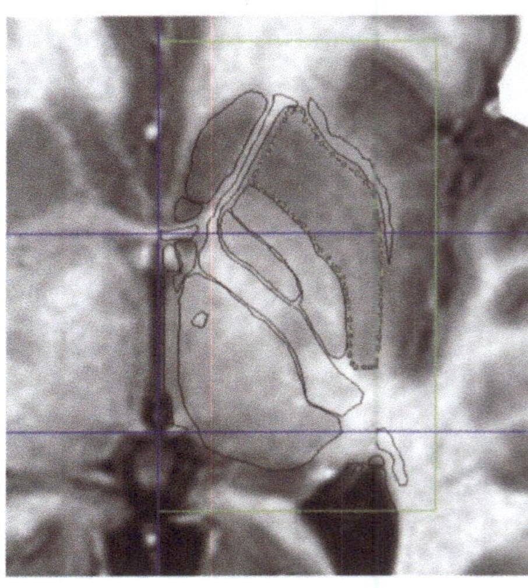

Fig. 6. Outlining the structures of interest using Bezier's ▷ curves drawing method

# 3D Plate Reconstructions: NURBS Modeling

Non-uniform rational B-splines, or NURBS, are some of the most commonly used geometric primitives in 3D modeling software today. With NURBS, free-form curves and surfaces as well as more traditional shapes, such as conics or quadrics can be clearly specified. NURBS were developed as a method of precisely specifying curves and surfaces for use by computer-controlled machines capable of producing shapes in 3D. With this technique, 3D models have smoother borders due to the analytic tessellation and are a very different from polygonal models, which are generally faceted. These properties of NURBS make it possible to create organic volumes such as brain deep gray nuclei.

The modeling procedure of our atlas follows essentially six steps:

1. Creation of a 2D NURBS curve adapted to the boundary of the structure for each MRI slice (Fig. 7)
2. Positioning each curve in the correct 3D space coordinates (Fig. 8)
3. Creation of a NURBS 3D surface by interpolating all bidimensional curves (Fig.8)
4. Rendering of objects by a raytrace method (Fig.8)
5. Positioning and regulation of the scene lights (Fig.8)
6. Producing the frame of each scene view (Fig.9)

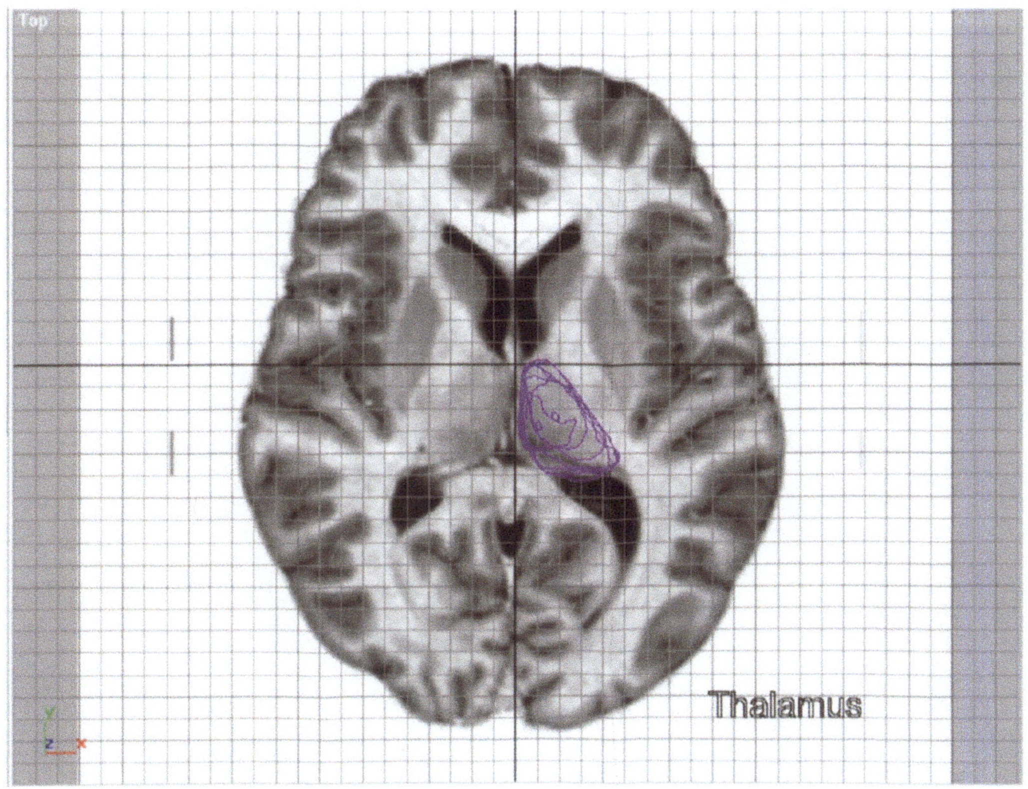


**Fig. 7.** Creation of a two-dimensional, adapted NURBS curve (Thalamus)

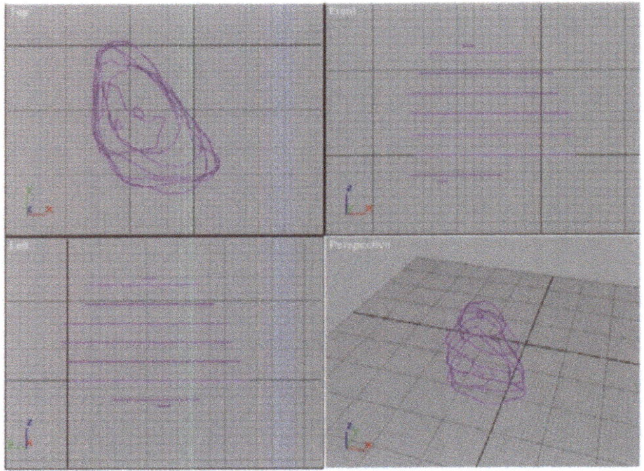

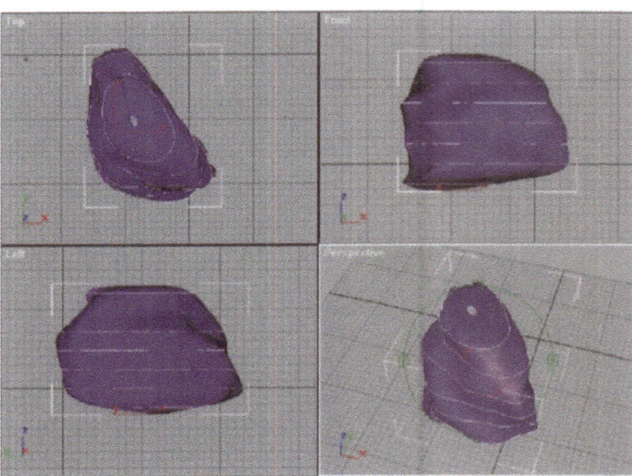

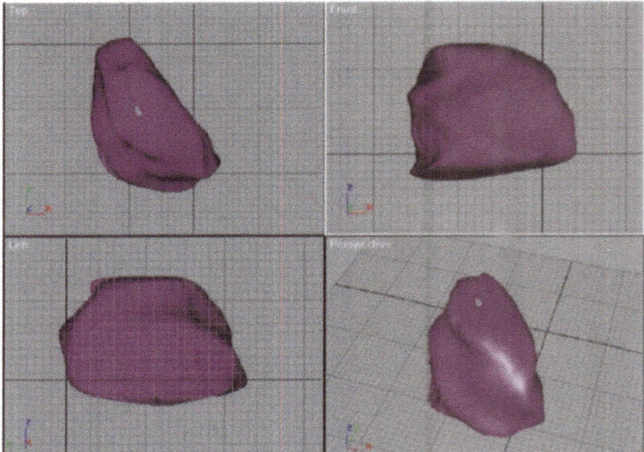

**Fig. 8.** Creation and rendering of a three-dimensional, adapted NURBS surface (Thalamus)

**Fig. 9.** Definitive three-dimensional image (thalamic region)

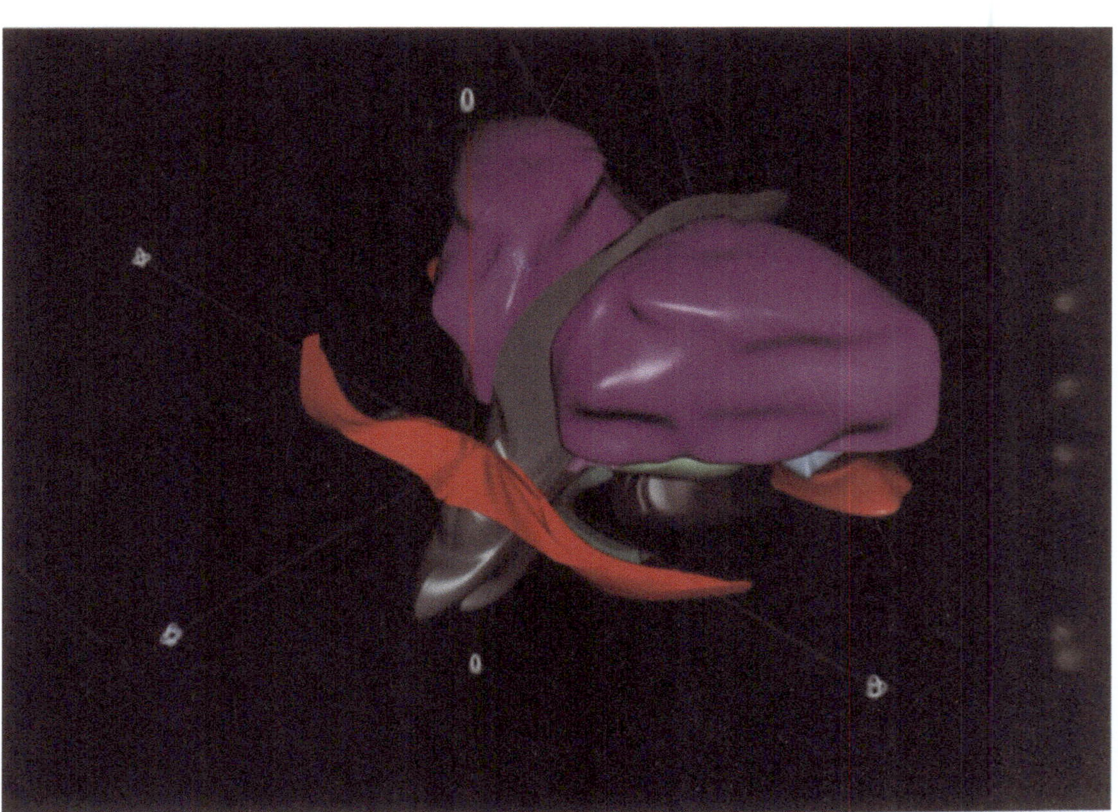

# Example of How To Use the Atlas

Although it is possible to use the present atlas with conventionally oriented CT scans and MRI images, the authors emphasize the importance of making a great effort to obtain ca-cp-oriented neuroradiological images, because, only in this way can optimal precision be gained from the atlas. With MRI images, this is very simple; in fact, the anterior and posterior commissure are almost always visible on a T1-weighted median sagittal slice. In contrast, on CT scan the orbitomeatal orientation (frequently used by neuroradiologists) is only rarely parallel to ca-cp plane; moreover, the commissures are not clearly visible in CT slices. Therefore, for a better CT scan orientation, in the author's experience, it is useful to tilt the gantry until it is parallel to a ideal line which joins the tuberculum sellae and the inferior part of internal occipital protuberance (both quite visible in the topogram).

As mentioned above, the interindividual anatomical variations may induce a greater or lesser loss in precision; nevertheless, a proportion between the two intercommissural distances (atlas - patient) can help to minimize this problem.

The following example (Fig.10) shows how to use the atlas for localizing the subthalamic nucleus of Luis (STN) in an axial MRI slice.

**Fig. 10.** Example of how to use the system

*Step 1:* Selection of patient's MRI slice corresponding to ca-cp-plane

**Step 2:** Measuring ca-cp distance (in this case was 24 mm)

*Step 3:* Calculating the magnification factor between patient and atlas images utilizing the intercommissural distance
(24 : 28 = 0.86)

▷

*Step 4:* Selection of corresponding axial atlas plates for STN and rela- ▽
tives coordinates (Ax-3, Cor-15, Sag 11)

*Step 5:* Converting coordinates in patient's coordinates
(-3 x 0.86 = 2.6; -16 x 0.86 = -13,8; 11 x 0.86 = 9.5)

*Step 6:* Application of the calculated coordinates on patient's image

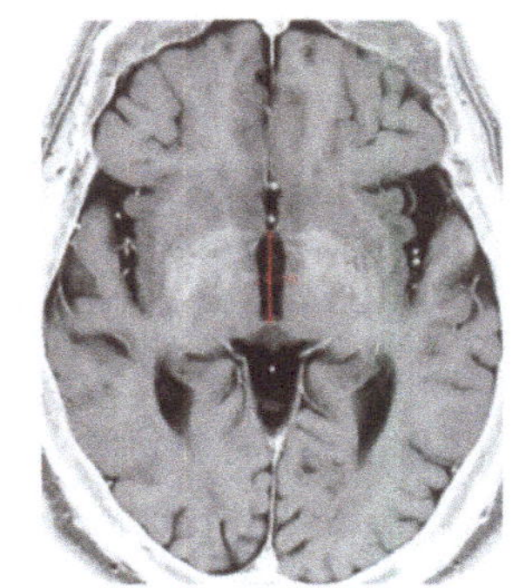

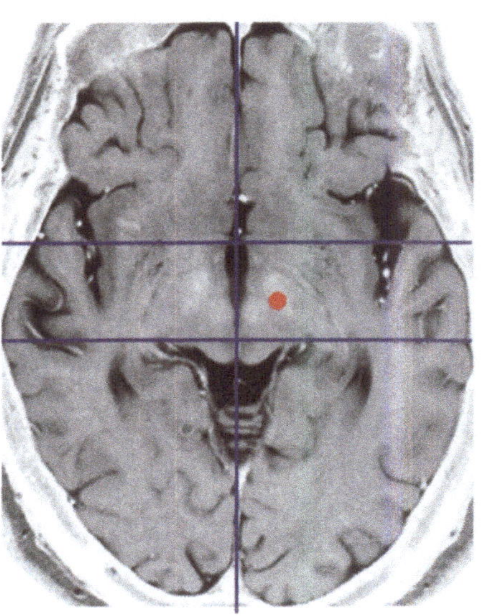

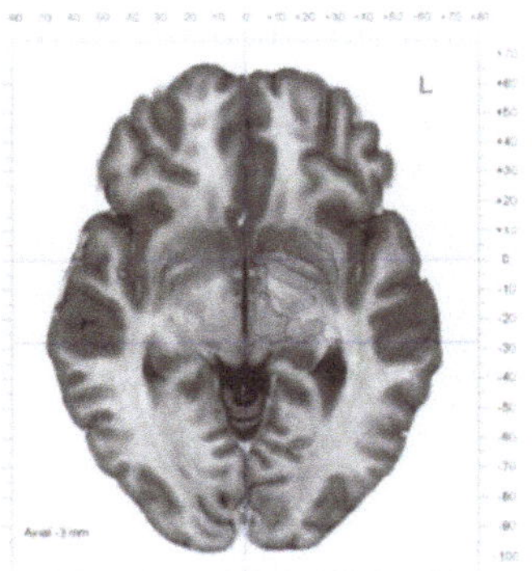

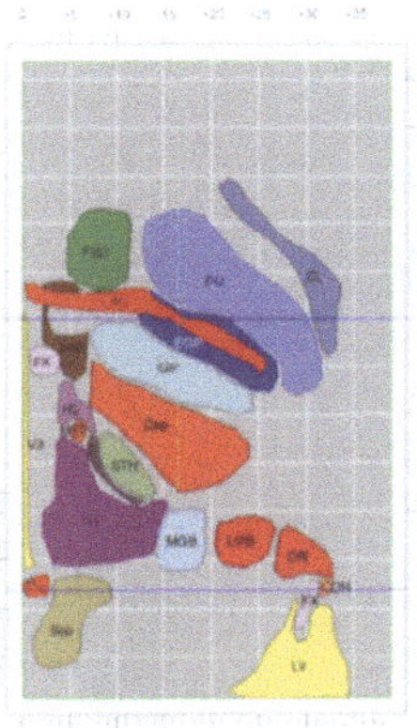

# Axial Sections

Plates 1-17

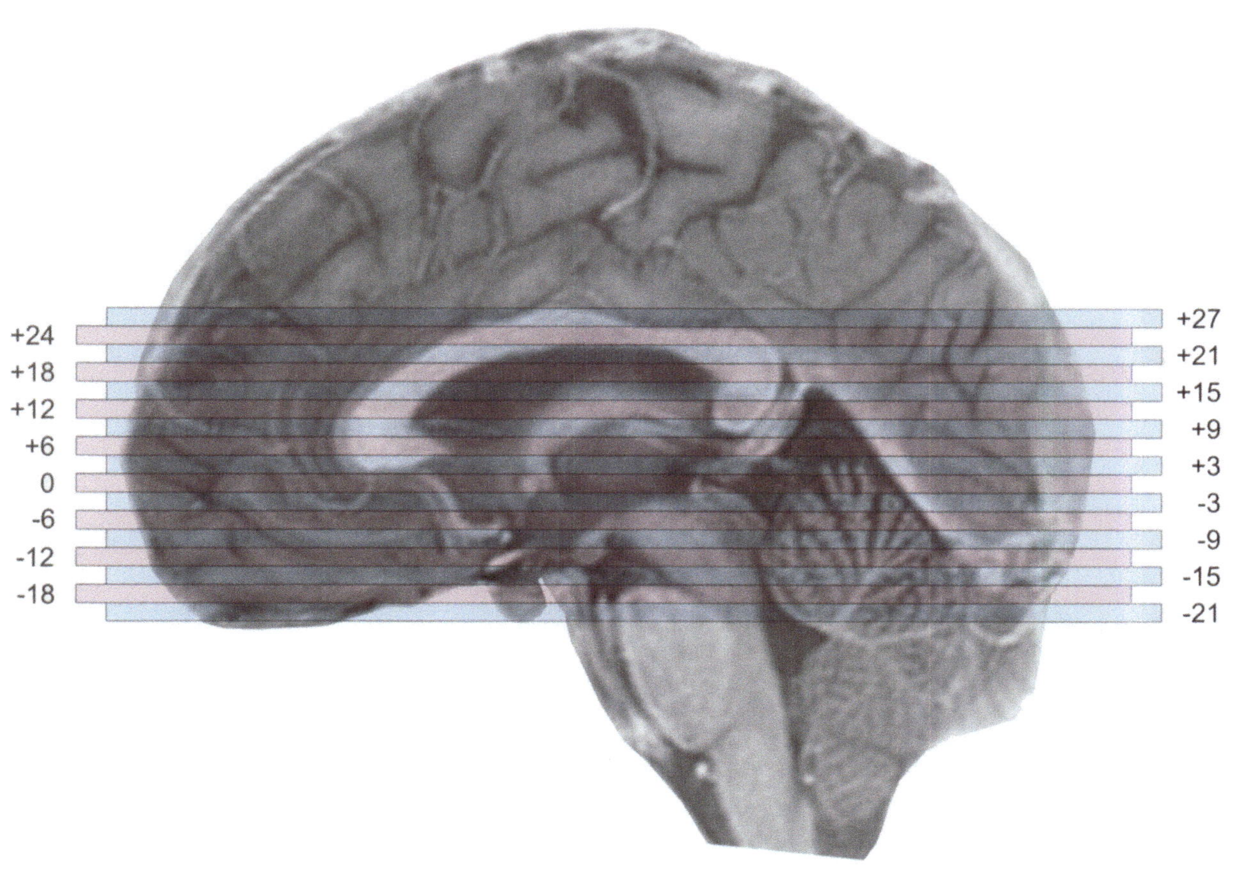

+24
+18
+12
+6
0
-6
-12
-18
+27
+21
+15
+9
+3
-3
-9
-15
-21


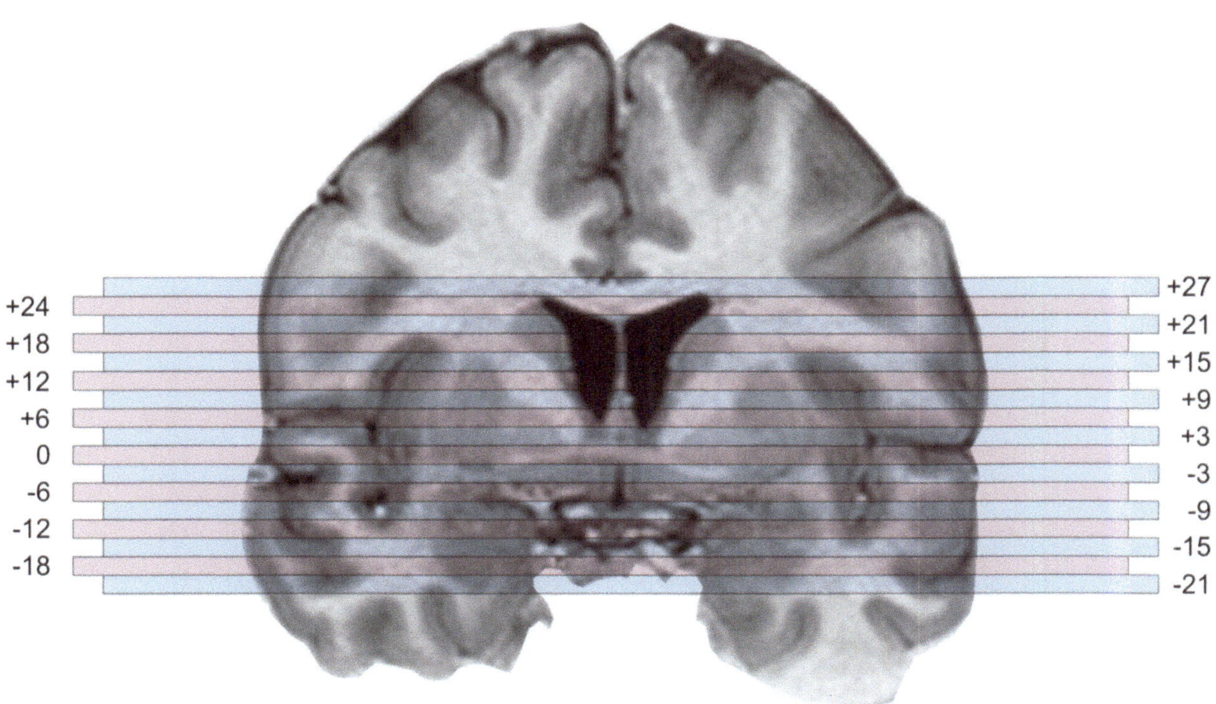

+24
+18
+12
+6
0
-6
-12
-18
+27
+21
+15
+9
+3
-3
-9
-15
-21

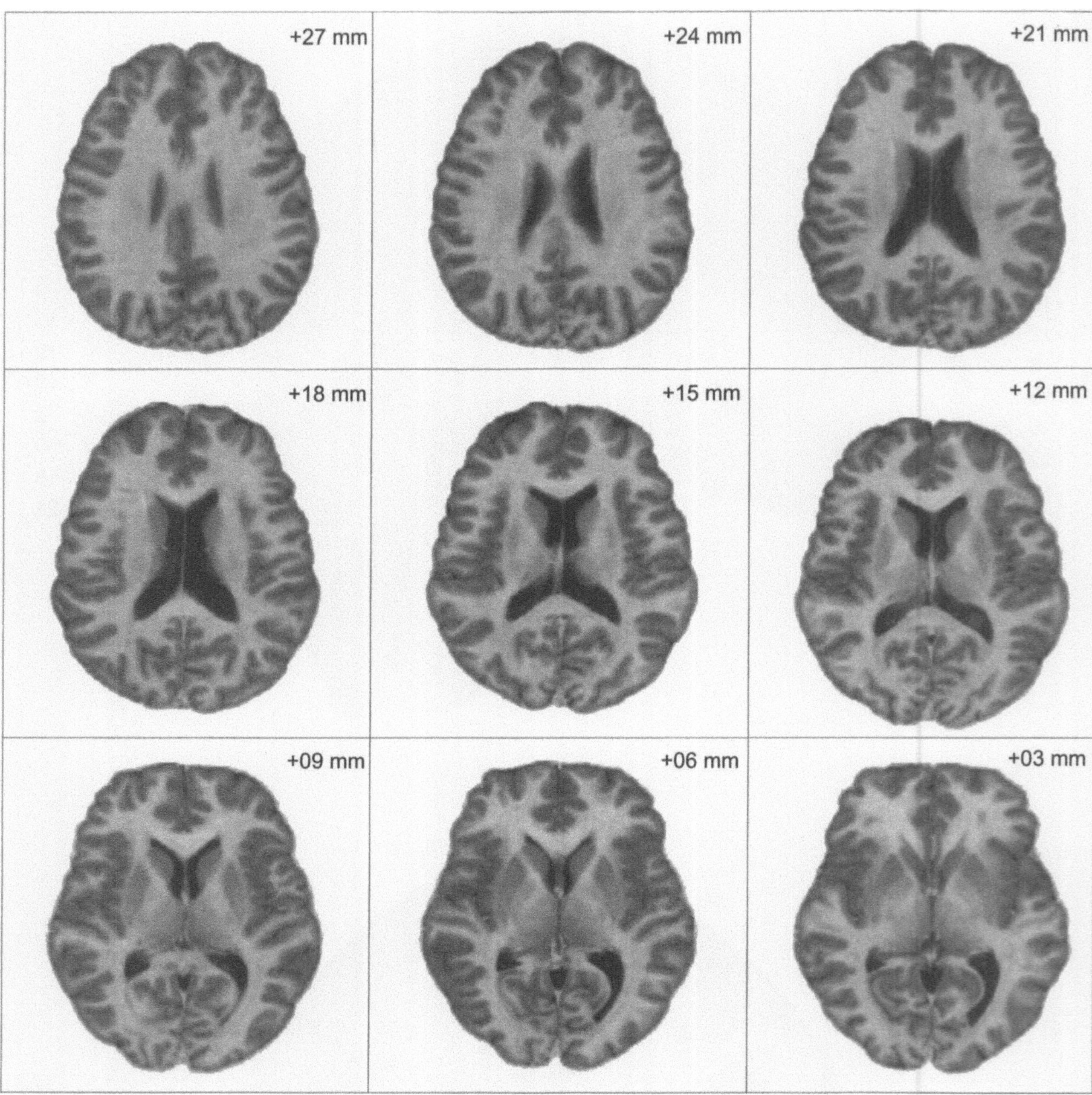
+27 mm
+24 mm
+21 mm
+18 mm
+15 mm
+12 mm
+09 mm
+06 mm
+03 mm

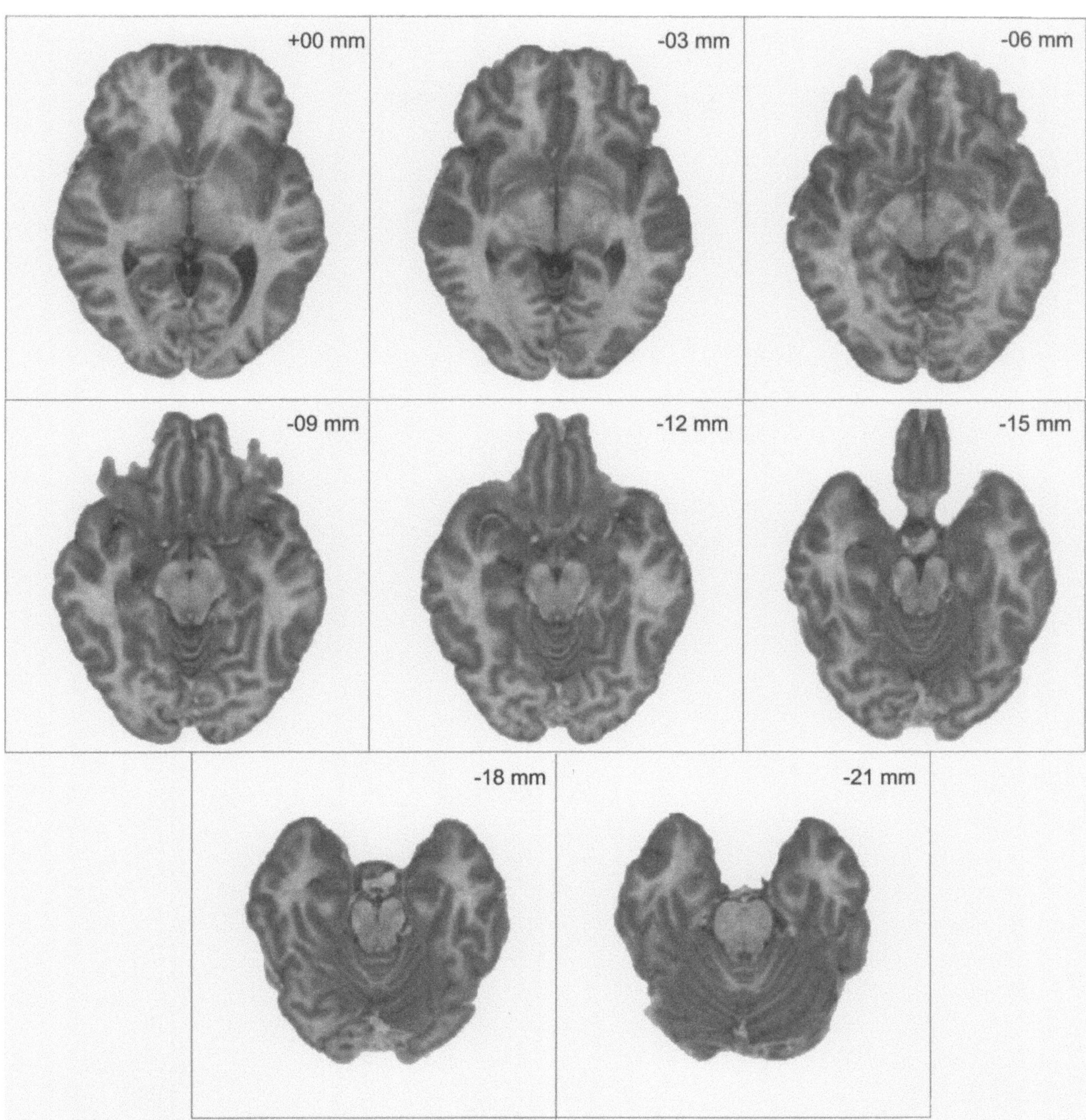

# Abbreviation – Nomenclature – Color Codes

| | | |
|---|---|---|
| **AC** | Anterior Commissure | |
| **AL** | Ansa Lenticularis | |
| **AN** | Amigdaloid Nucleus | |
| **CC** | Corpus Callosum | |
| **CDN** | Caudate Nucleus | |
| **Cep** | Cerebral peduncle | |
| **CL** | Claustrum | |
| **DE** | Diencephalon | |
| **EGP** | Ext.globus  pallidum | |
| **FSC** | Fundus striati, caudati | |
| **FX** | Fornix | |
| **H2** | H2 Forel's field | |
| **HY** | Hyppocampus | |
| **IC** | Internal Capsula | |

| | | |
|---|---|---|
| **Ico** | Inferior colliculus | |
| **IGP** | Int.  Globus Pallidum | |
| **LGB** | Lat. Geniculate Body | |
| **LV** | Lateral Ventricles | |
| **MB** | Mammillary Body | |
| **MGB** | Med. Genic. Body | |
| **MTT** | Mammillo thal. tract | |
| **OC** | Optic Chiasm | |
| **OR** | Optic Radiation | |
| **OT** | Optic Tract | |
| **PC** | Post. Commissure | |
| **PG** | Pineal Gland | |
| **PHN** | Paraventricular Hypothalamic Nuclei | |

| | | |
|---|---|---|
| **PU** | Putamen | |
| **RN** | Red Nucleus | |
| **TH** | Thalamus | |
| **Sco** | Superior Colliculus | |
| **SN** | Substantia Nigra | |
| **STN** | Subthalamic Nucleus | |
| **V3** | Third ventricle | |
| **ZI** | Zona Incerta | |

# Plate 1a

-80 -70 -60 -50 -40 -30 -20 -10 0 +10 +20 +30 +40 +50 +60 +70 +80
+70
+60
+50
+40
+30
+20
+10
0
-10
-20
-30
-40
-50
-60
-70
-80
-90
-100
L
Axial +27 mm

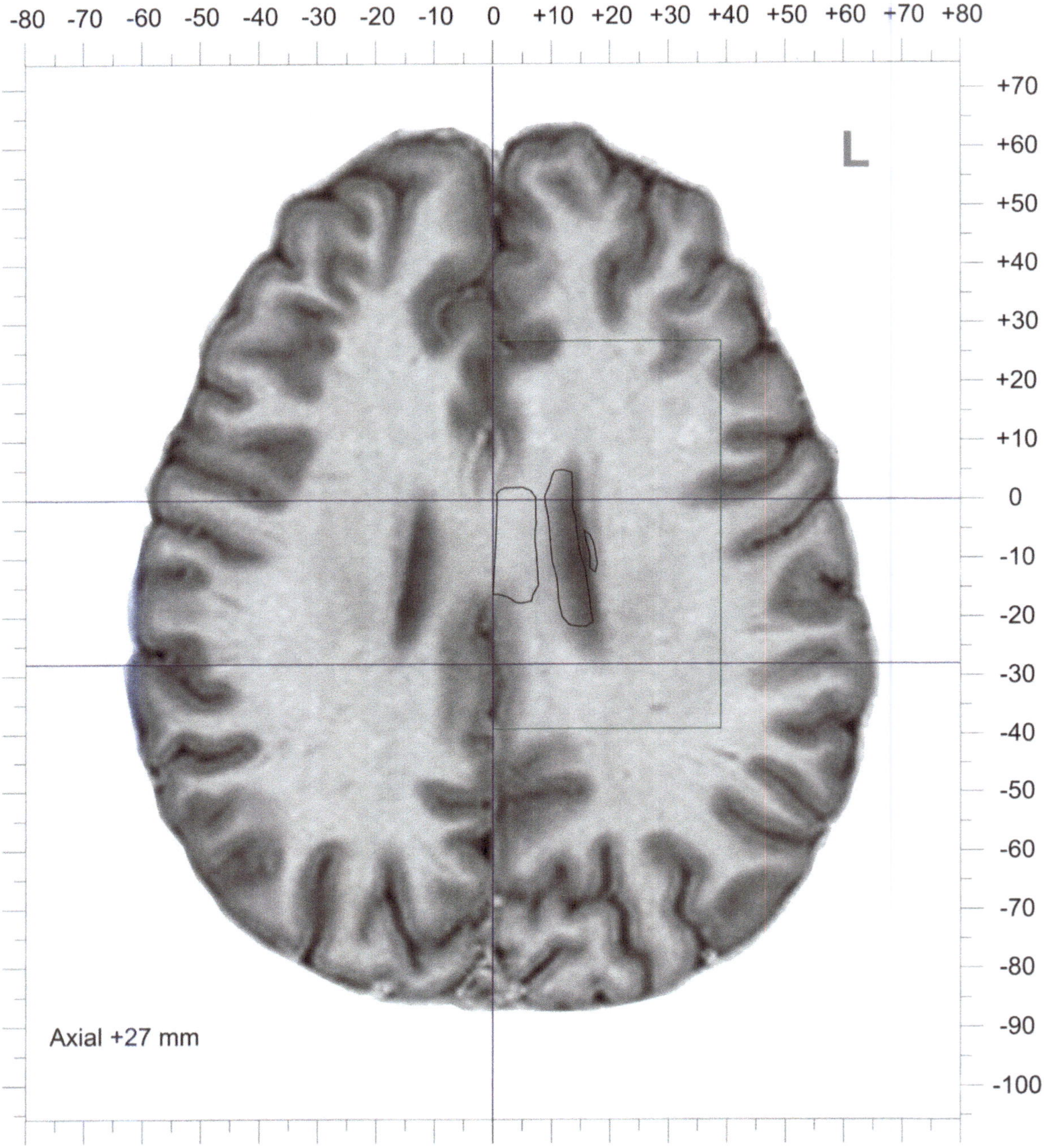

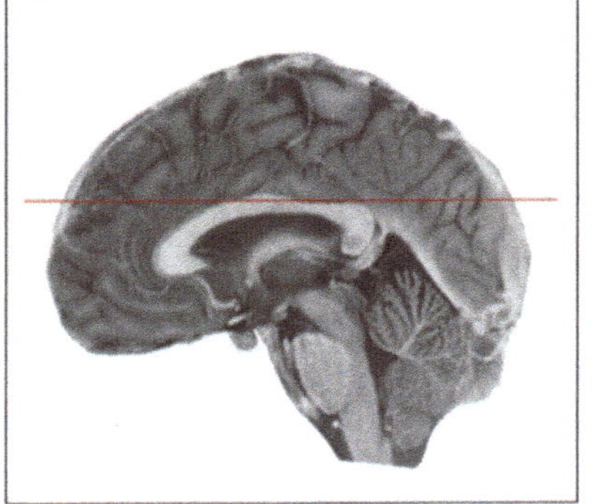

## Plate 1b

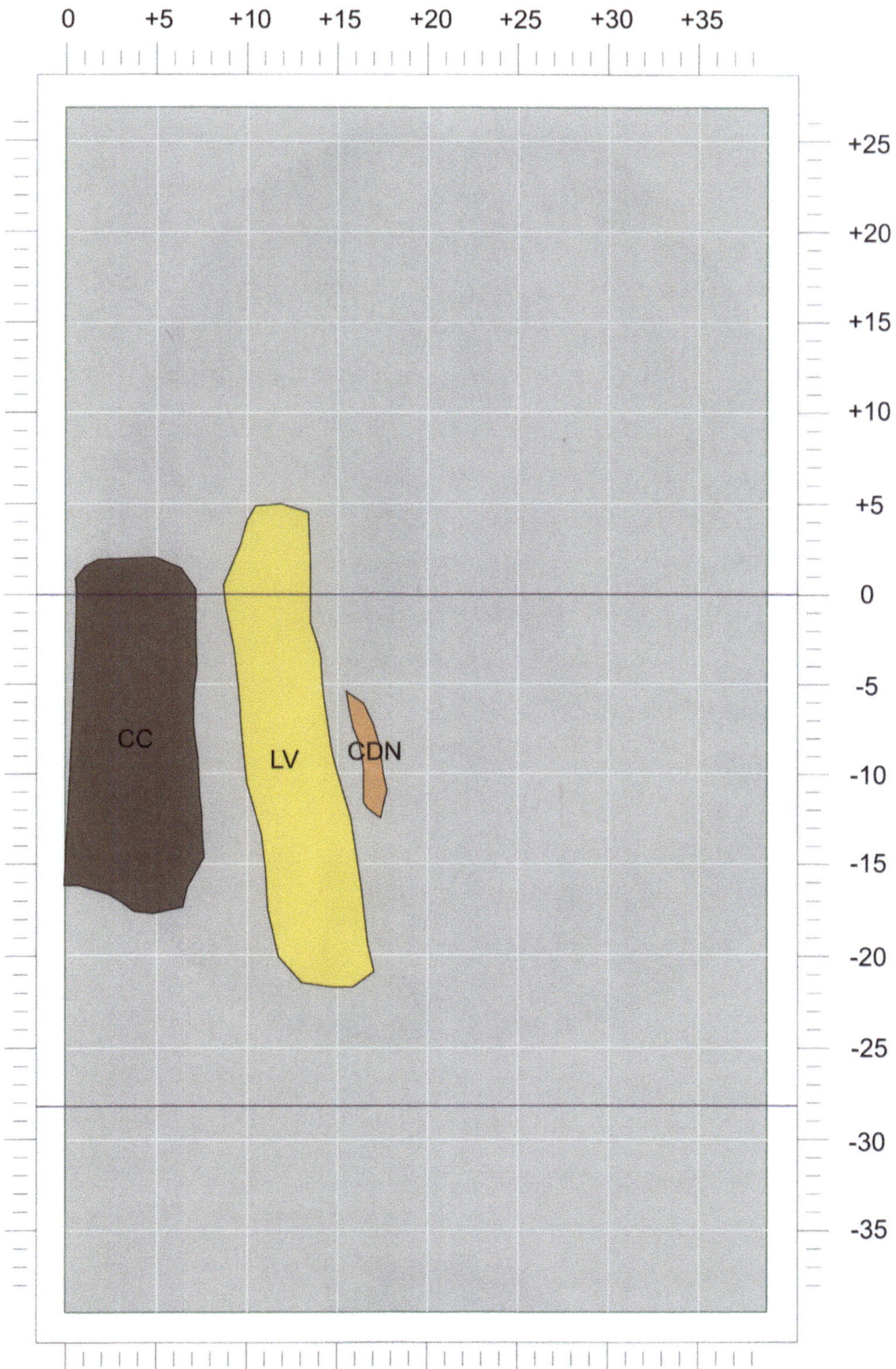

# Plate 2a

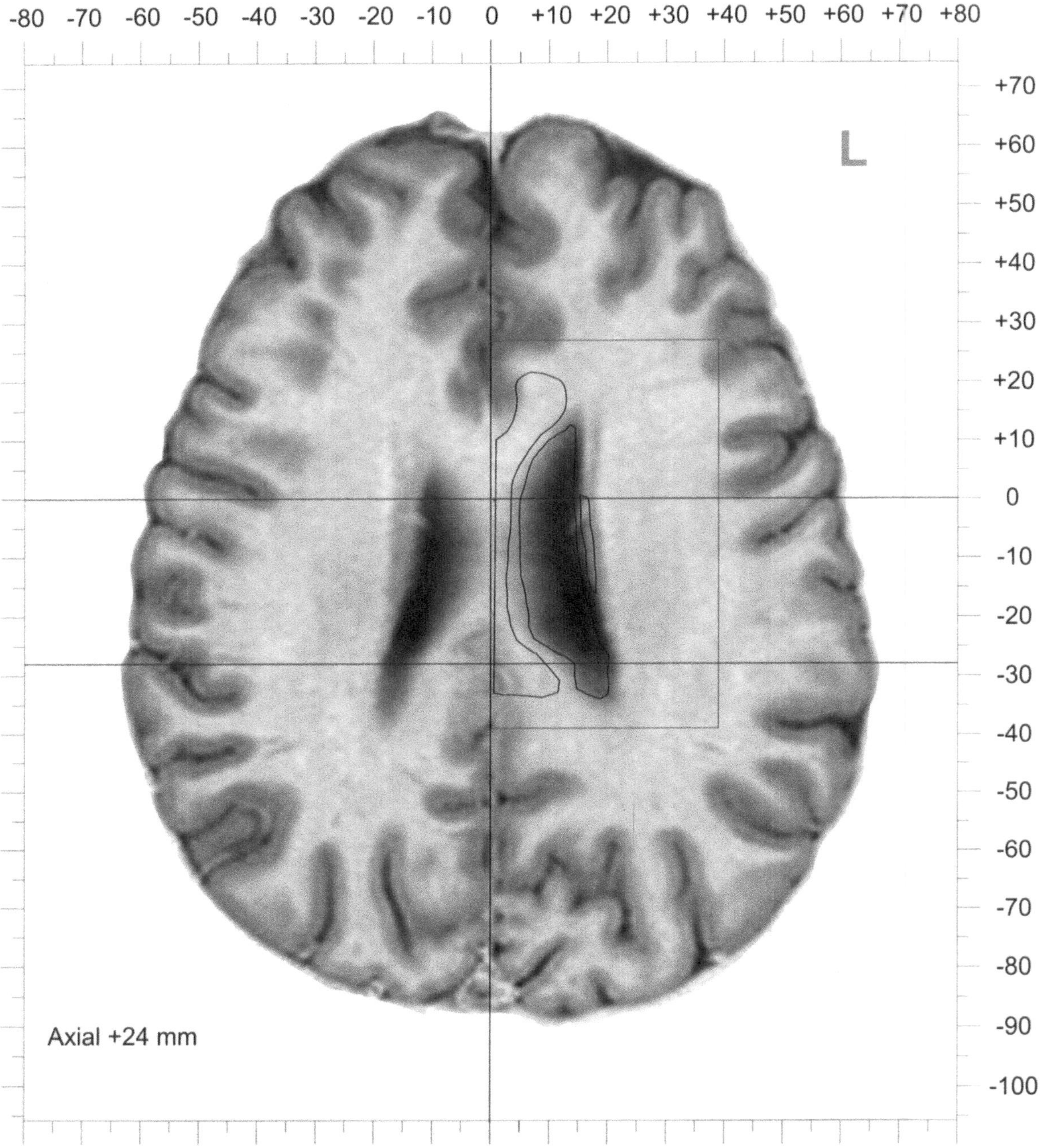

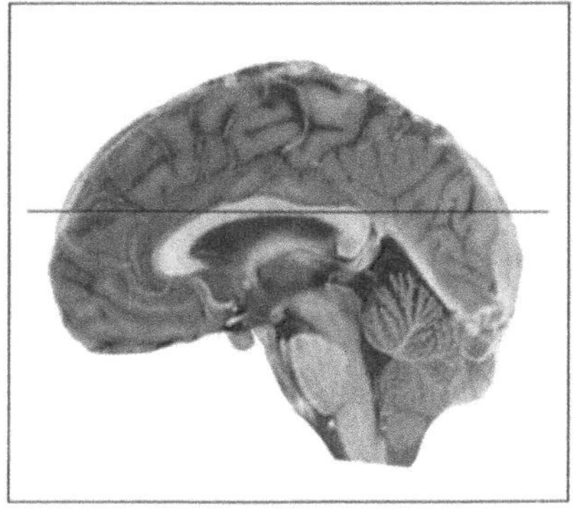

Axial +24 mm

L

-80  -70  -60  -50  -40  -30  -20  -10  0  +10  +20  +30  +40  +50  +60  +70  +80

+70  +60  +50  +40  +30  +20  +10  0  -10  -20  -30  -40  -50  -60  -70  -80  -90  -100

## Plate 2b

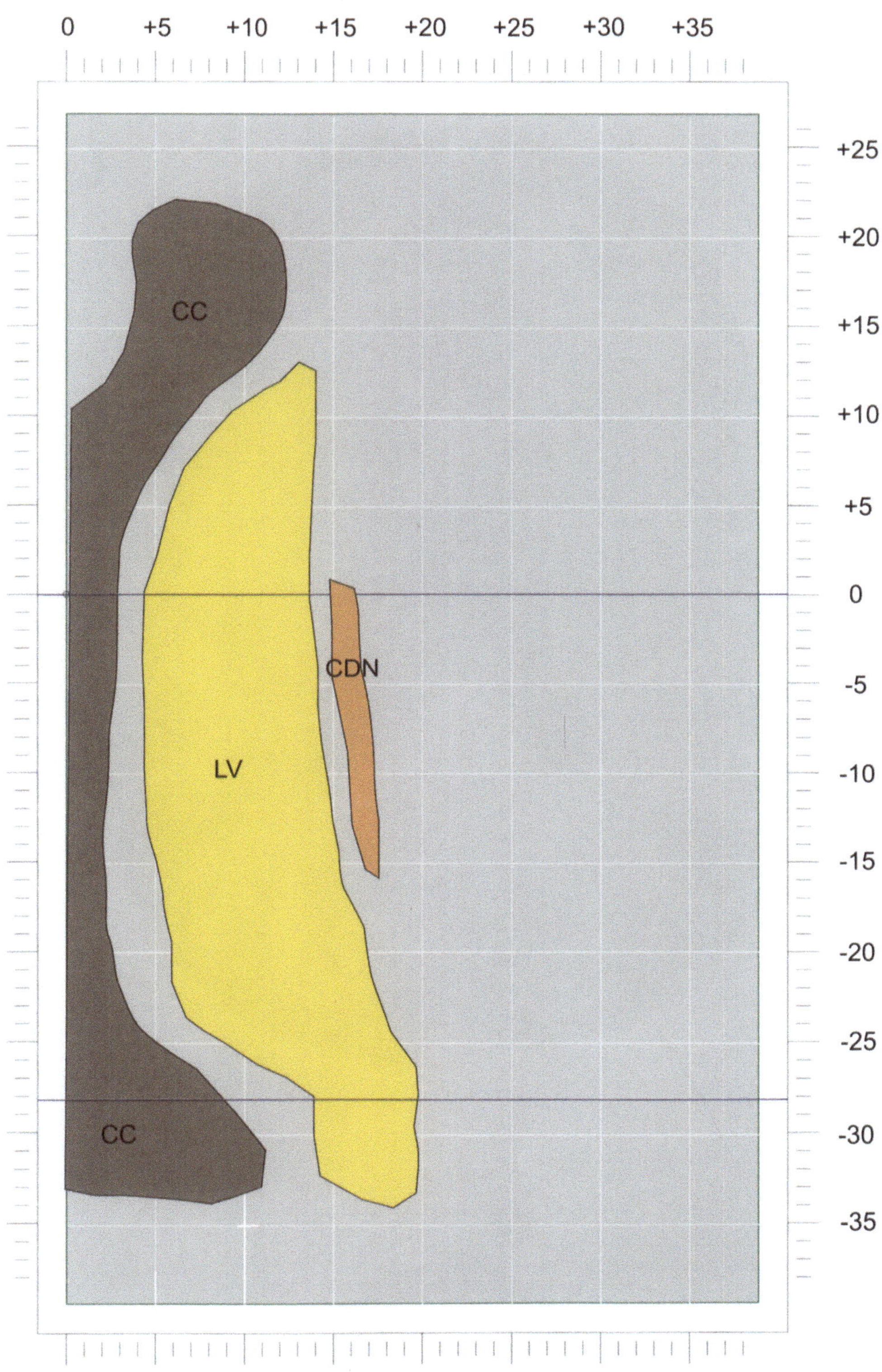


Axial +24 mm

## Plate 3a

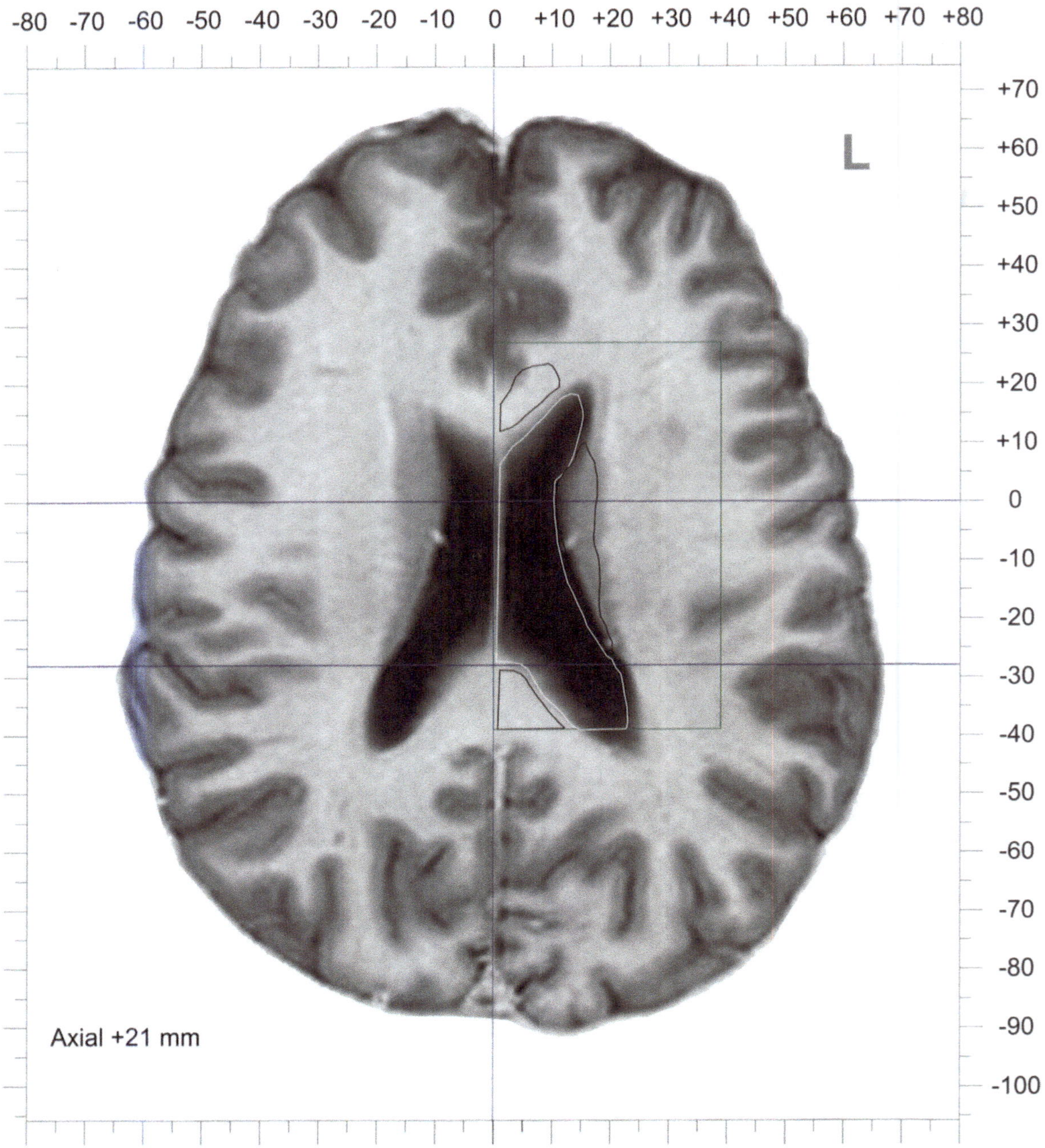

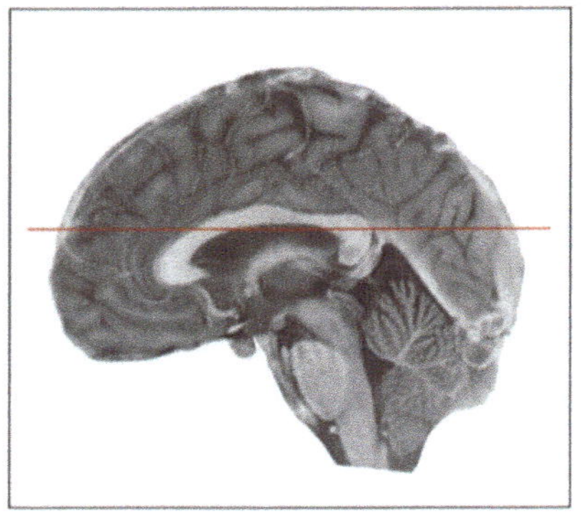

# Plate 3b

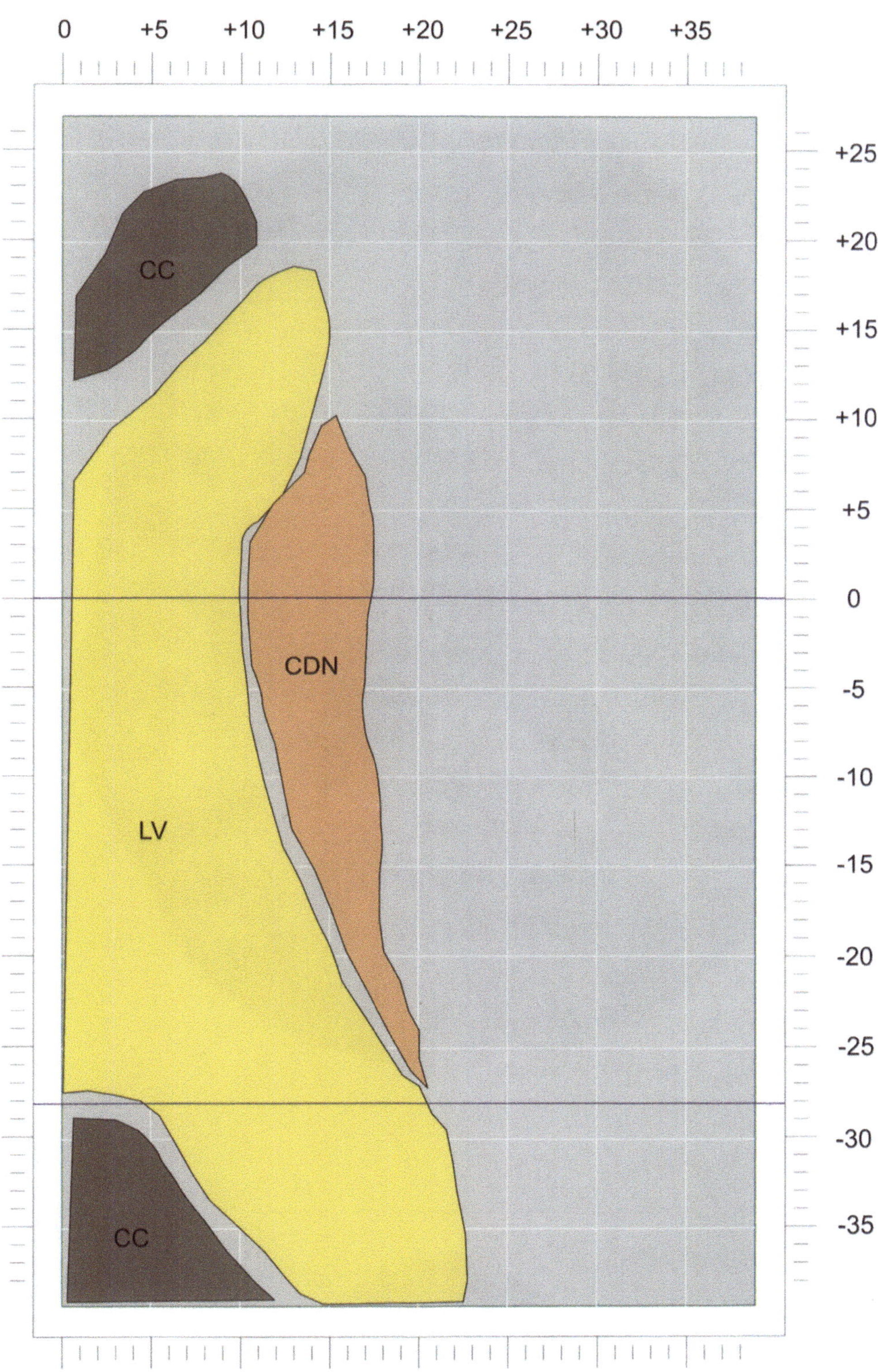


Axial +21 mm

# Plate 4a

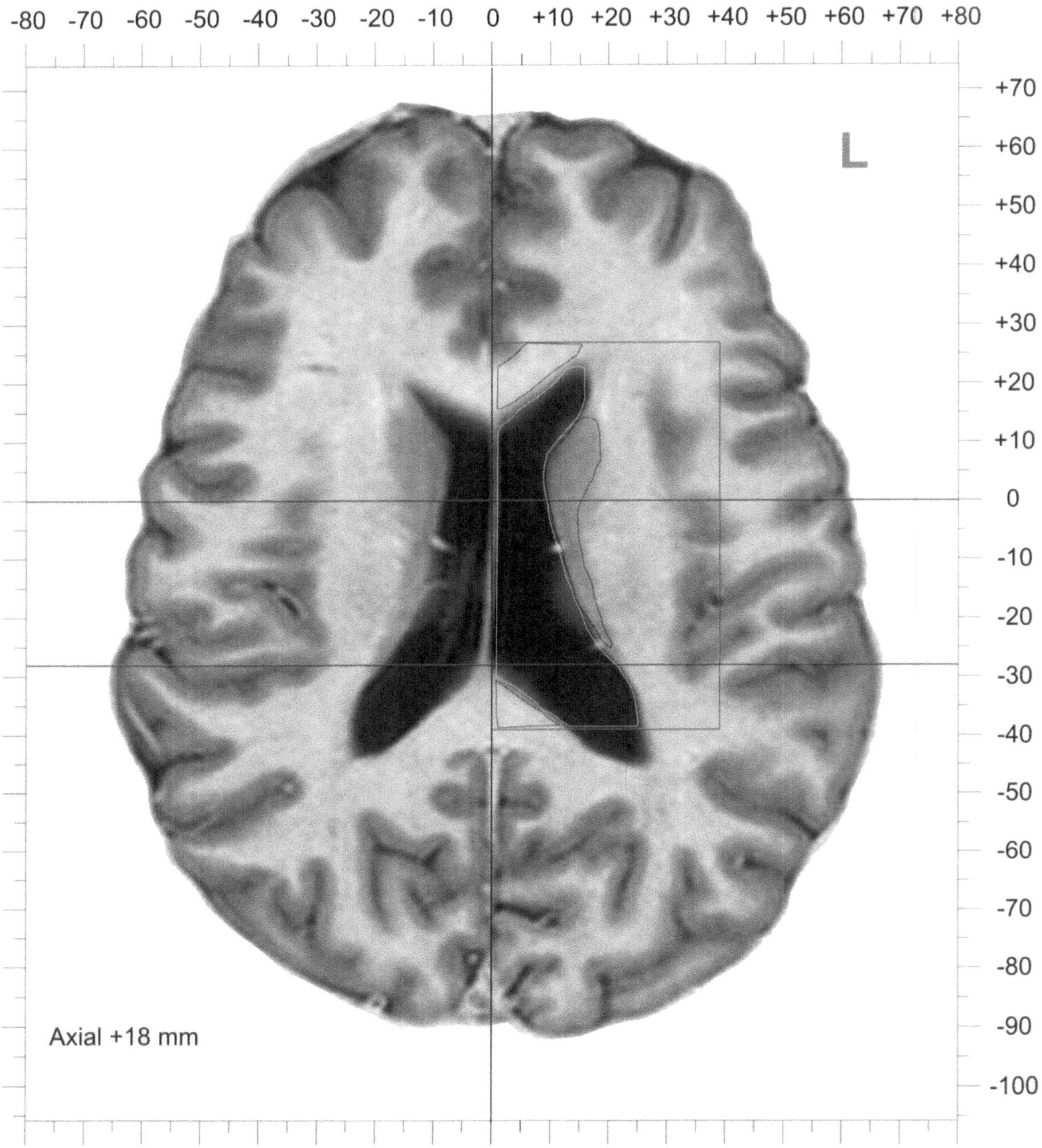

-80  -70  -60  -50  -40  -30  -20  -10   0   +10  +20  +30  +40  +50  +60  +70  +80

+70
+60
+50
+40
+30
+20
+10
0
-10
-20
-30
-40
-50
-60
-70
-80
-90
-100

L

Axial +18 mm

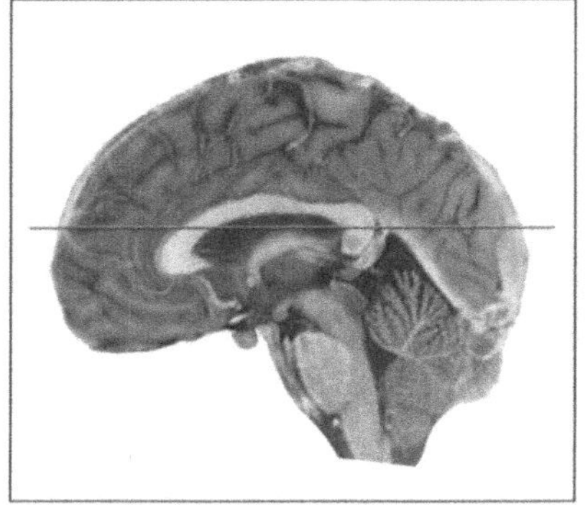

## Plate 4b

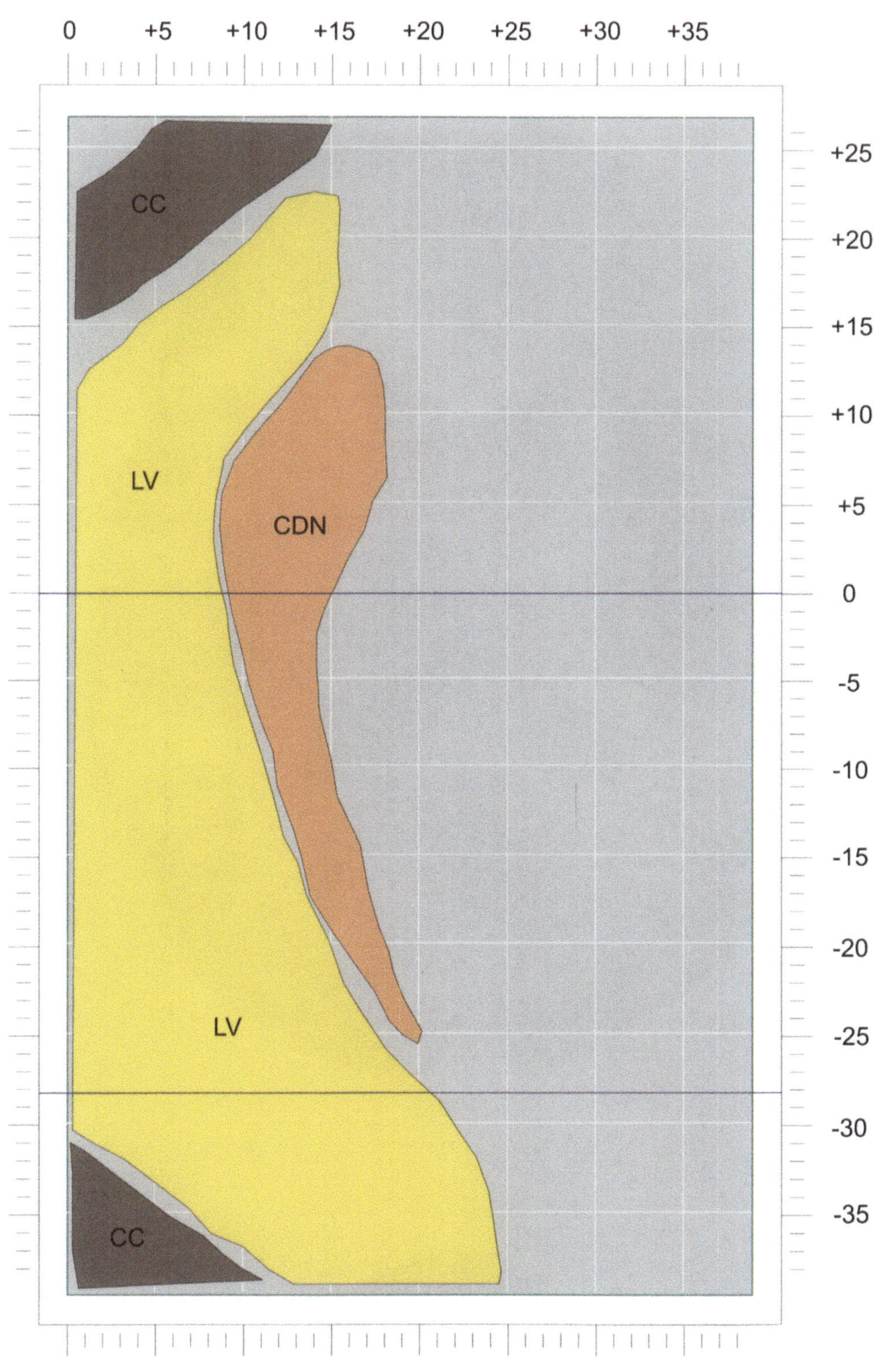



Axial +18 mm

# Plate 5a

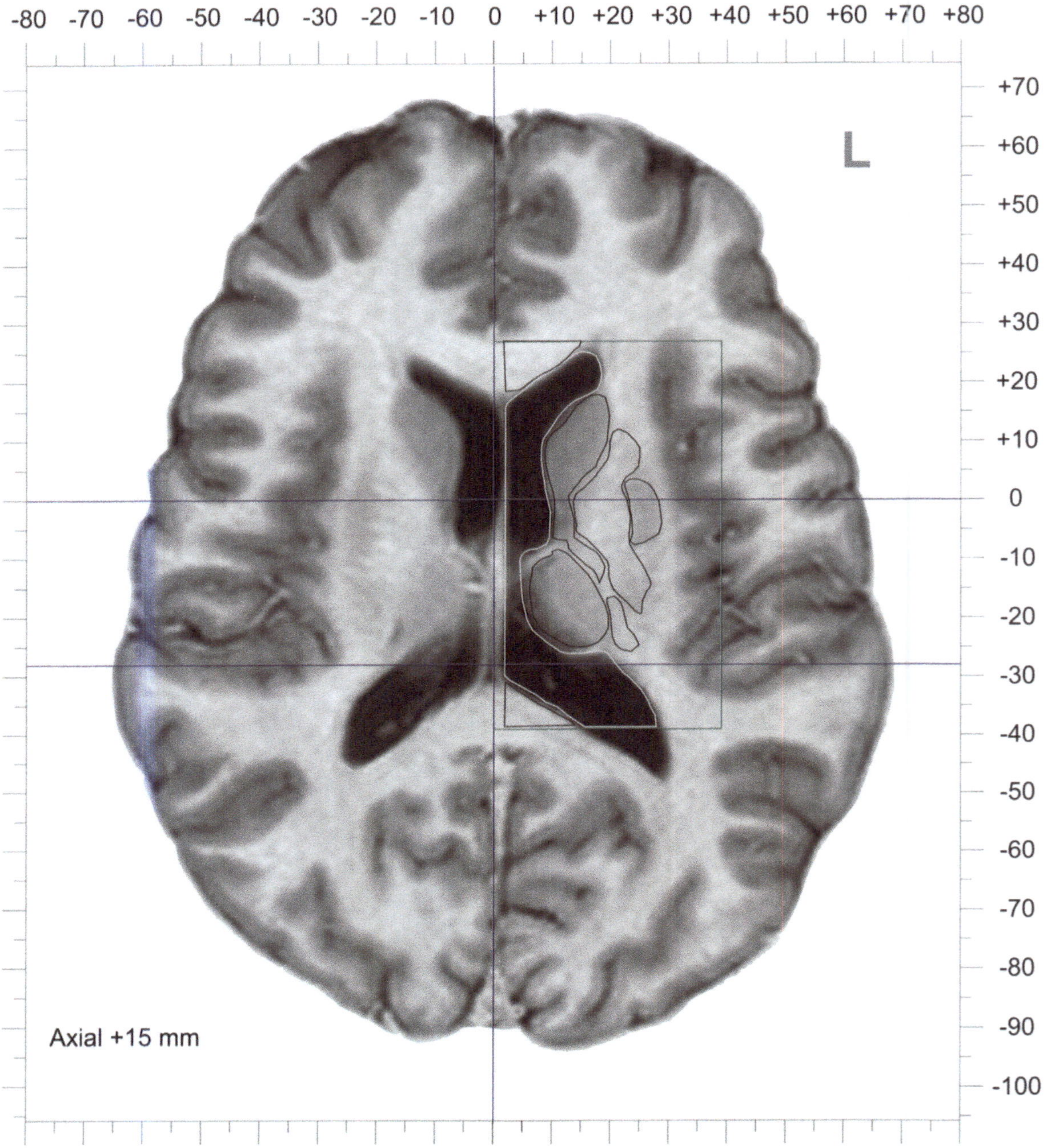

-80  -70  -60  -50  -40  -30  -20  -10   0   +10  +20  +30  +40  +50  +60  +70  +80

+70
+60
+50
+40
+30
+20
+10
0
-10
-20
-30
-40
-50
-60
-70
-80
-90
-100

L

Axial +15 mm

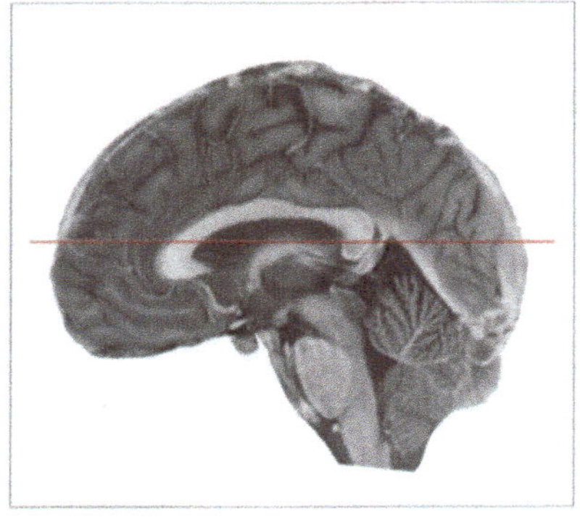

## Plate 5b

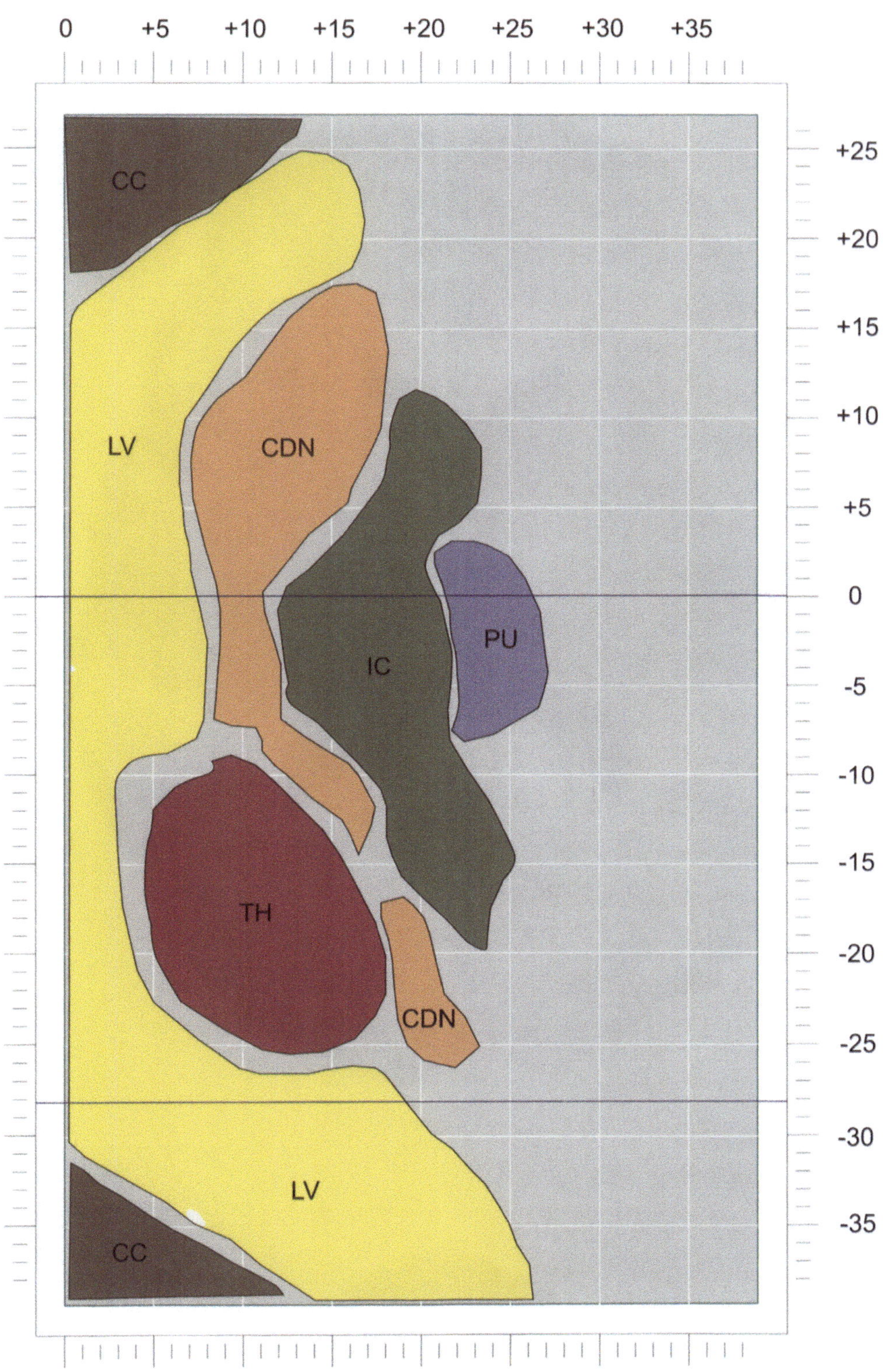


Axial +15 mm

## Plate 6a

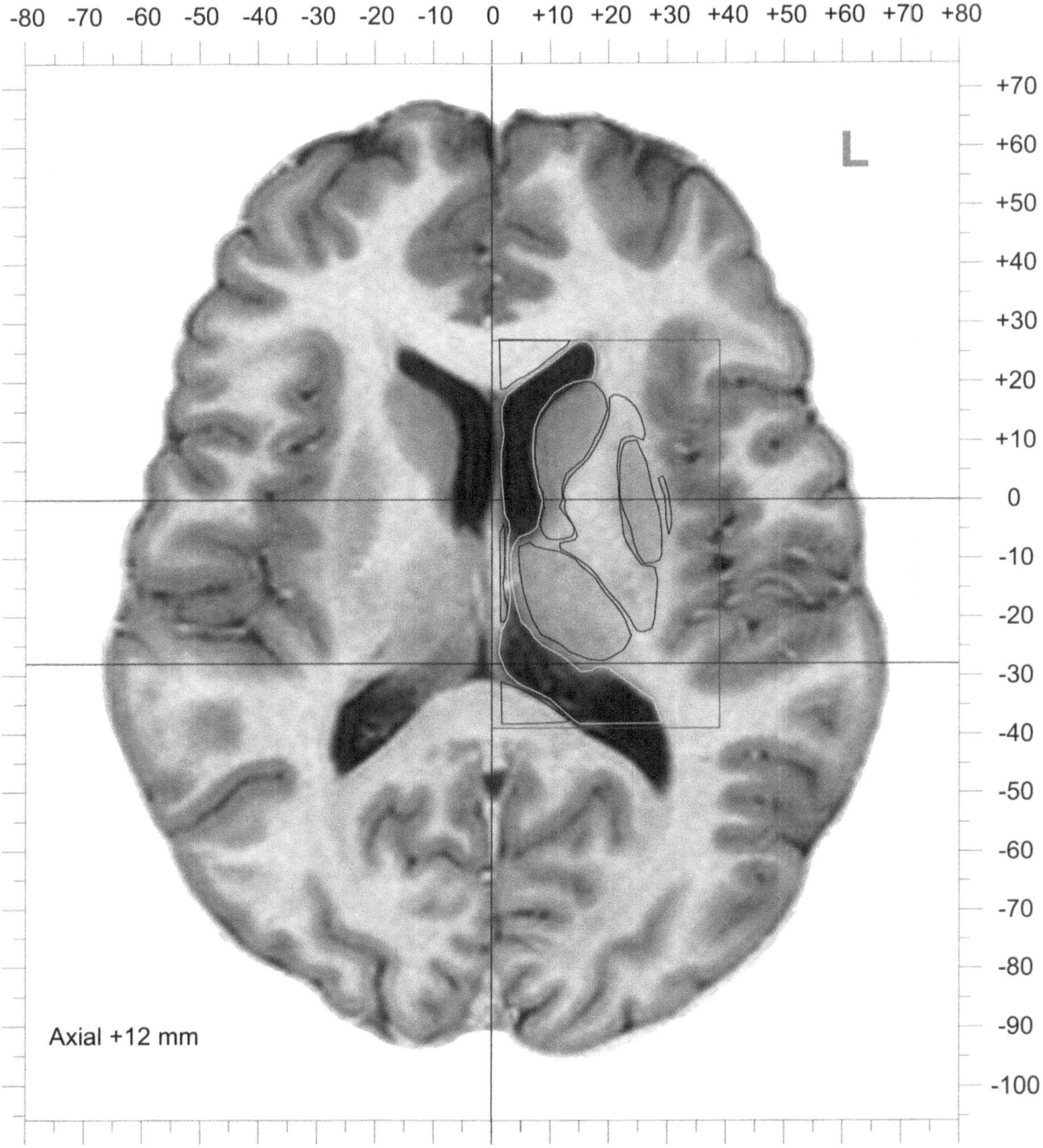

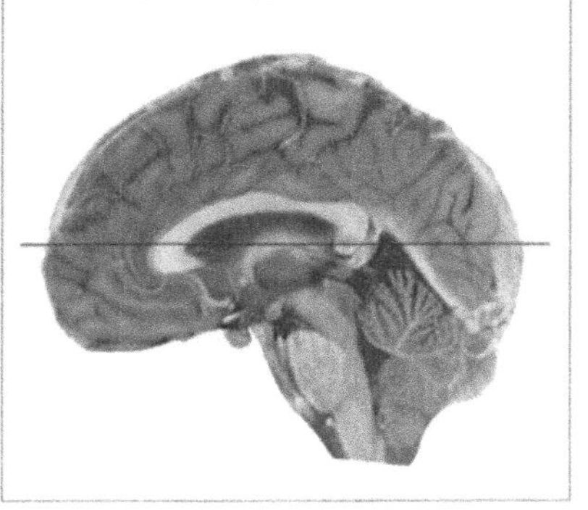

Axial +12 mm

## Plate 6b

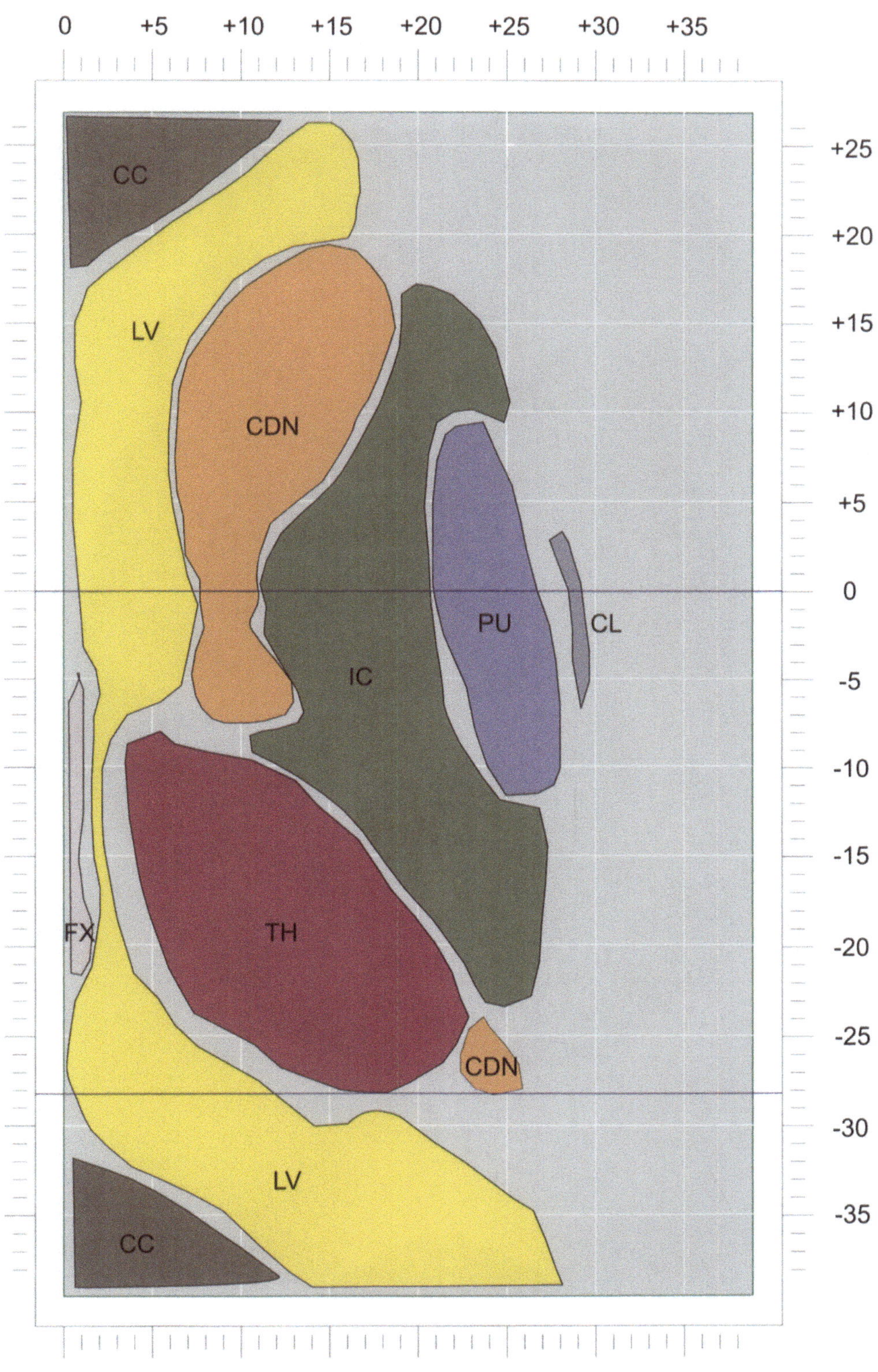


Axial +12 mm

# Plate 7a

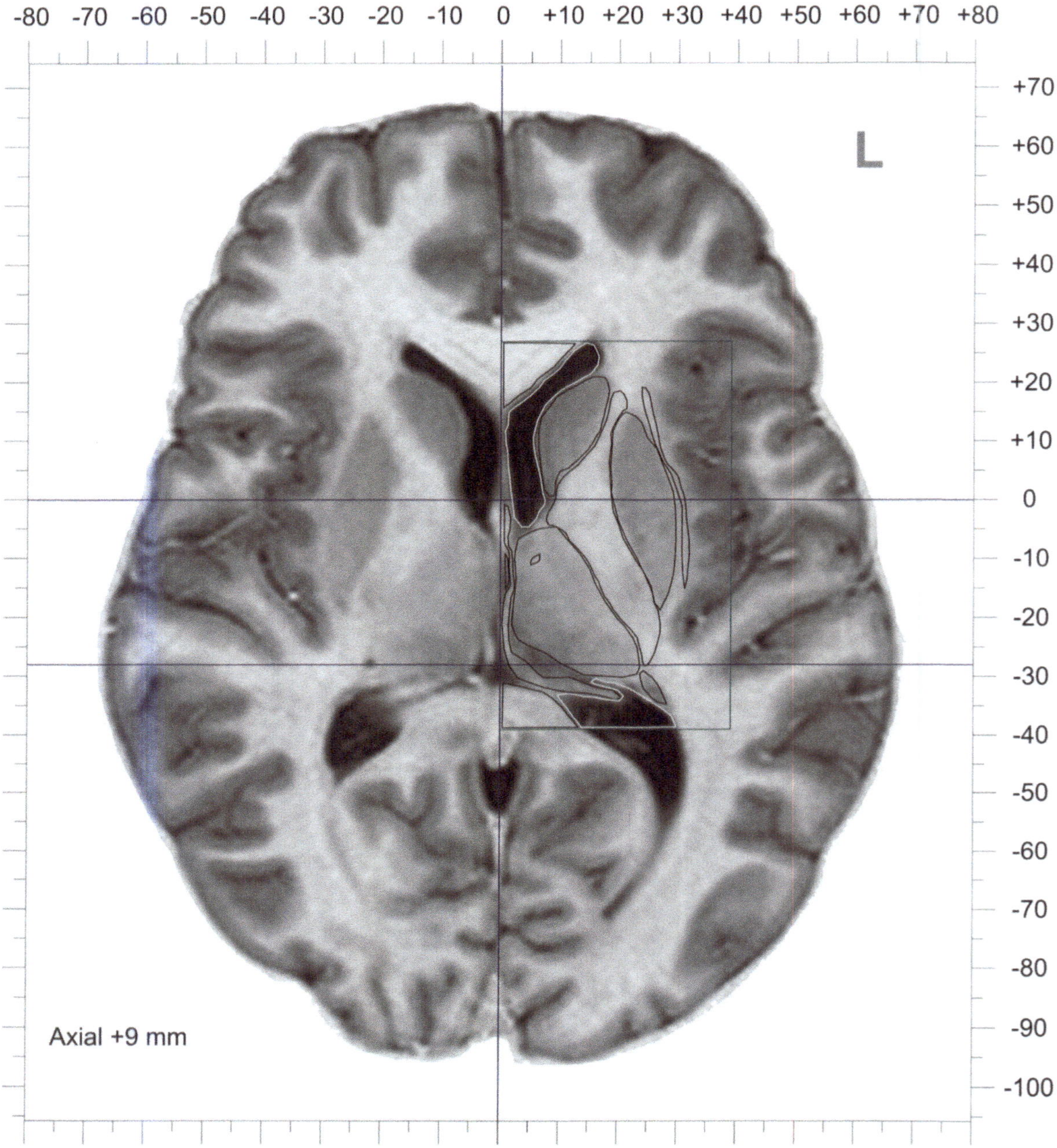

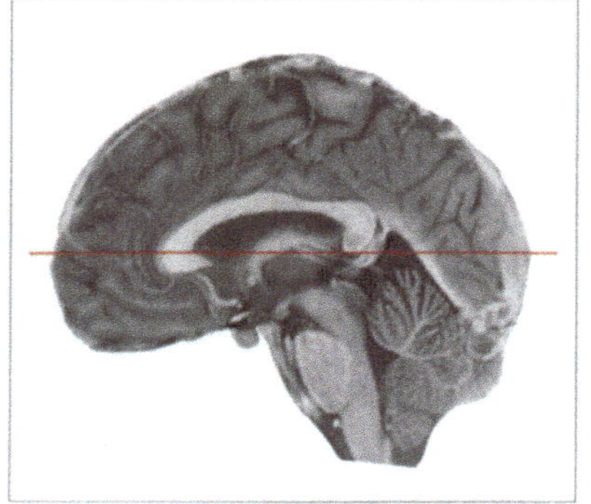

Axial +9 mm

## Plate 7b

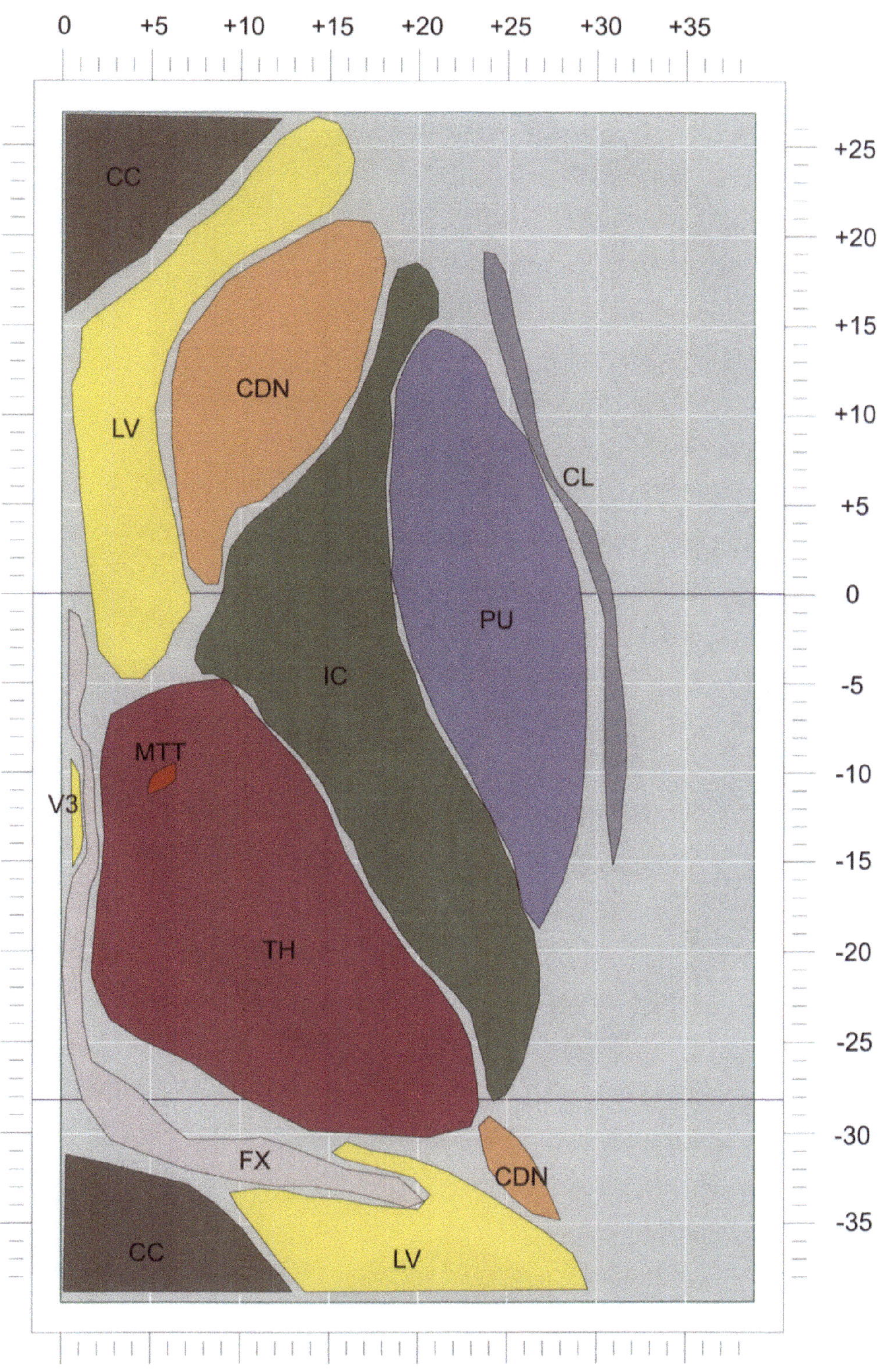


Axial +9 mm

# Plate 8a

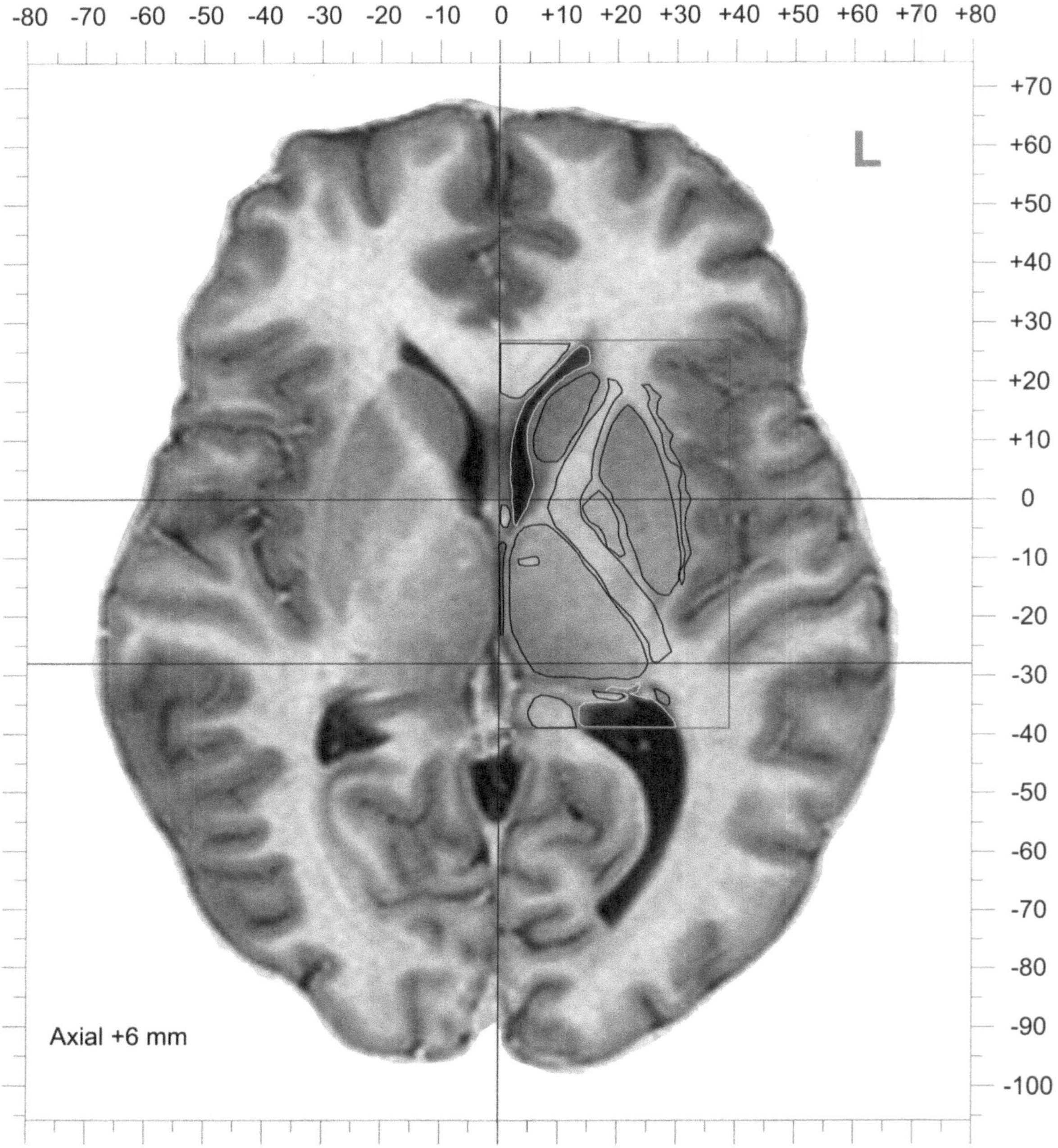

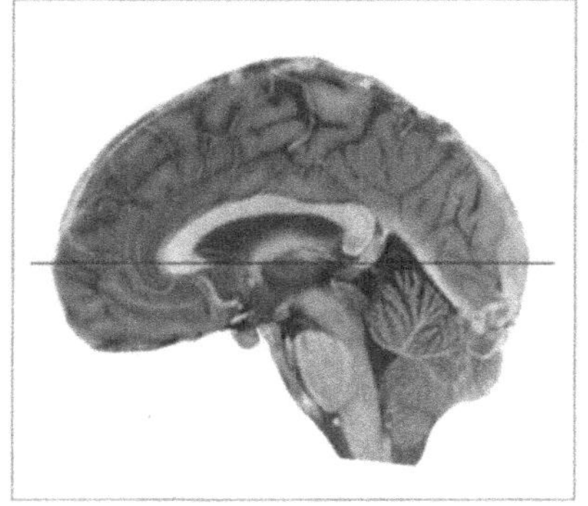

Axial +6 mm

## Plate 8b

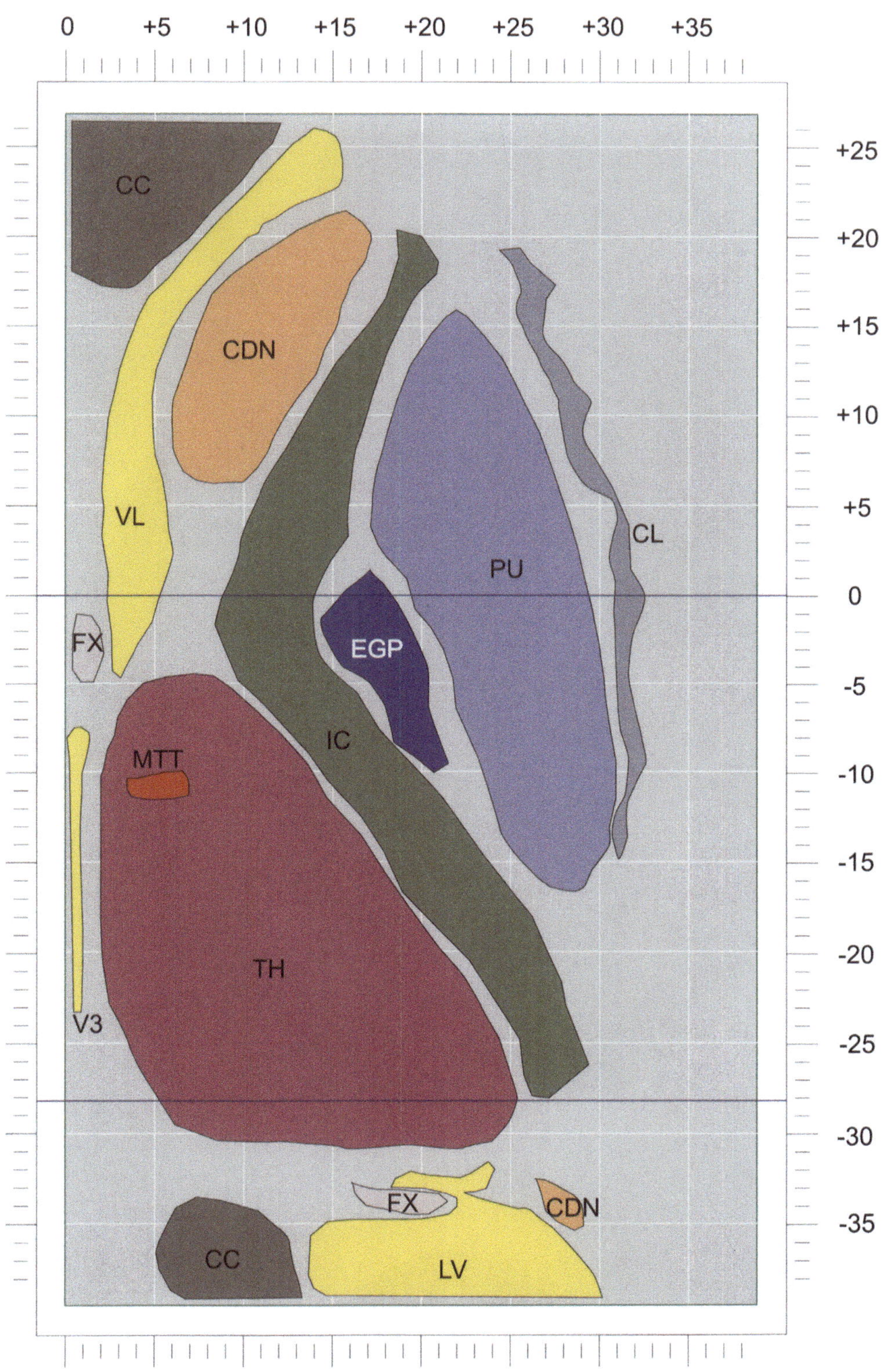


Axial +6 mm

# Plate 9a

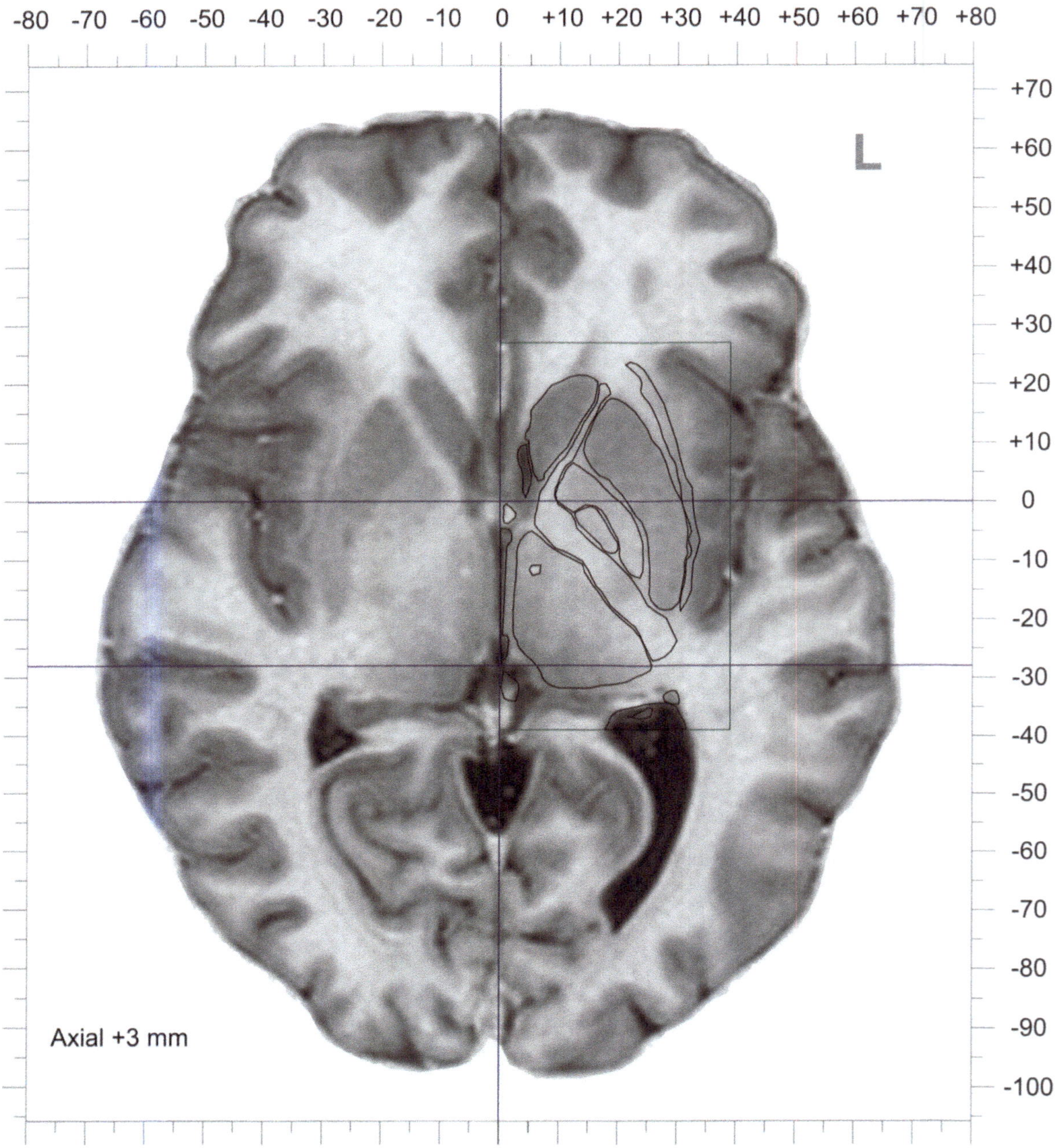

-80 -70 -60 -50 -40 -30 -20 -10 0 +10 +20 +30 +40 +50 +60 +70 +80
+70
+60
+50
+40
+30
+20
+10
0
-10
-20
-30
-40
-50
-60
-70
-80
-90
-100
L
Axial +3 mm

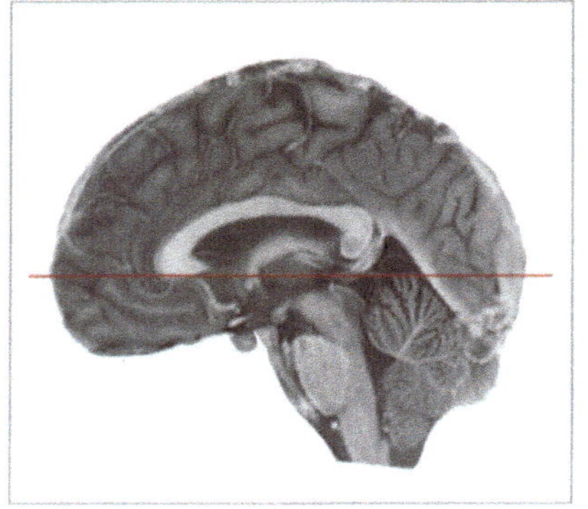

## Plate 9b

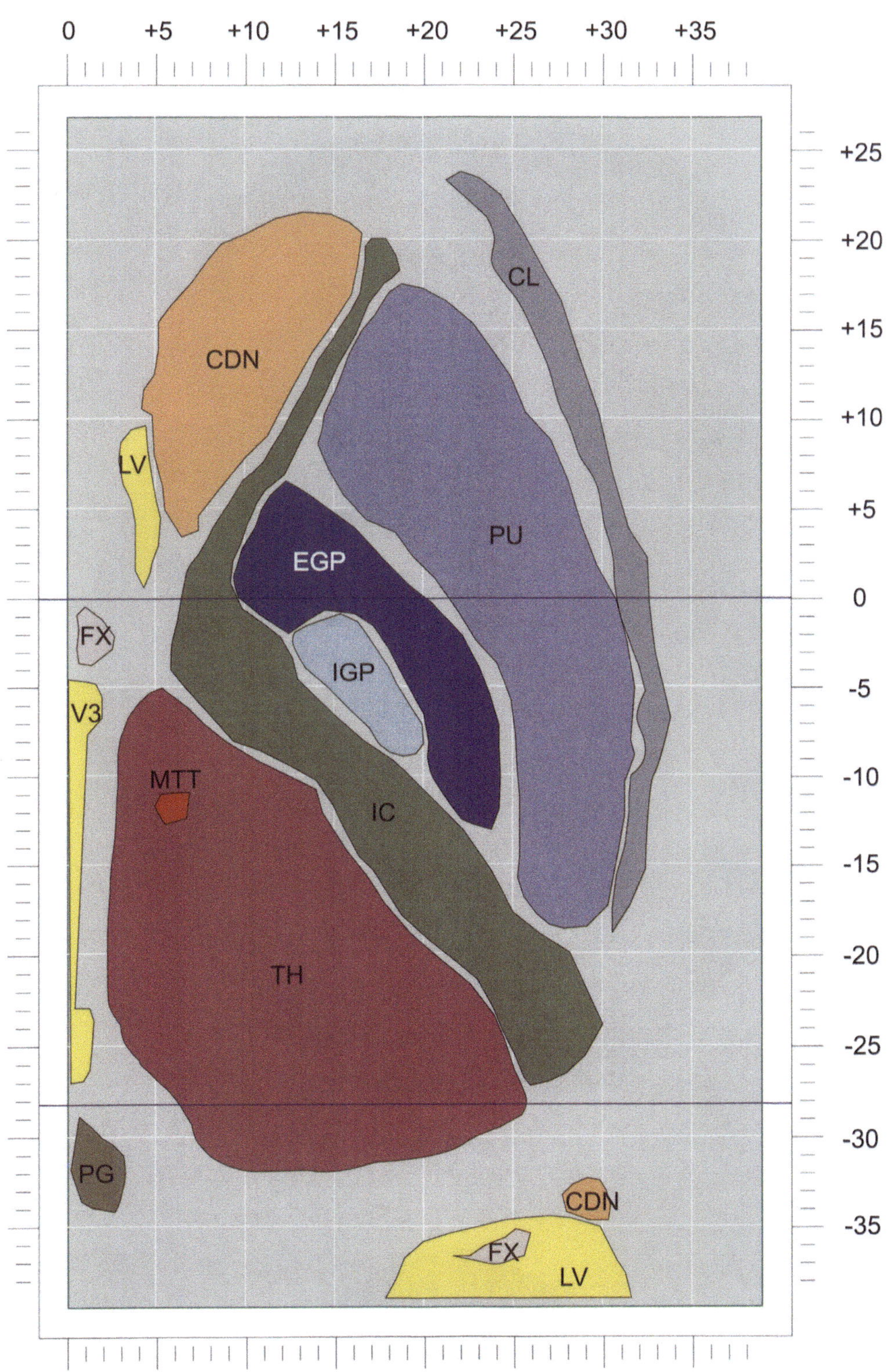


Axial +3 mm

## Plate 10a

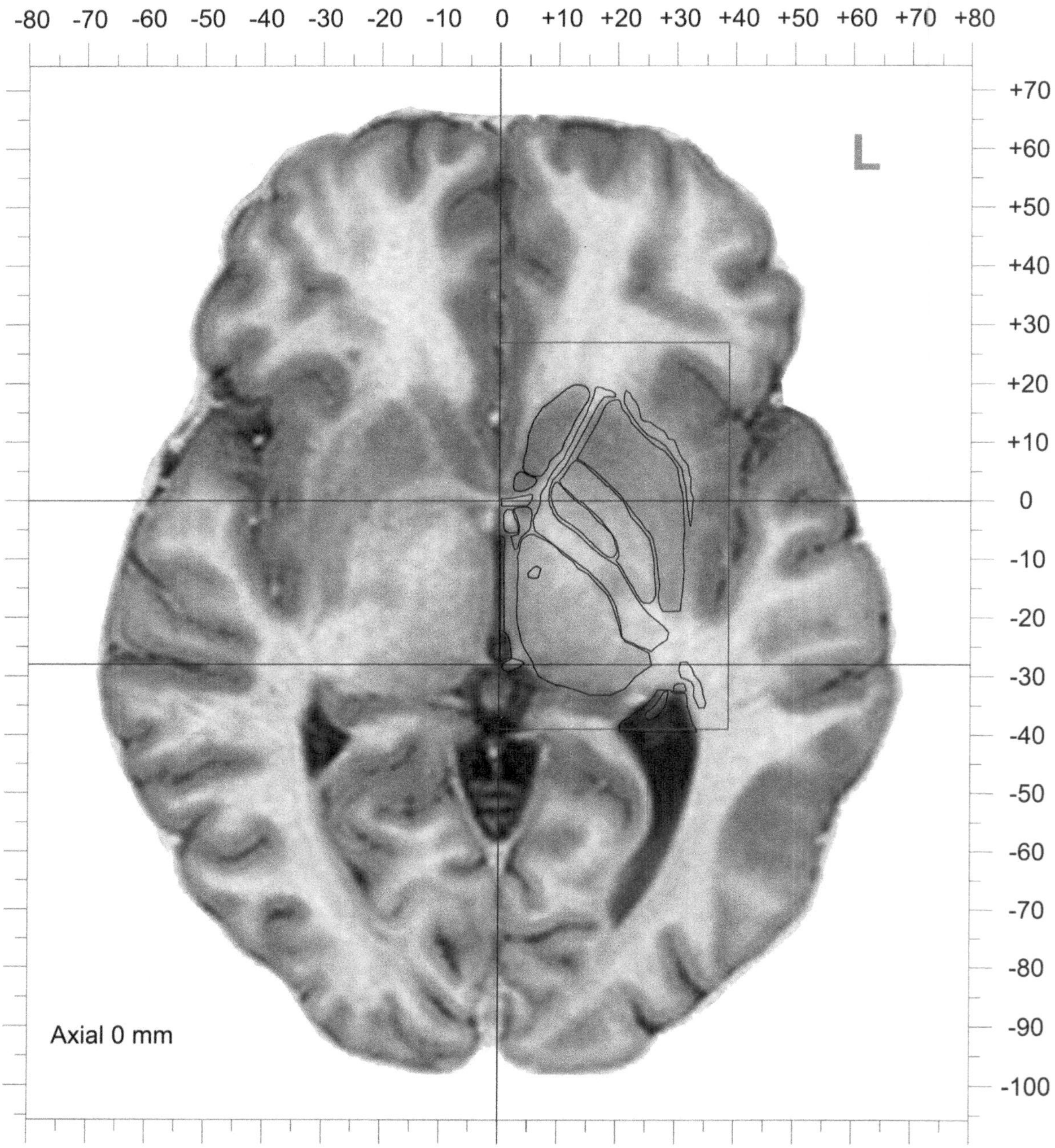

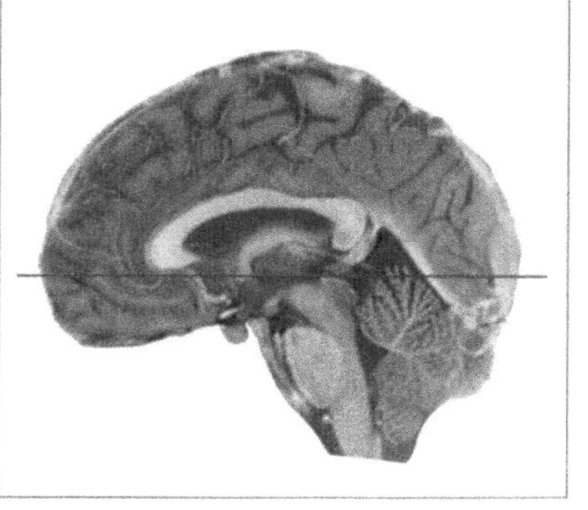

# Plate 10b

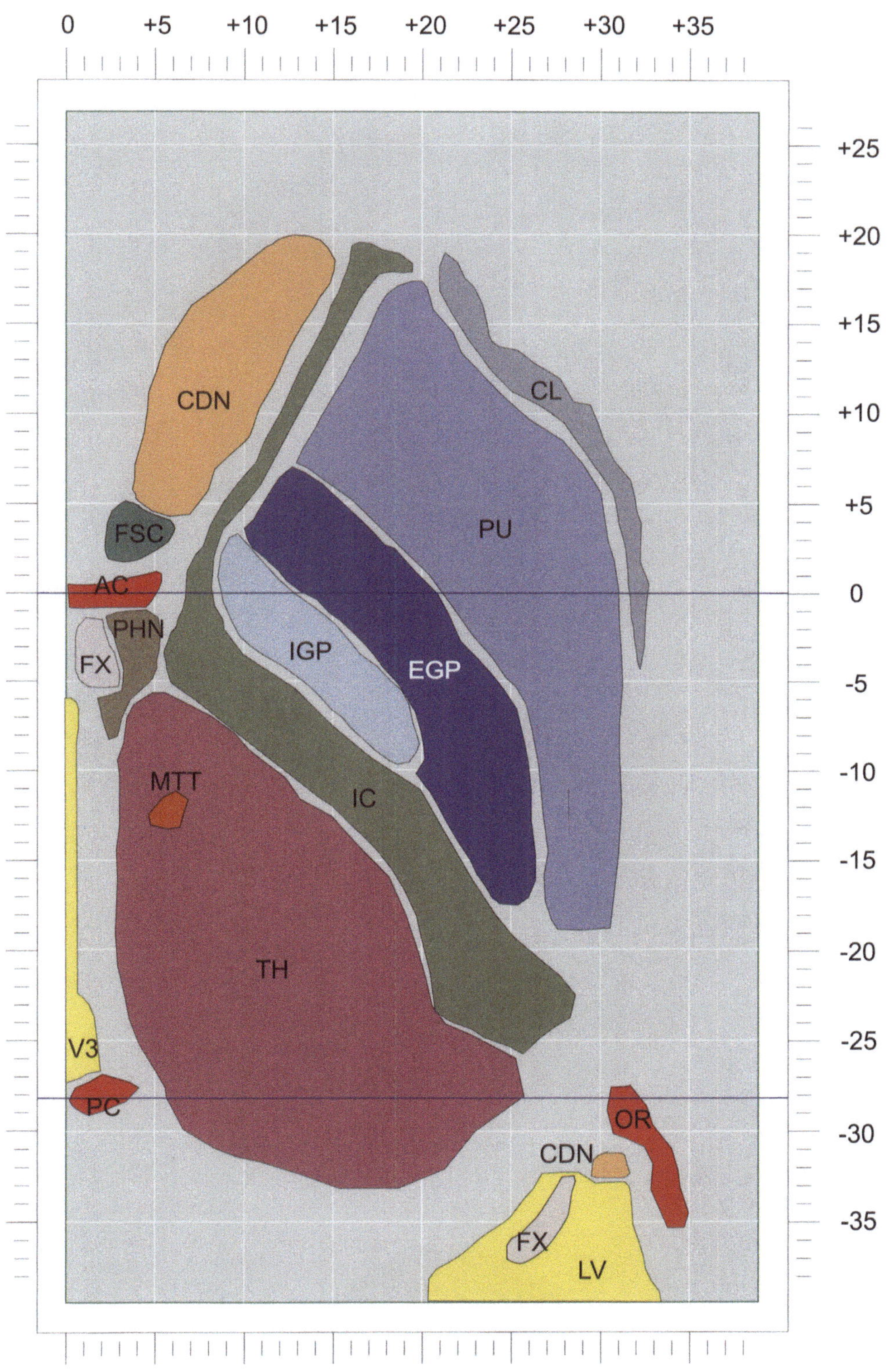


Axial 0 mm

## Plate 11a

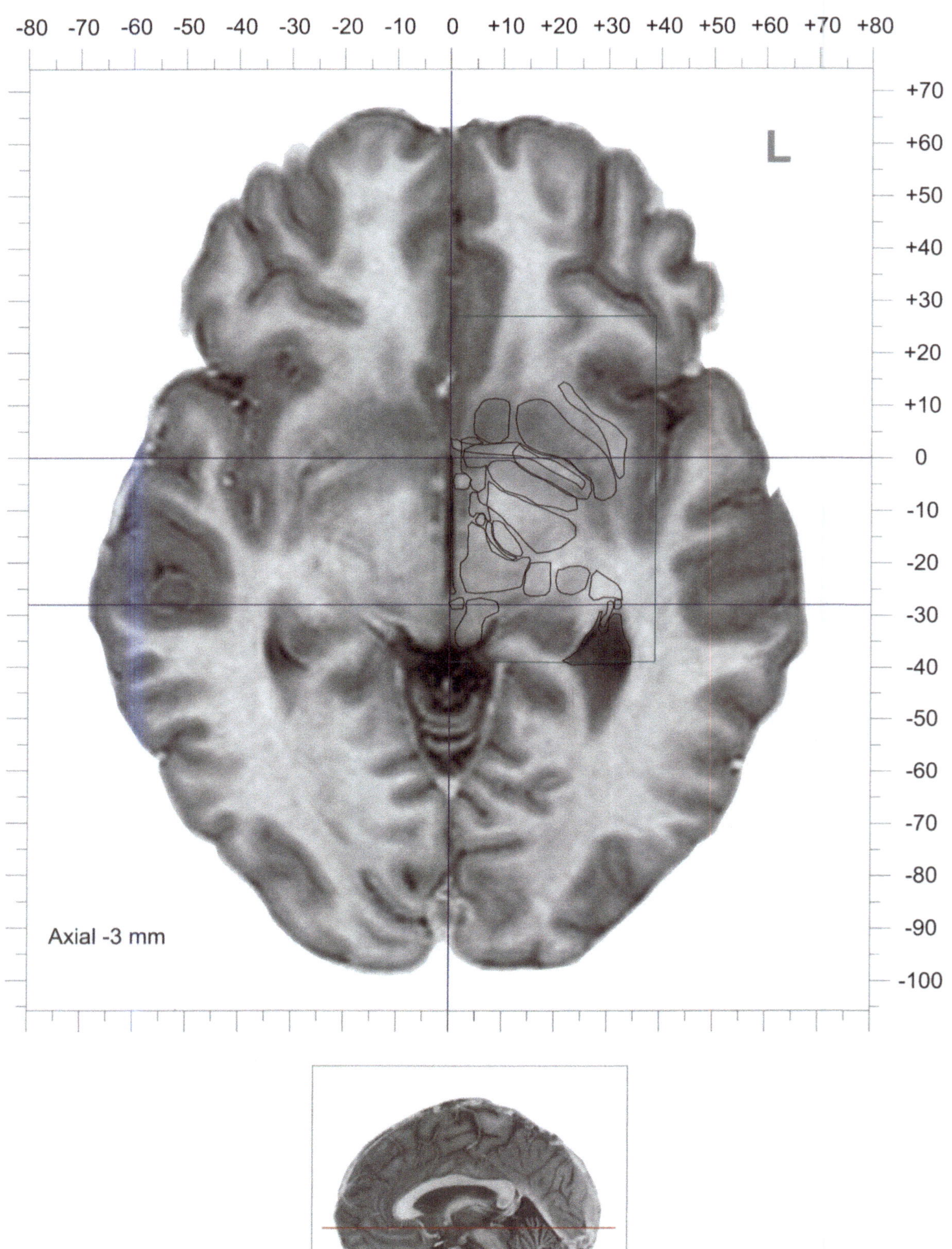

# Plate 11b

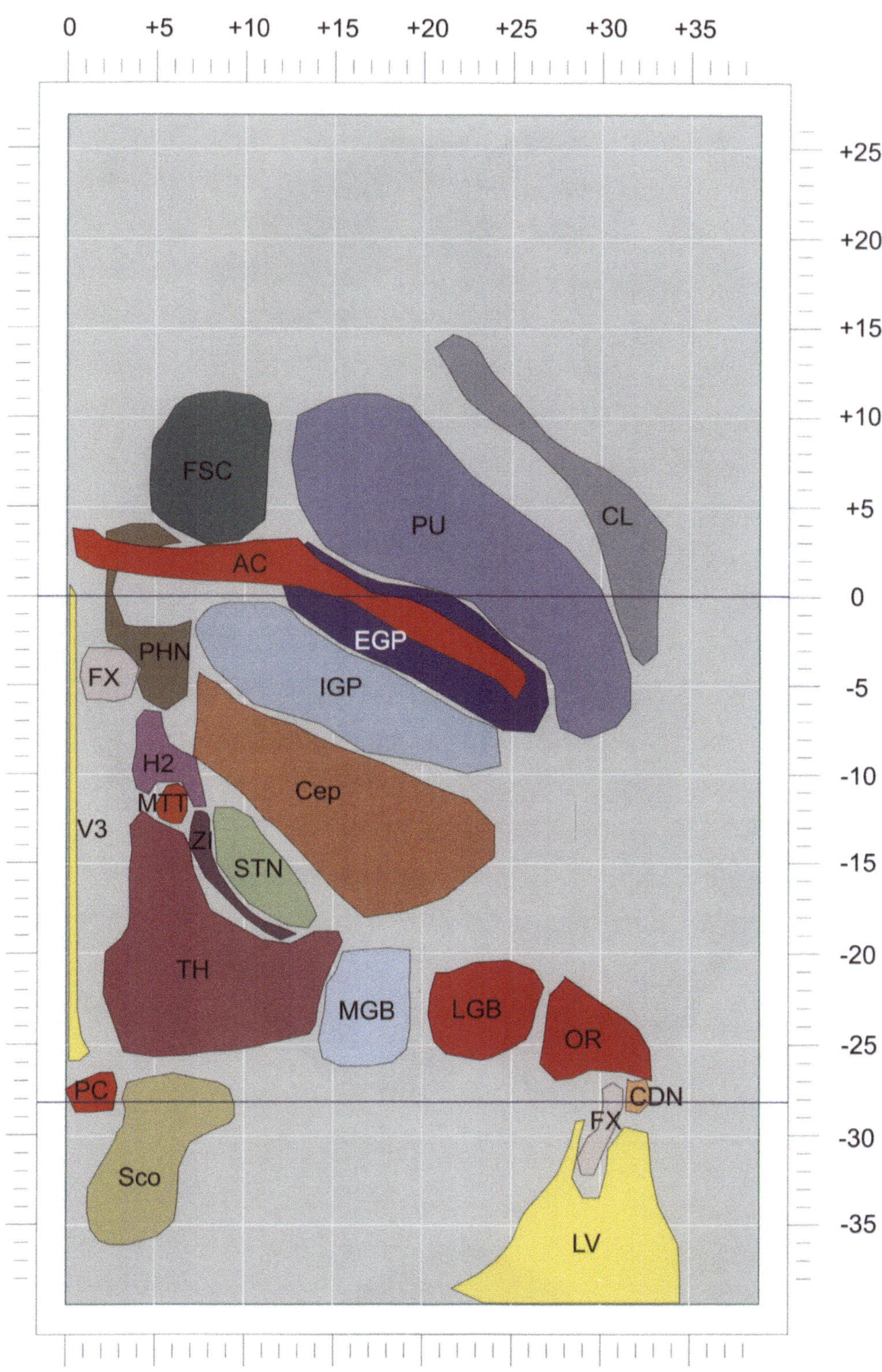


Axial -3 mm

# Plate 12a

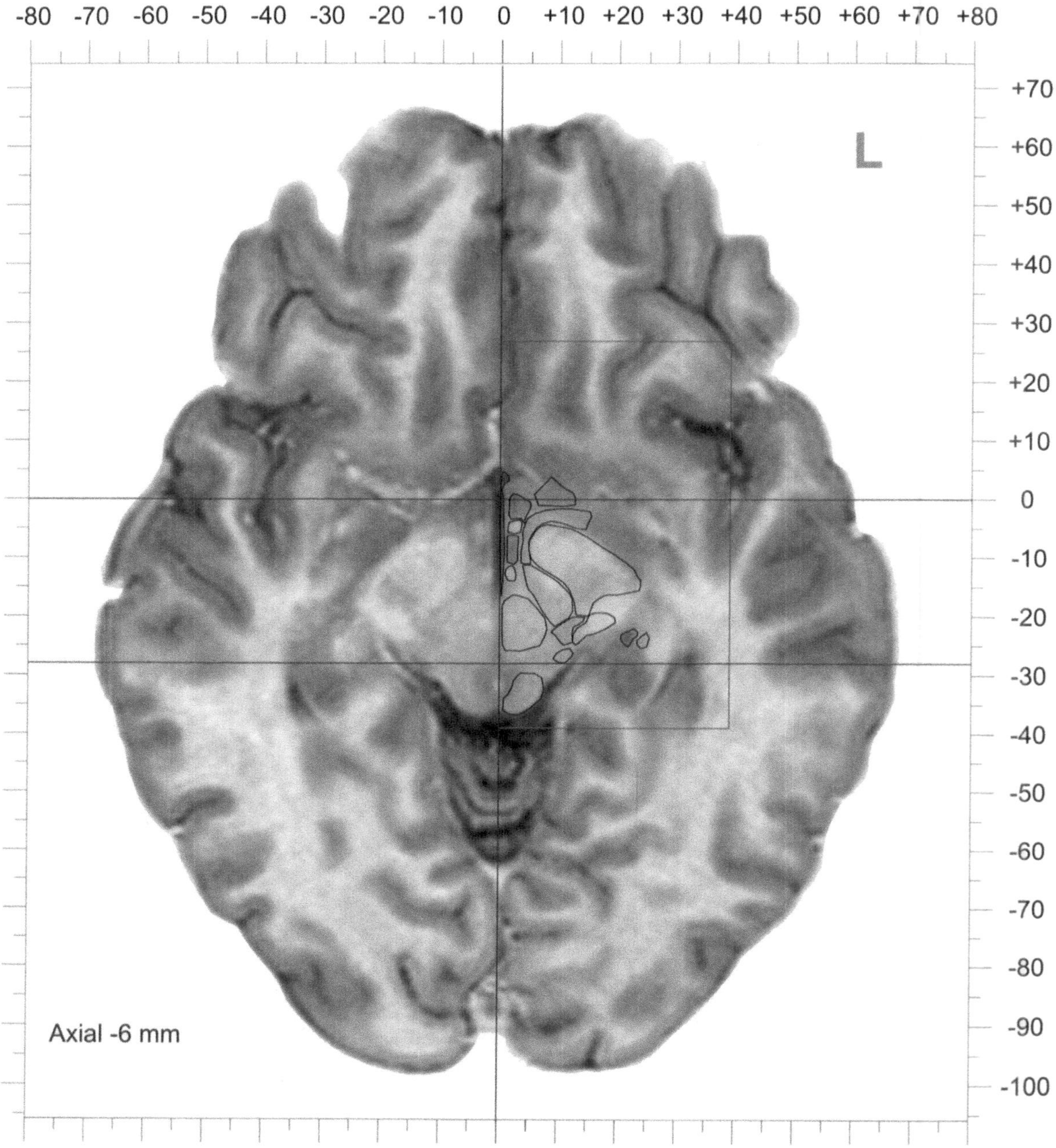

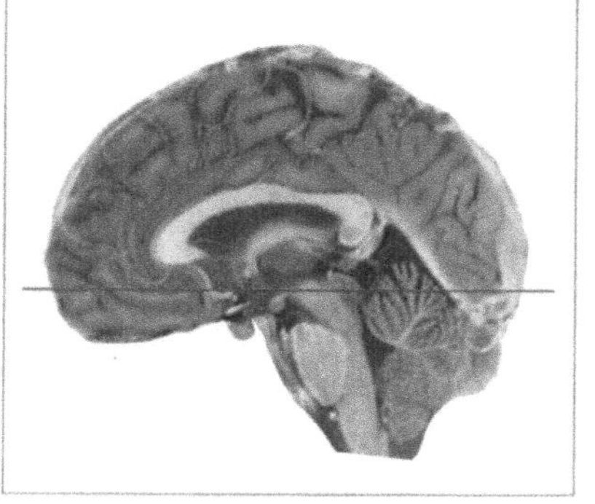

Axial -6 mm

## Plate 12b

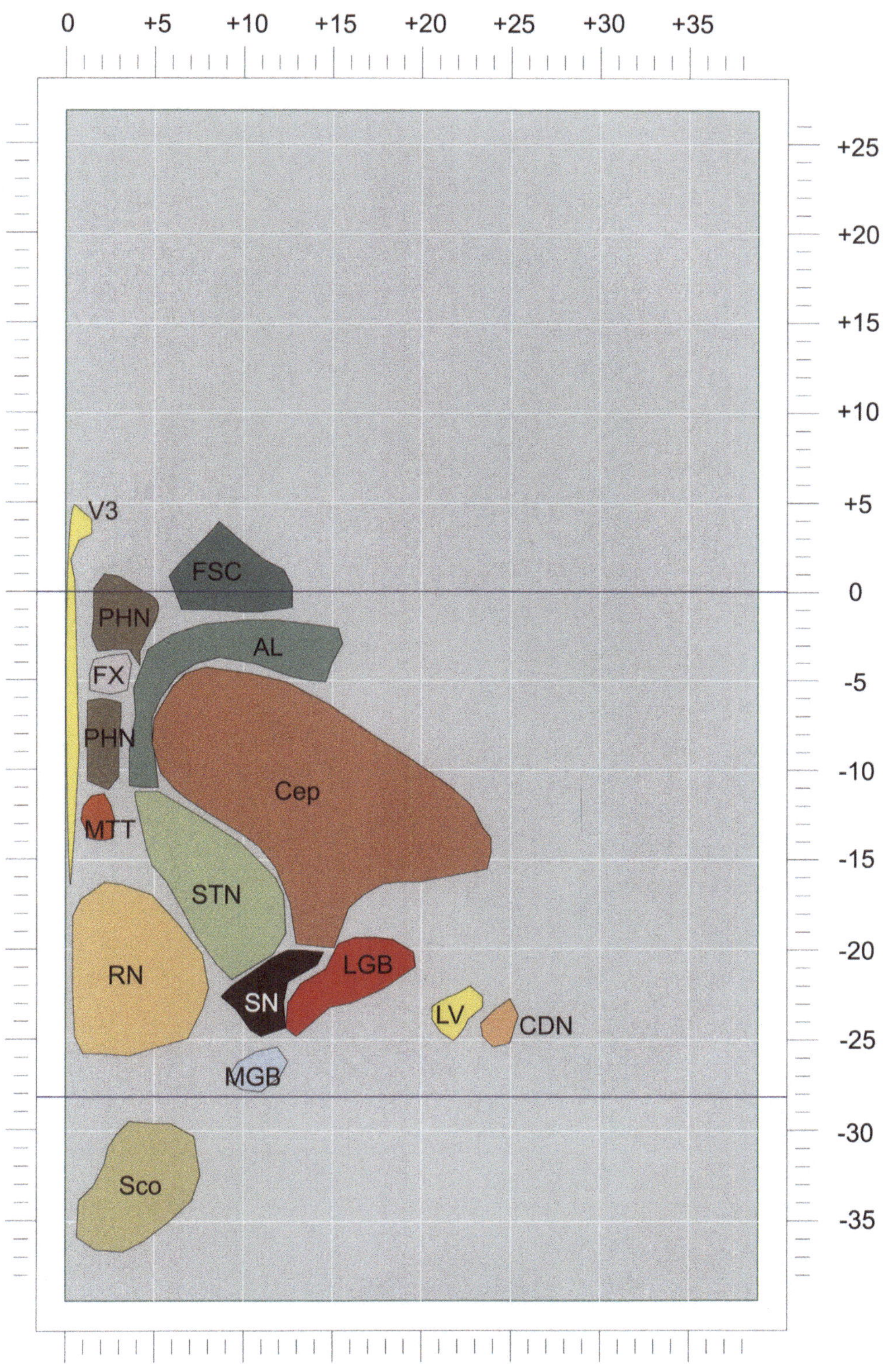


Axial -6 mm

# Plate 13a

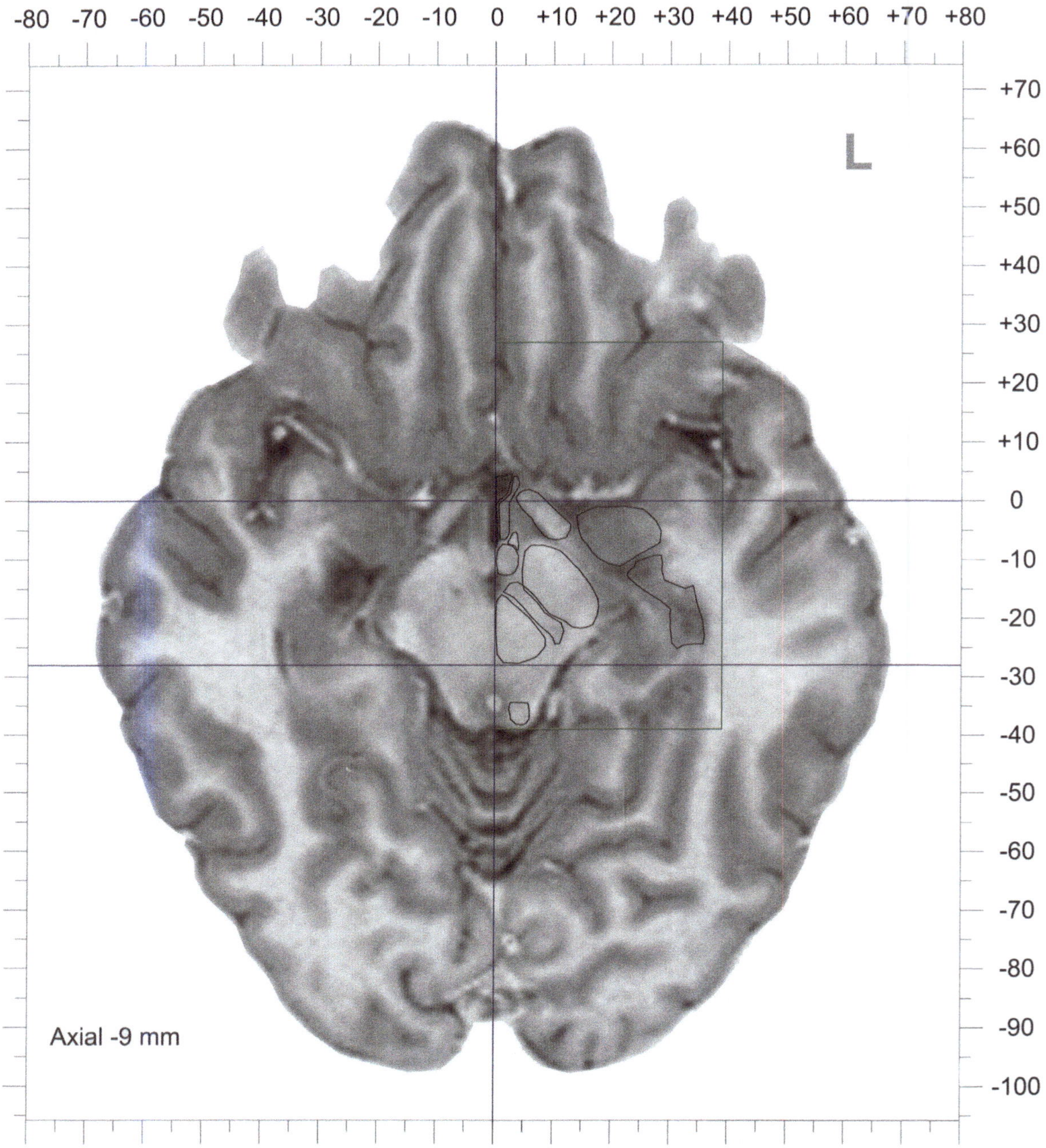

-80  -70  -60  -50  -40  -30  -20  -10   0   +10  +20  +30  +40  +50  +60  +70  +80

L

+70
+60
+50
+40
+30
+20
+10
0
-10
-20
-30
-40
-50
-60
-70
-80
-90
-100

Axial -9 mm

-80  -70  -60  -50  -40  -30  -20  -10   0   +10  +20  +30  +40  +50  +60  +70  +80

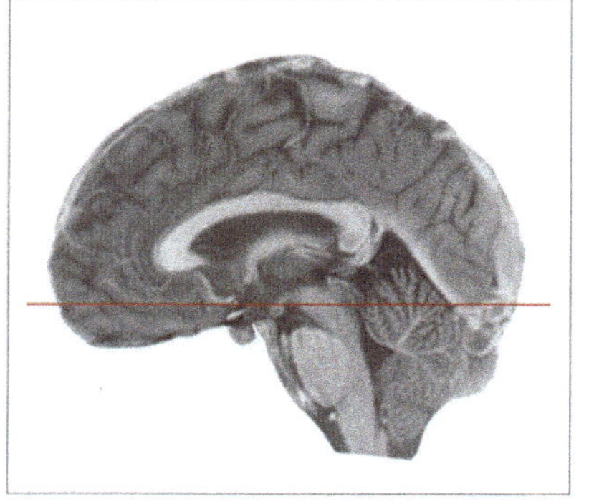

## Plate 13b

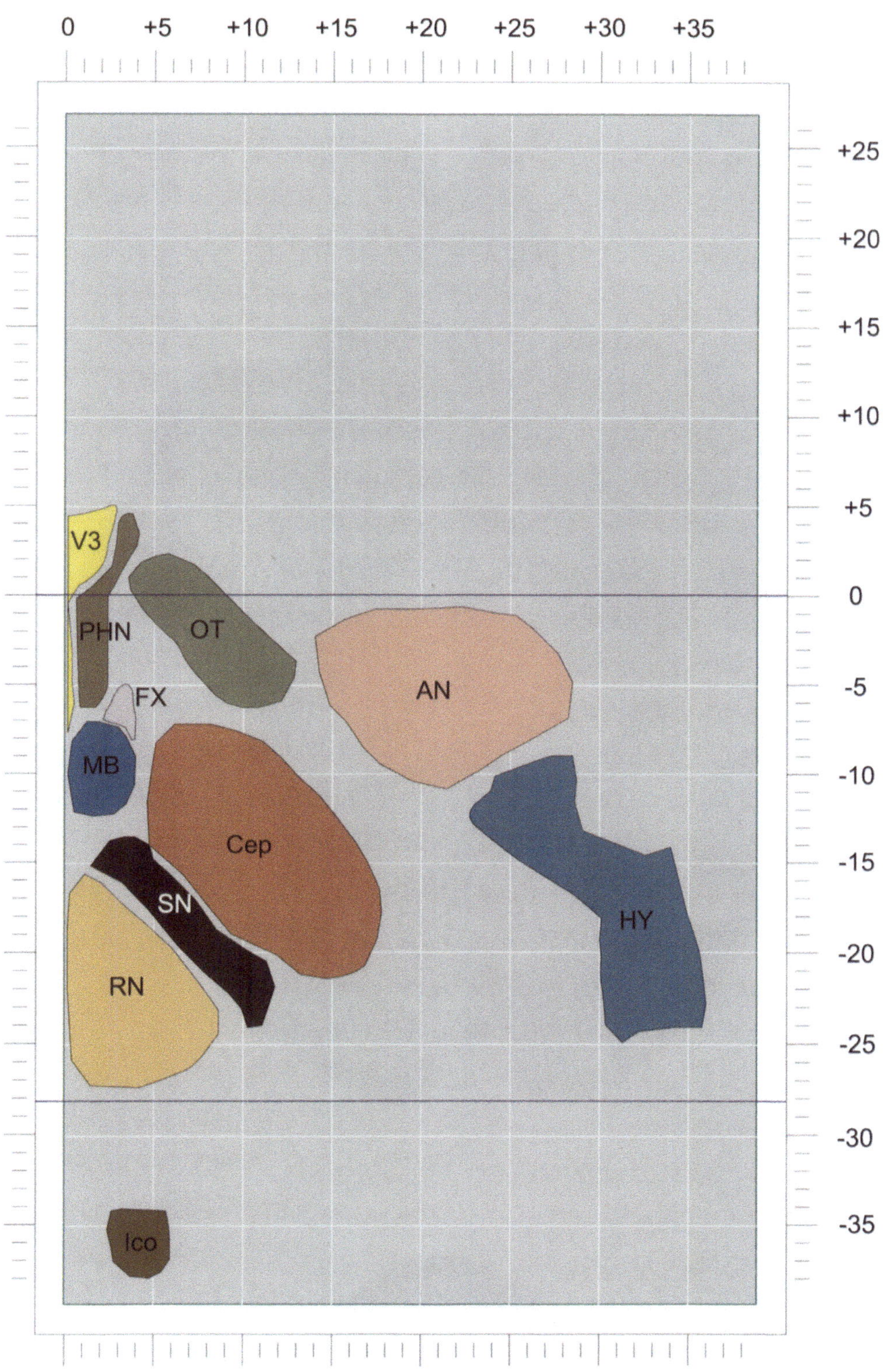


Axial -9 mm

# Plate 14a

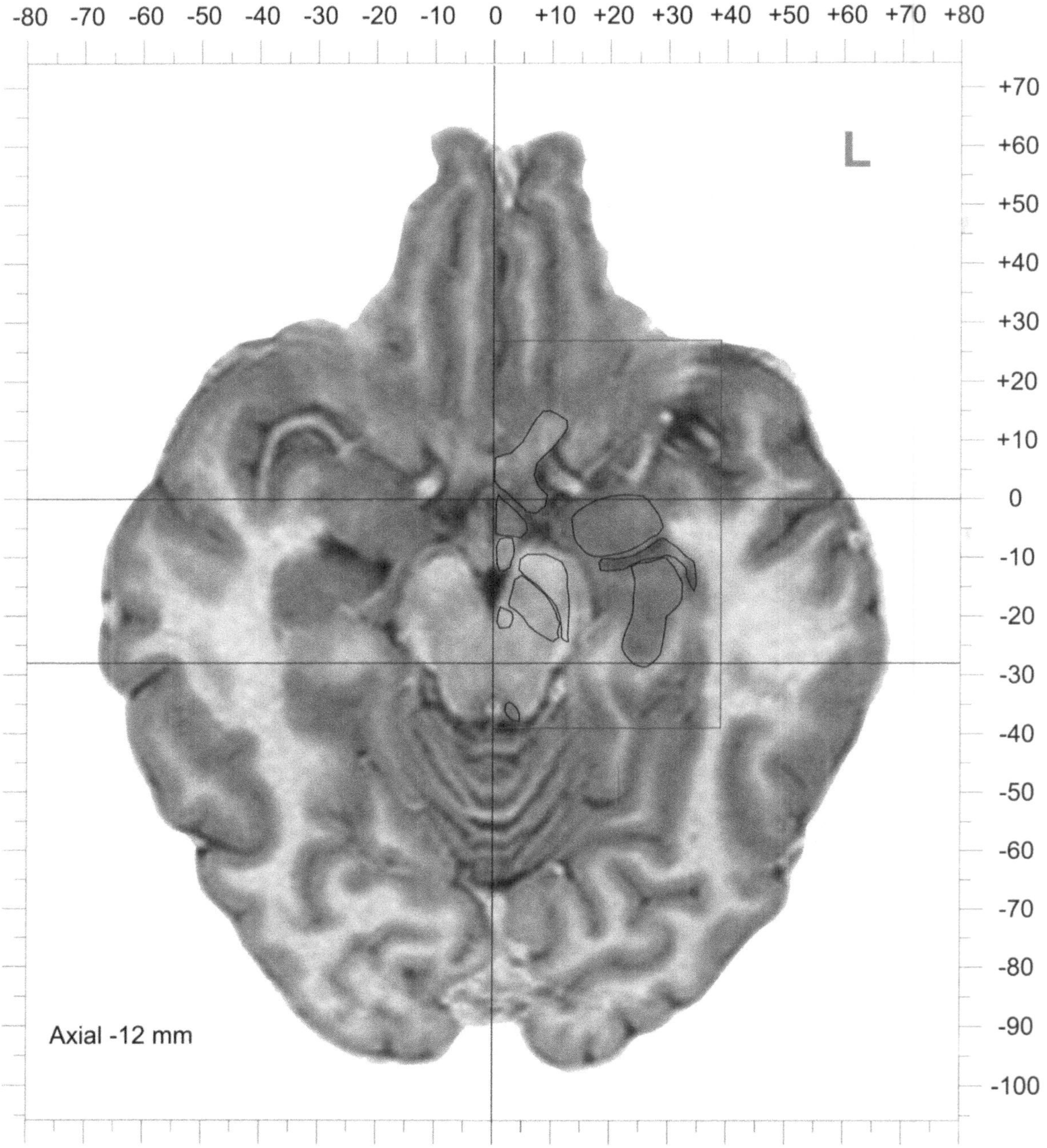

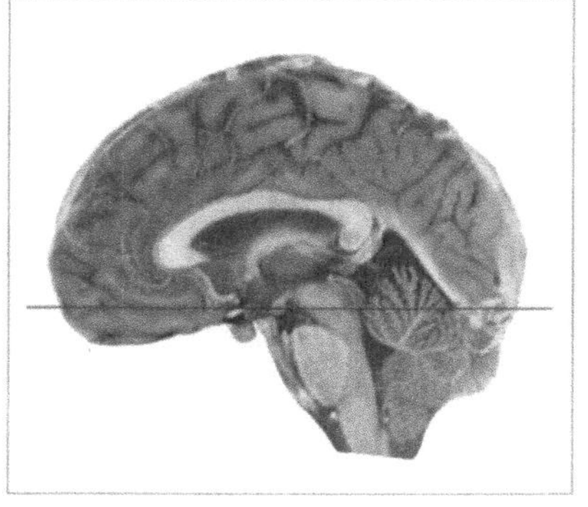

## Plate 14b

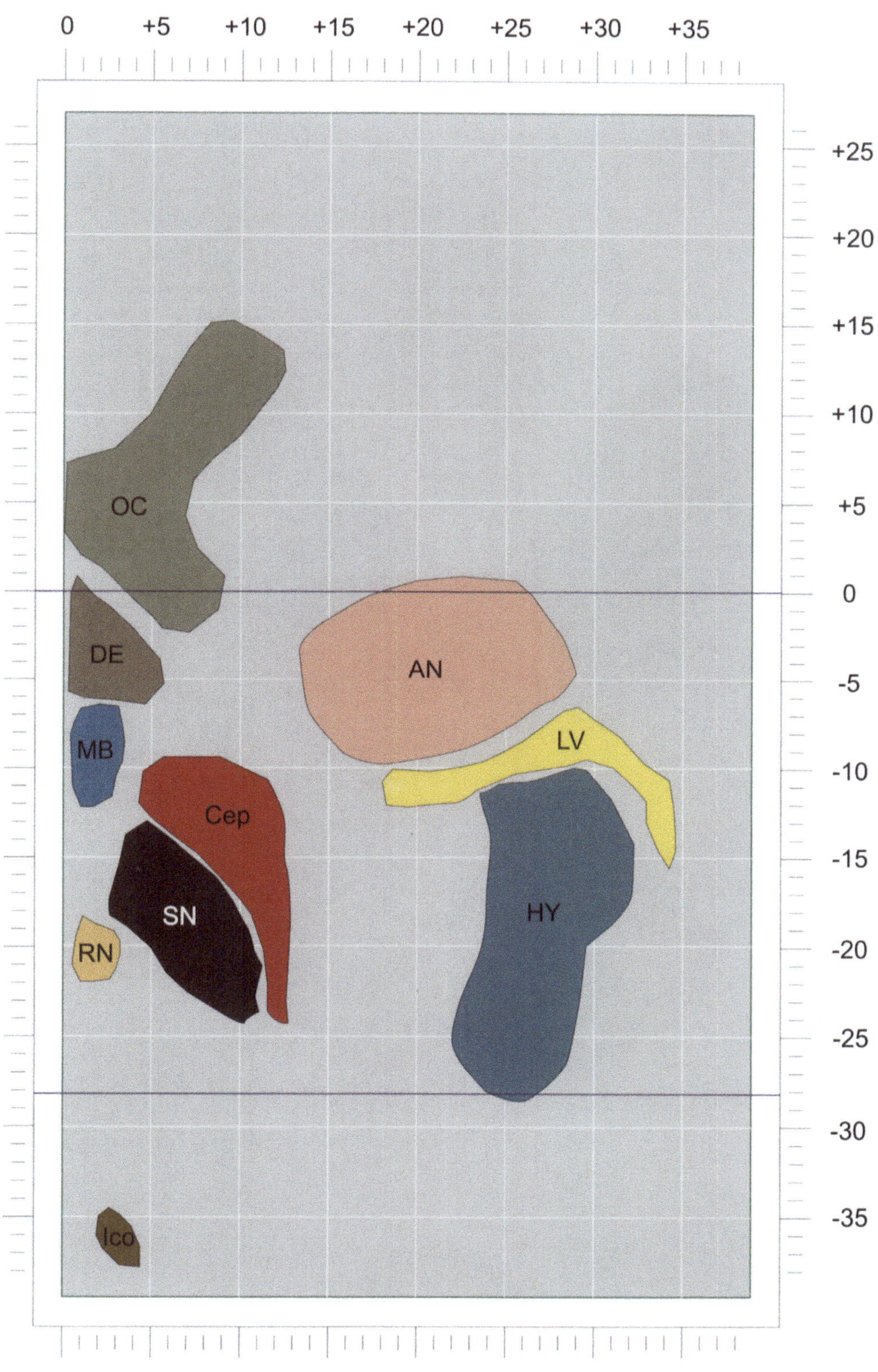


Axial -12 mm

## Plate 15a

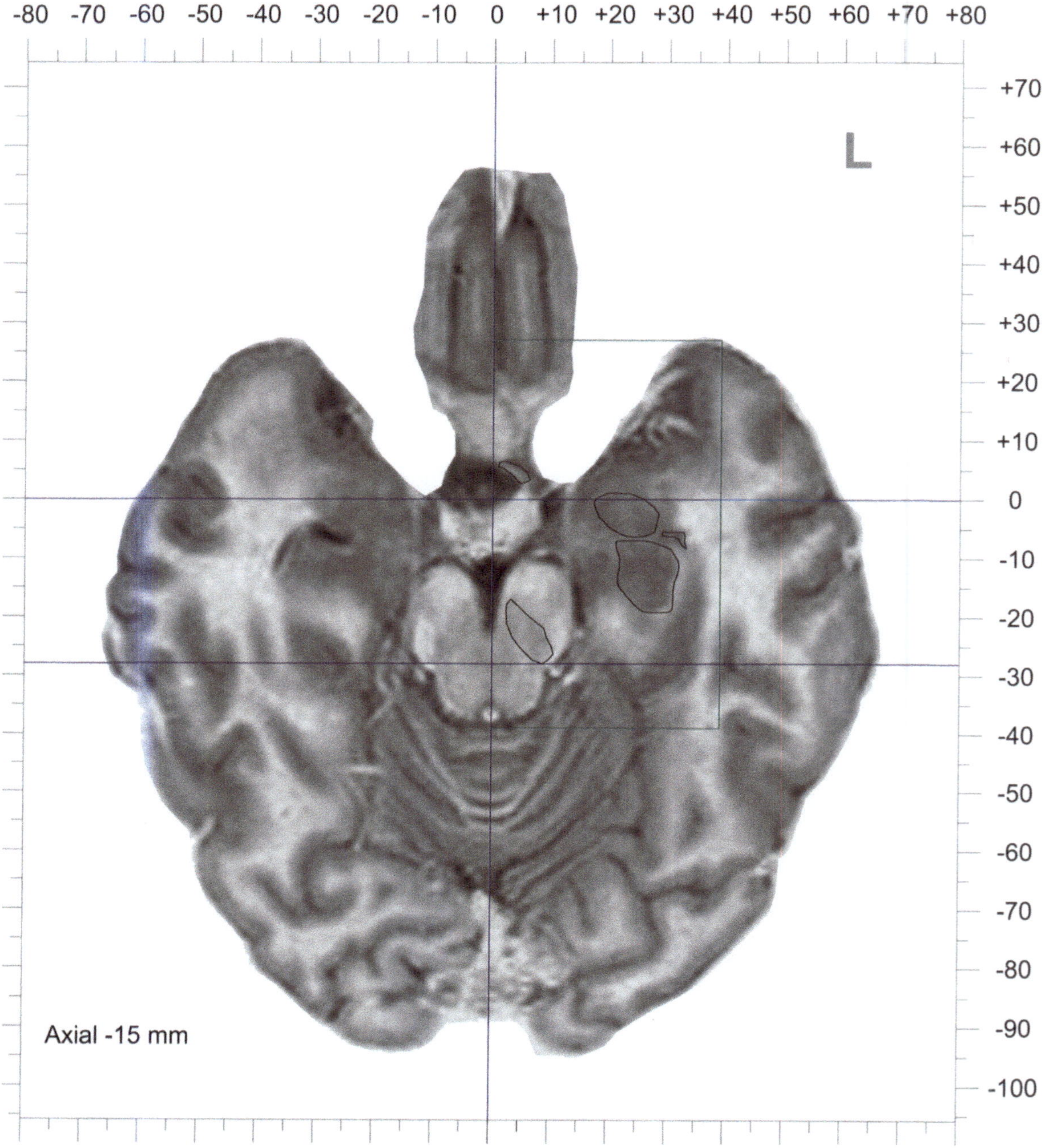

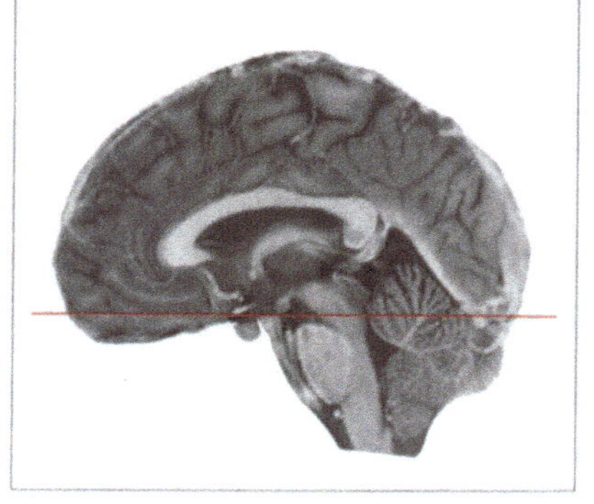

## Plate 15b

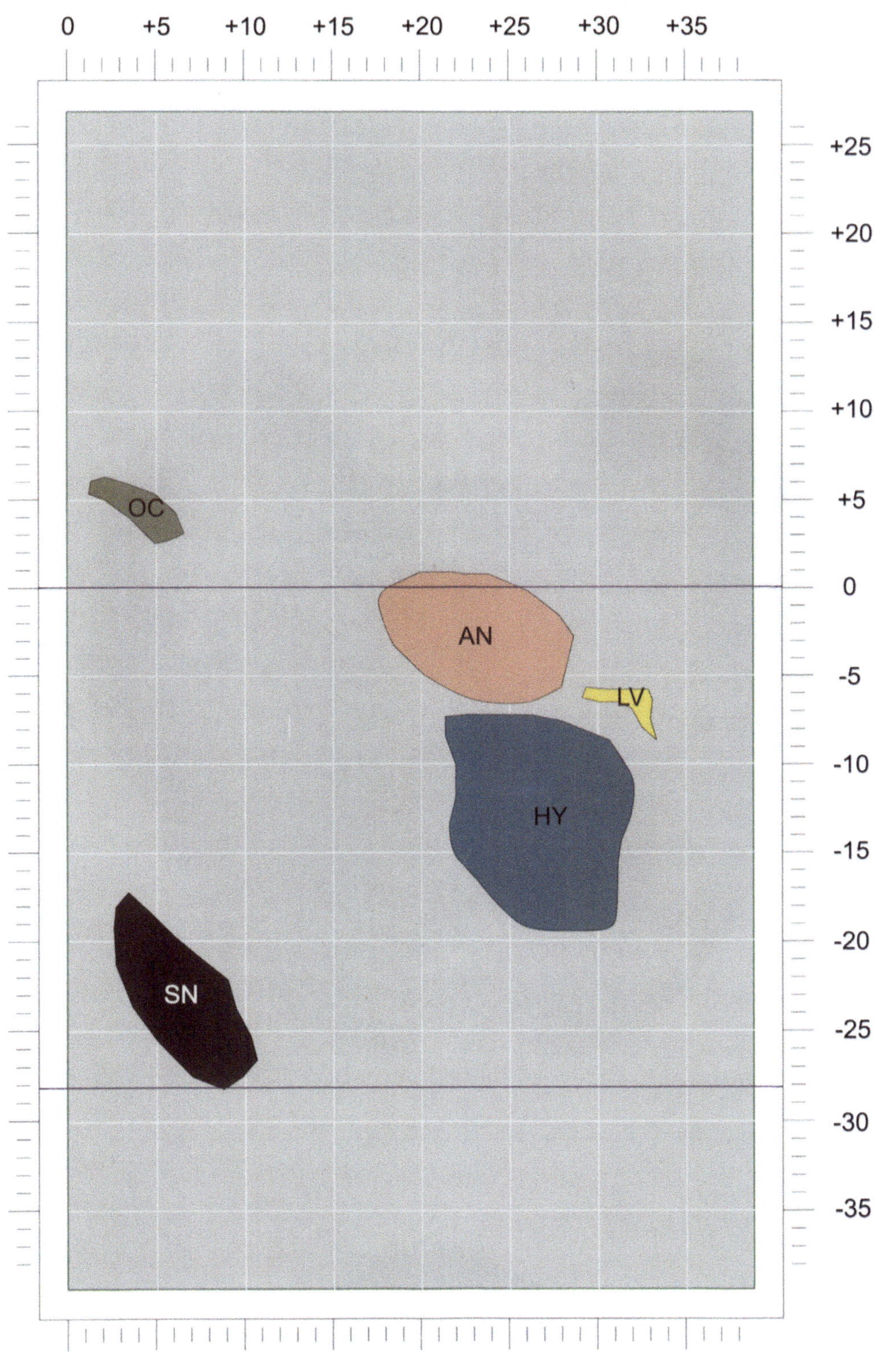


Axial -15 mm

# Plate 16a

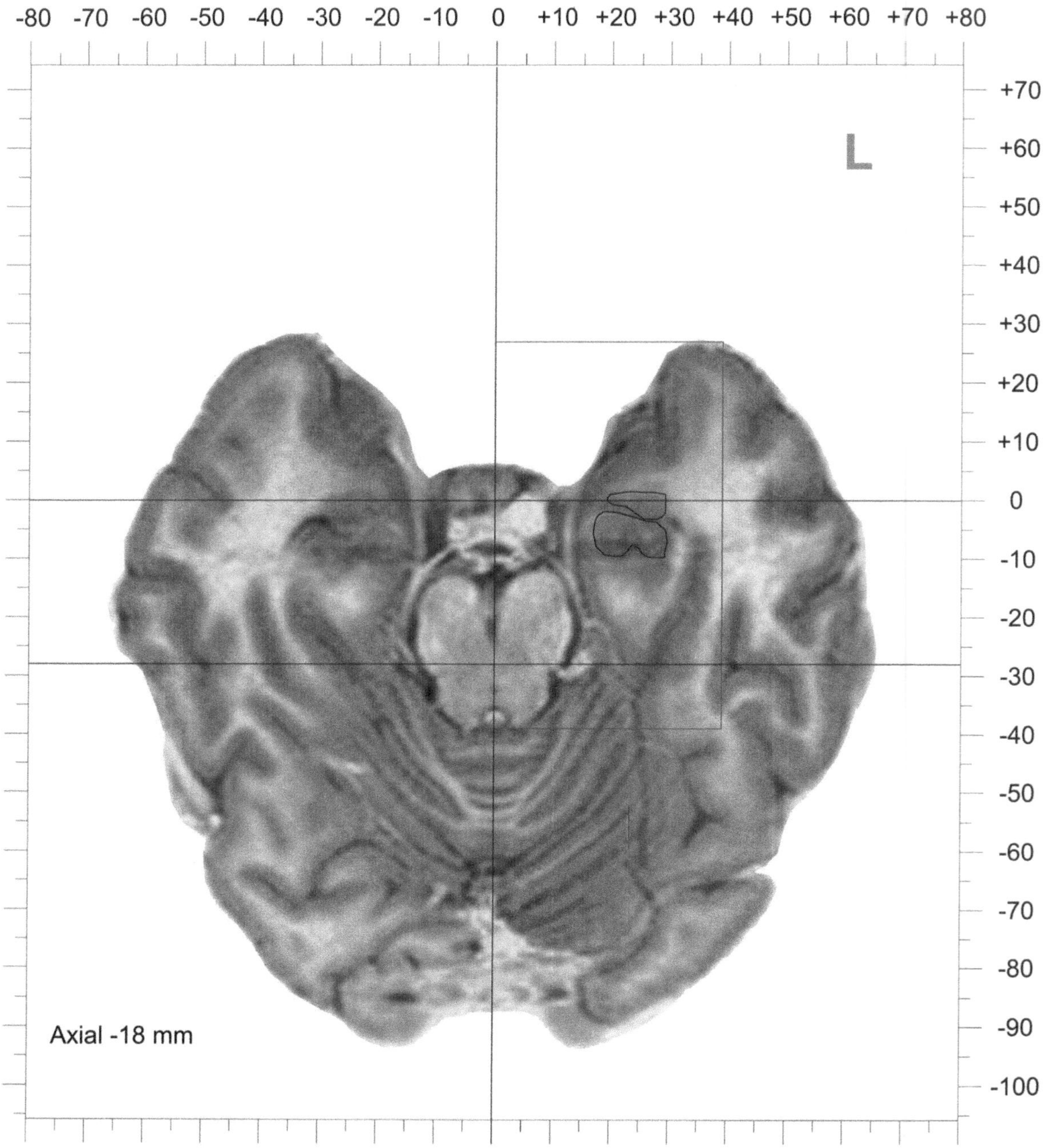

-80 -70 -60 -50 -40 -30 -20 -10 0 +10 +20 +30 +40 +50 +60 +70 +80
+70
+60
+50
+40
+30
+20
+10
0
-10
-20
-30
-40
-50
-60
-70
-80
-90
-100
L
Axial -18 mm

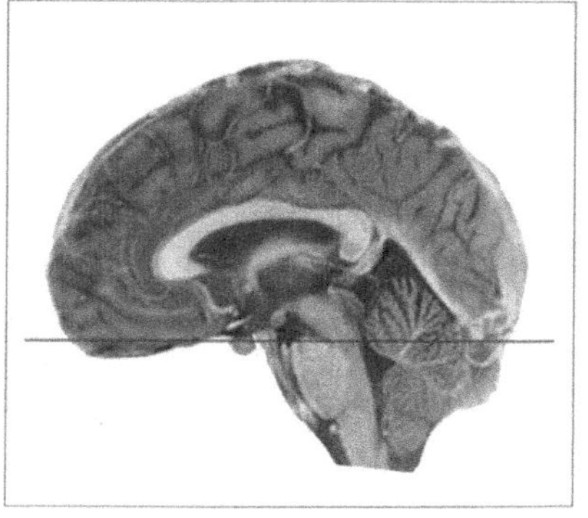

## Plate 16b

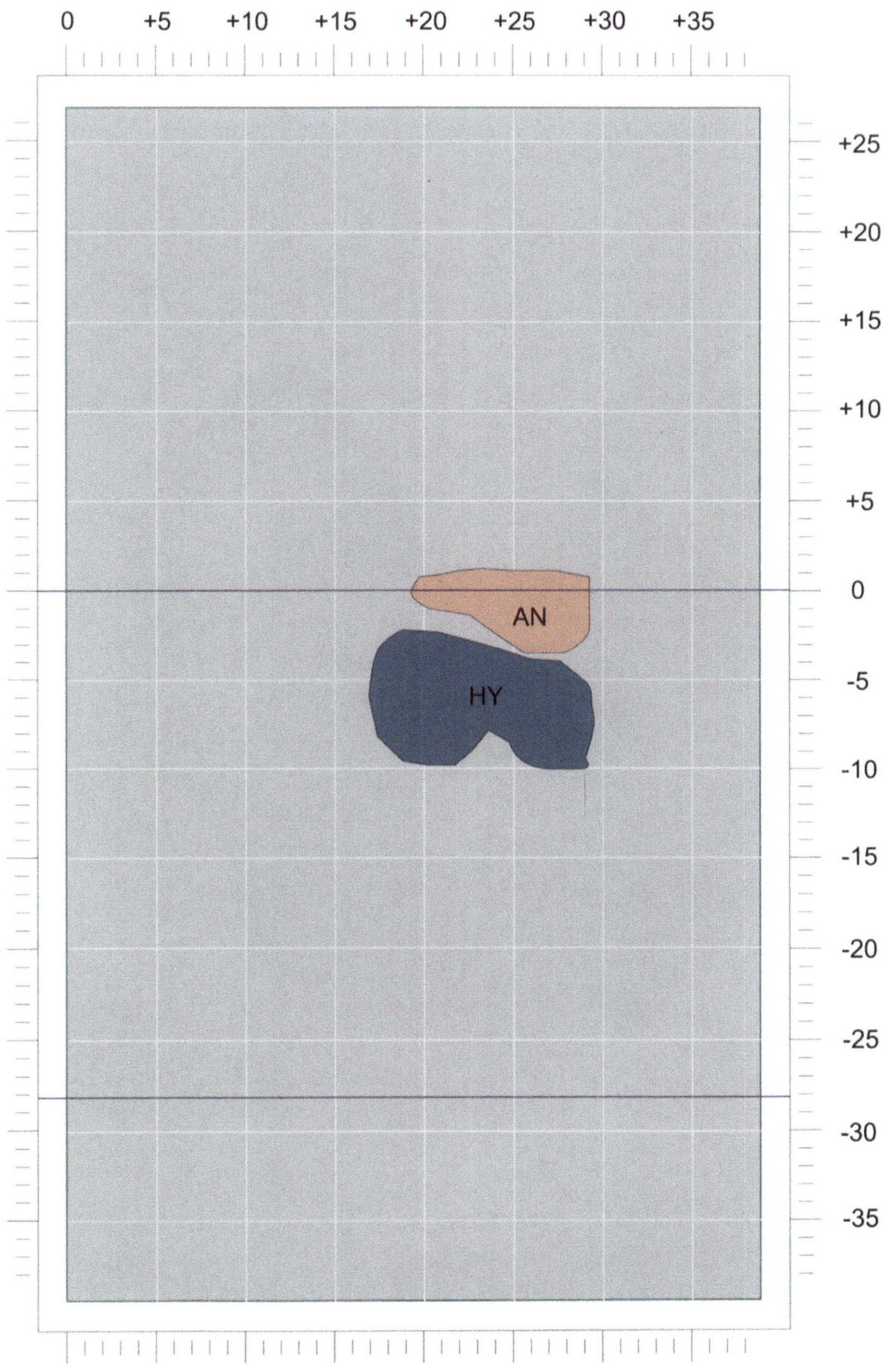



Axial -18 mm

## Plate 17a

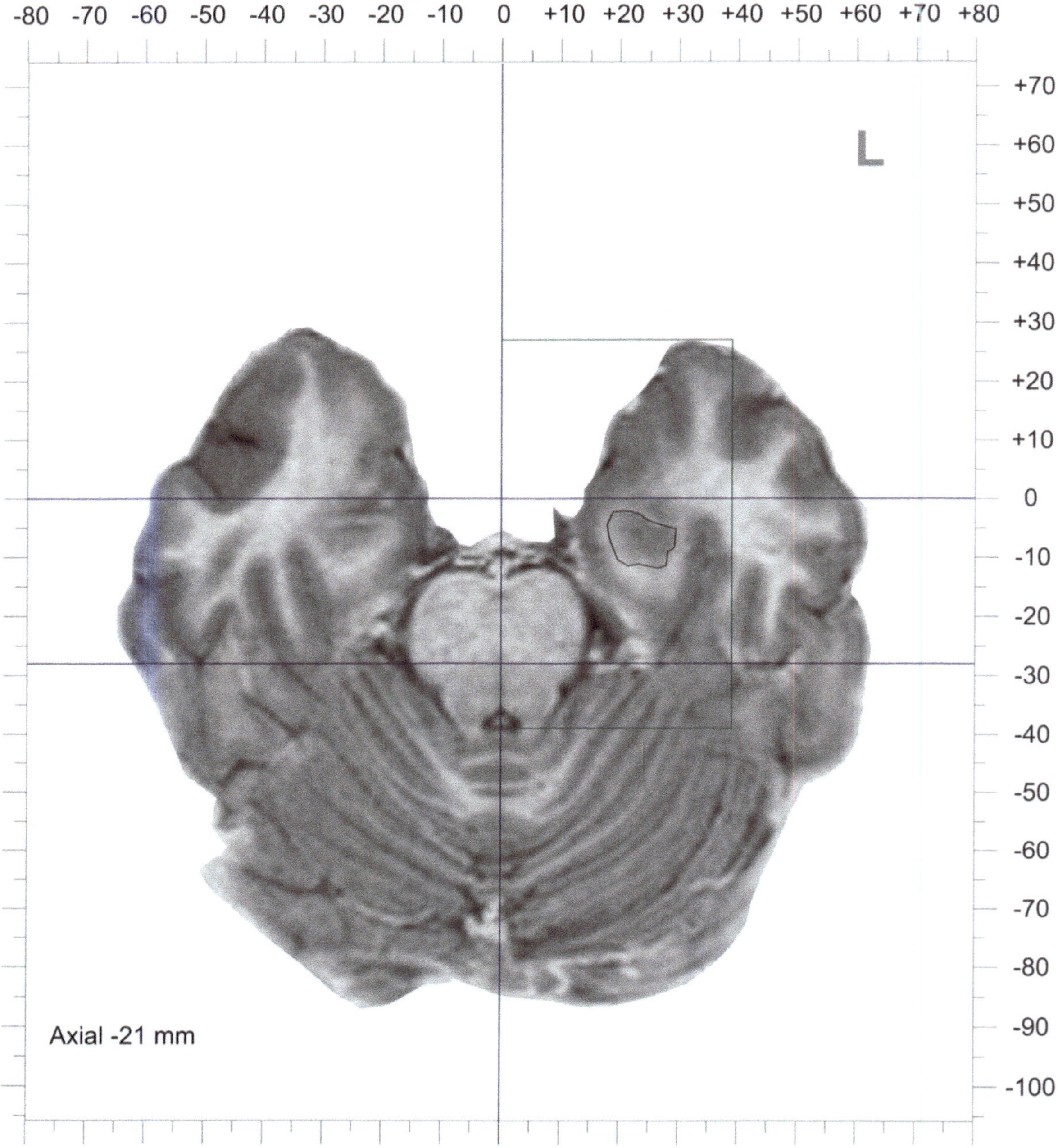

Axial -21 mm

L

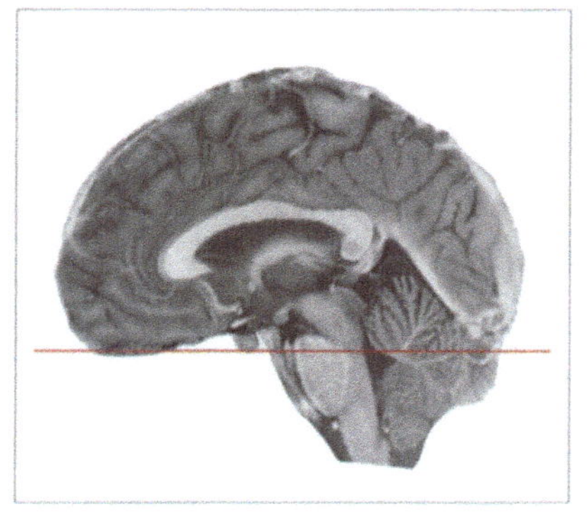

## Plate 17b

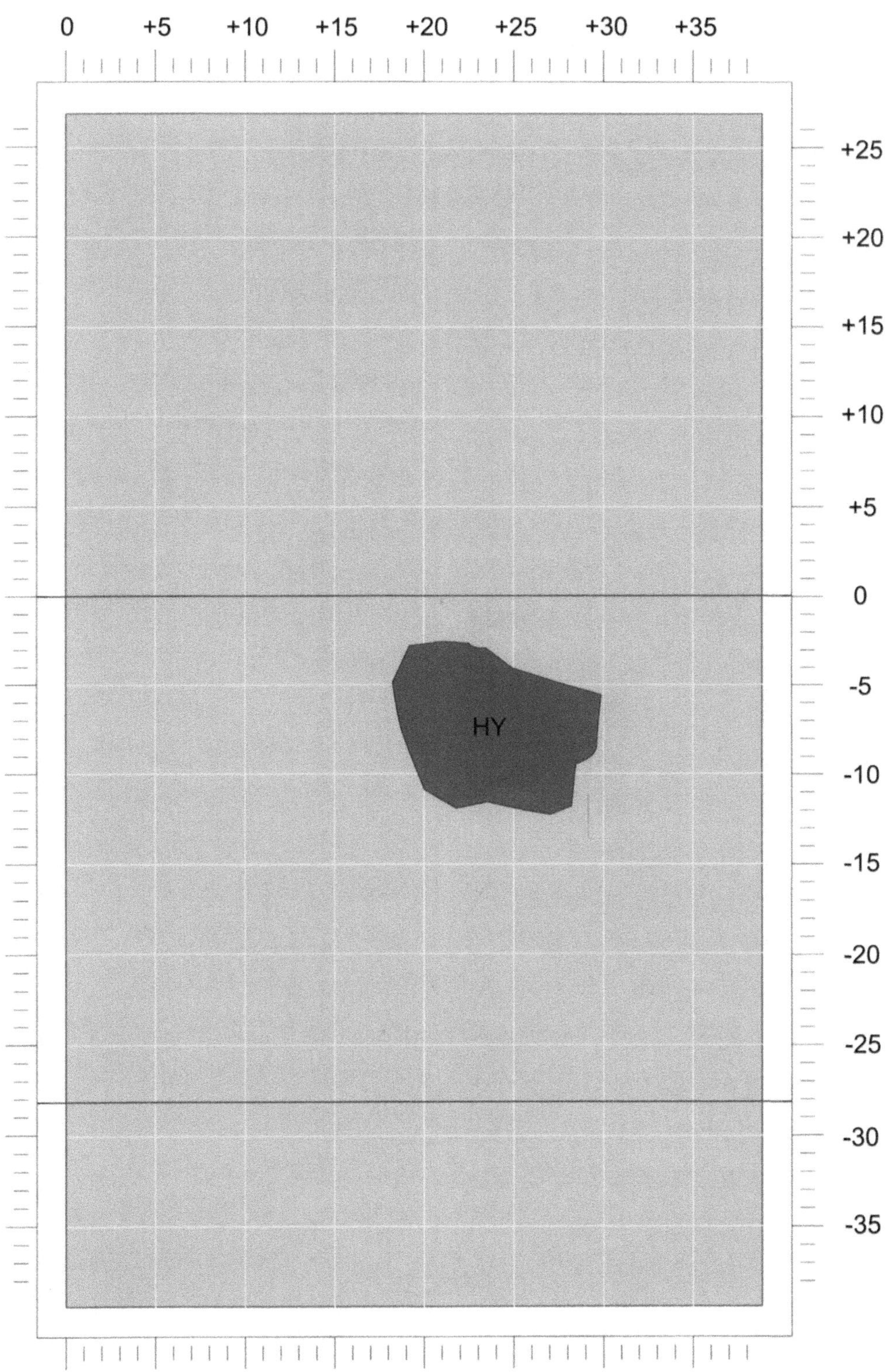


Axial -21 mm

# Coronal Sections

Plates 18-40

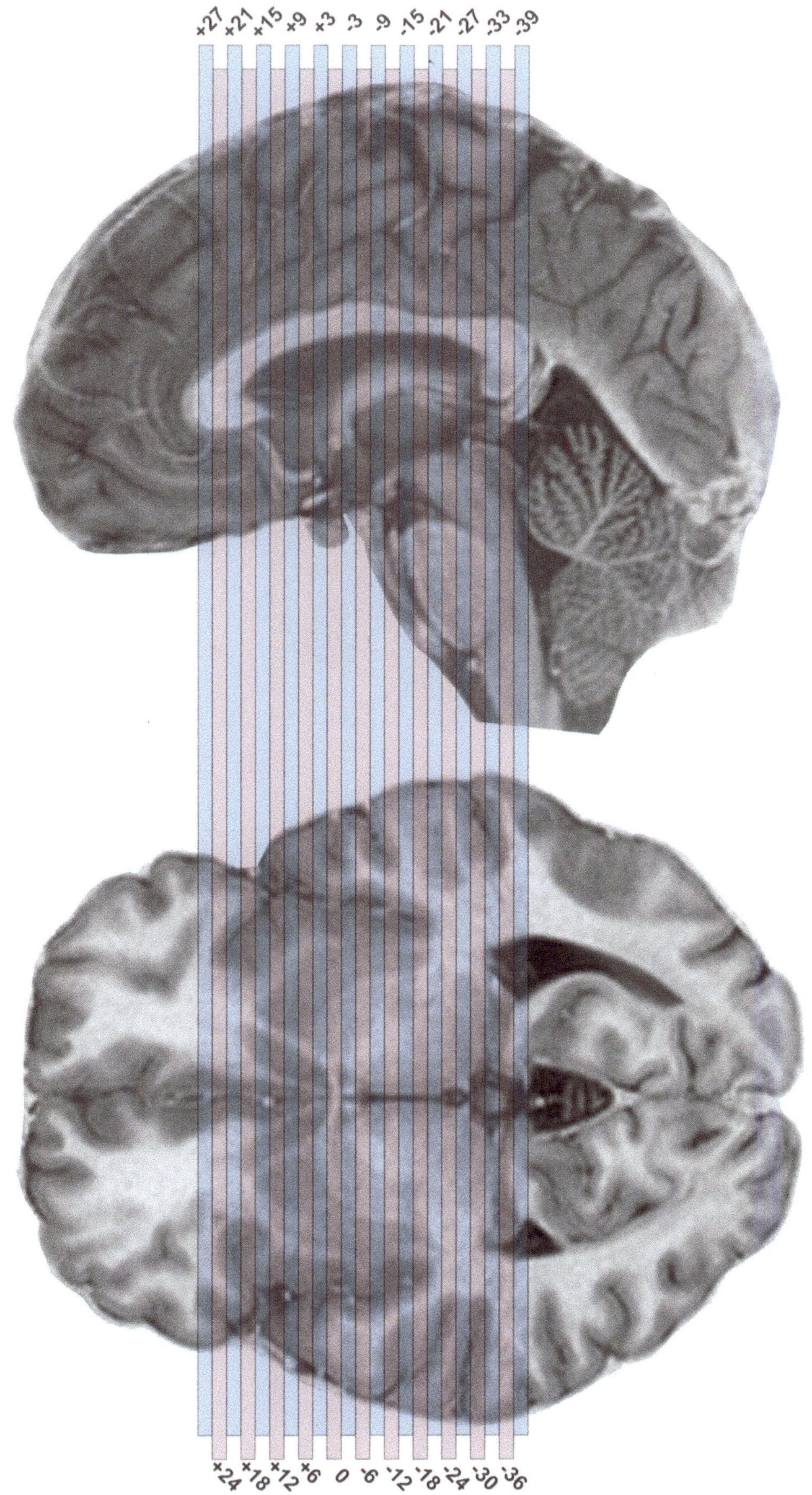

+27 +21 +15 +9 +3 -3 -9 -15 -21 -27 -33 -39
+24 +18 +12 +6 0 -6 -12 -18 -24 -30 -36

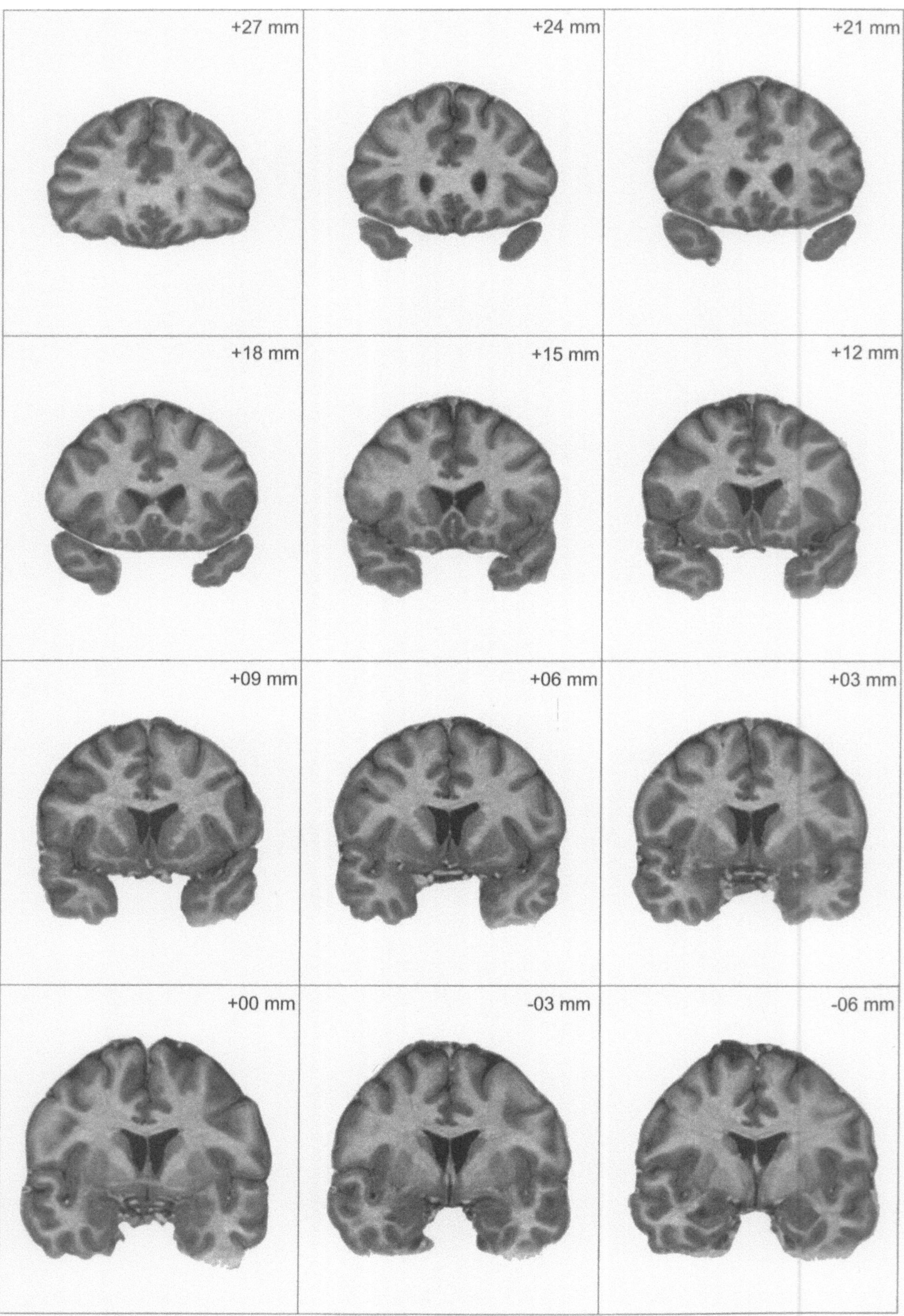

+27 mm
+24 mm
+21 mm
+18 mm
+15 mm
+12 mm
+09 mm
+06 mm
+03 mm
+00 mm
-03 mm
-06 mm

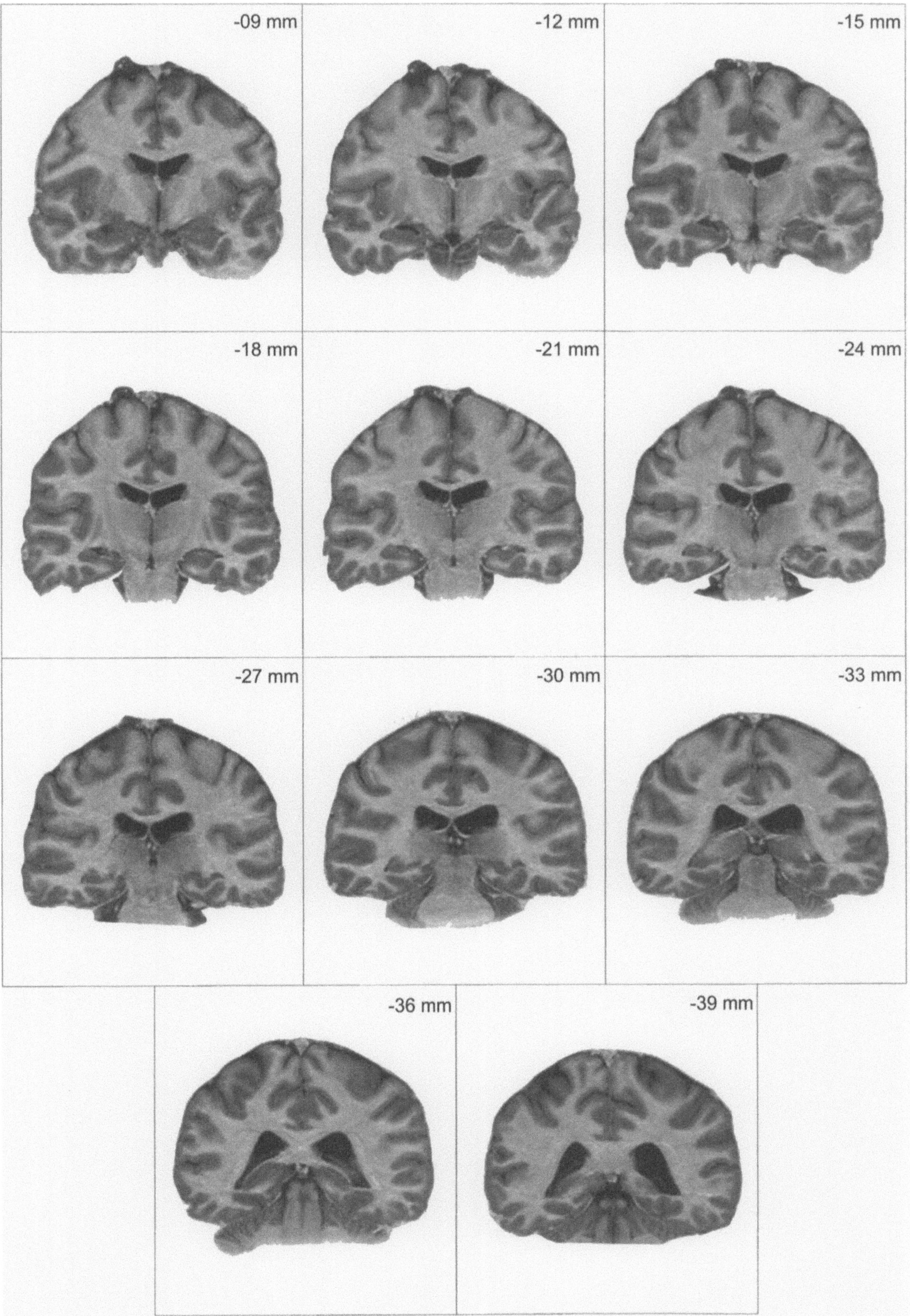

# Abbreviation – Nomenclature – Color Codes

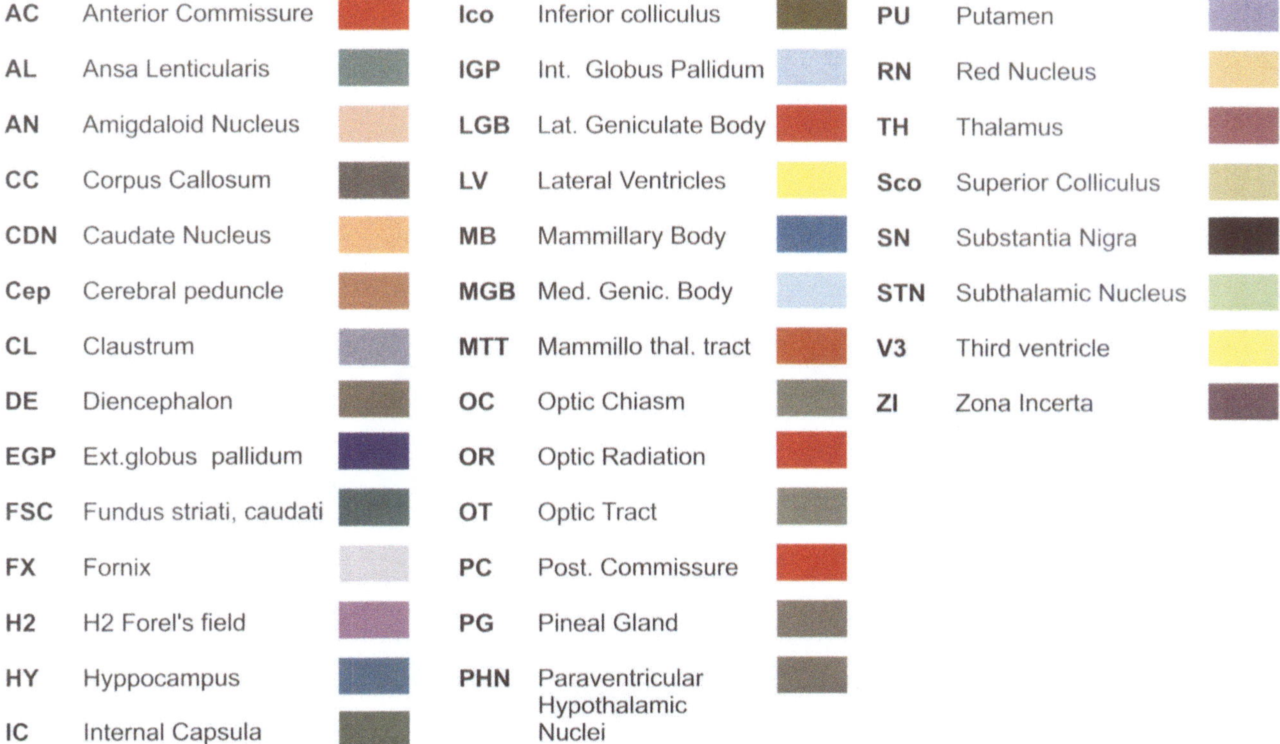

| | | | | | | | | |
|---|---|---|---|---|---|---|---|---|
| **AC** | Anterior Commissure | | **Ico** | Inferior colliculus | | **PU** | Putamen | |
| **AL** | Ansa Lenticularis | | **IGP** | Int. Globus Pallidum | | **RN** | Red Nucleus | |
| **AN** | Amigdaloid Nucleus | | **LGB** | Lat. Geniculate Body | | **TH** | Thalamus | |
| **CC** | Corpus Callosum | | **LV** | Lateral Ventricles | | **Sco** | Superior Colliculus | |
| **CDN** | Caudate Nucleus | | **MB** | Mammillary Body | | **SN** | Substantia Nigra | |
| **Cep** | Cerebral peduncle | | **MGB** | Med. Genic. Body | | **STN** | Subthalamic Nucleus | |
| **CL** | Claustrum | | **MTT** | Mammillo thal. tract | | **V3** | Third ventricle | |
| **DE** | Diencephalon | | **OC** | Optic Chiasm | | **ZI** | Zona Incerta | |
| **EGP** | Ext.globus pallidum | | **OR** | Optic Radiation | | | | |
| **FSC** | Fundus striati, caudati | | **OT** | Optic Tract | | | | |
| **FX** | Fornix | | **PC** | Post. Commissure | | | | |
| **H2** | H2 Forel's field | | **PG** | Pineal Gland | | | | |
| **HY** | Hyppocampus | | **PHN** | Paraventricular Hypothalamic Nuclei | | | | |
| **IC** | Internal Capsula | | | | | | | |

## Plate 18a

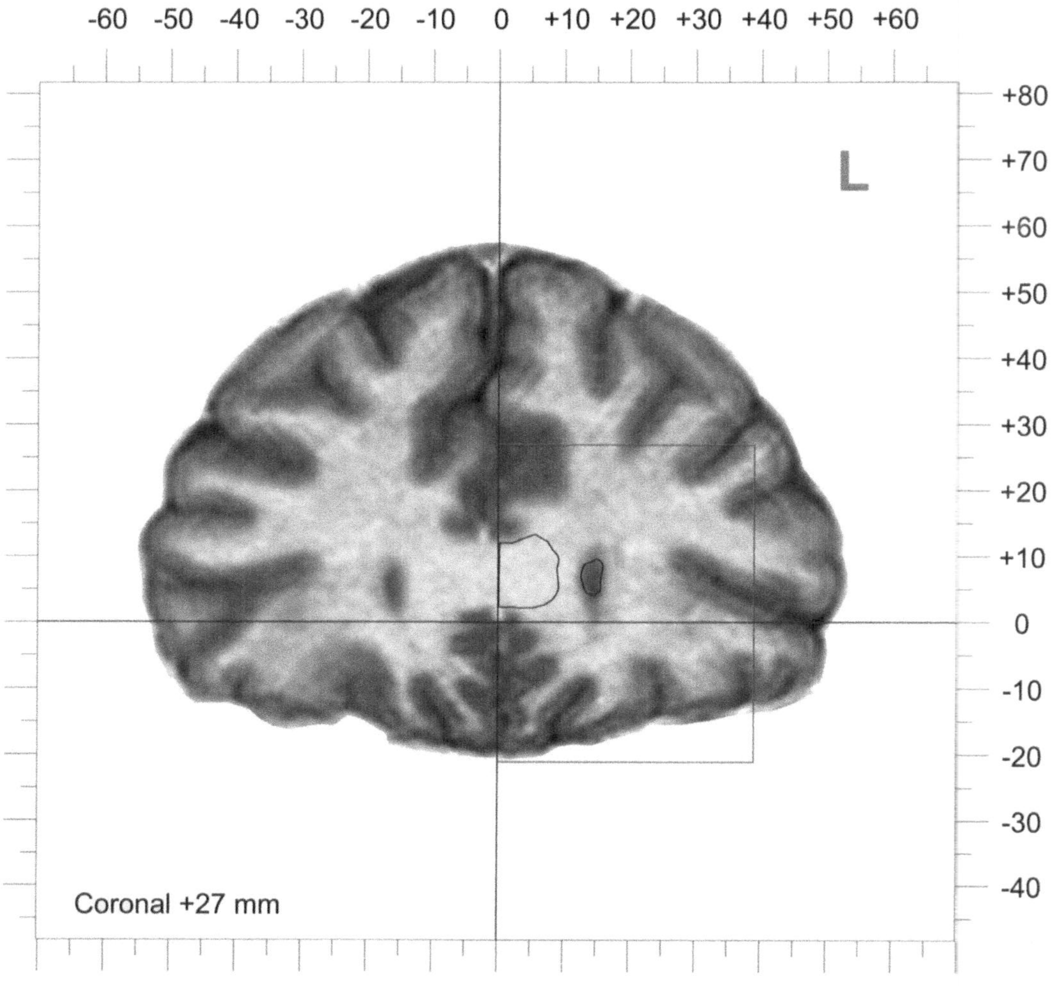


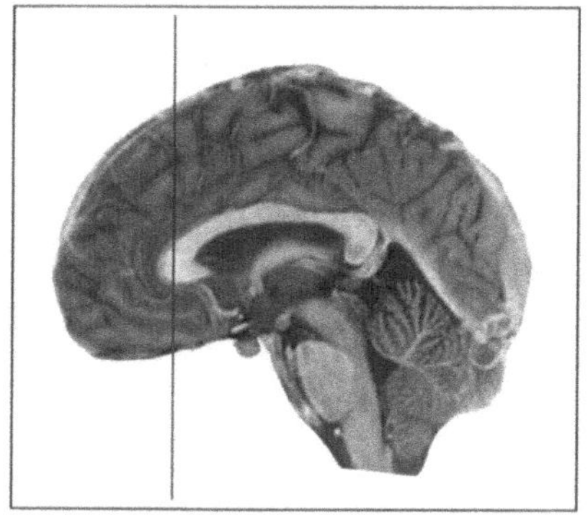

## Plate 18b

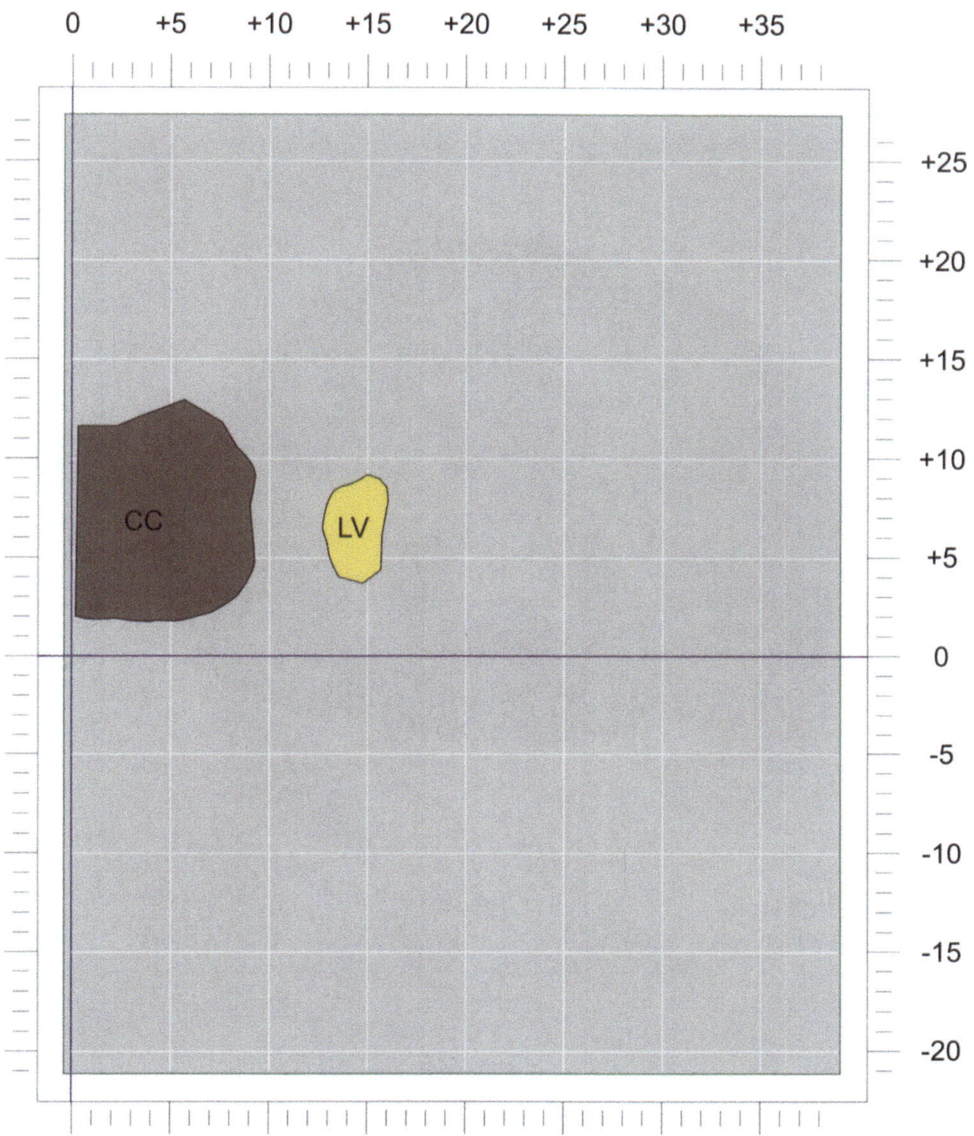


Coronal +27 mm

## Plate 19a

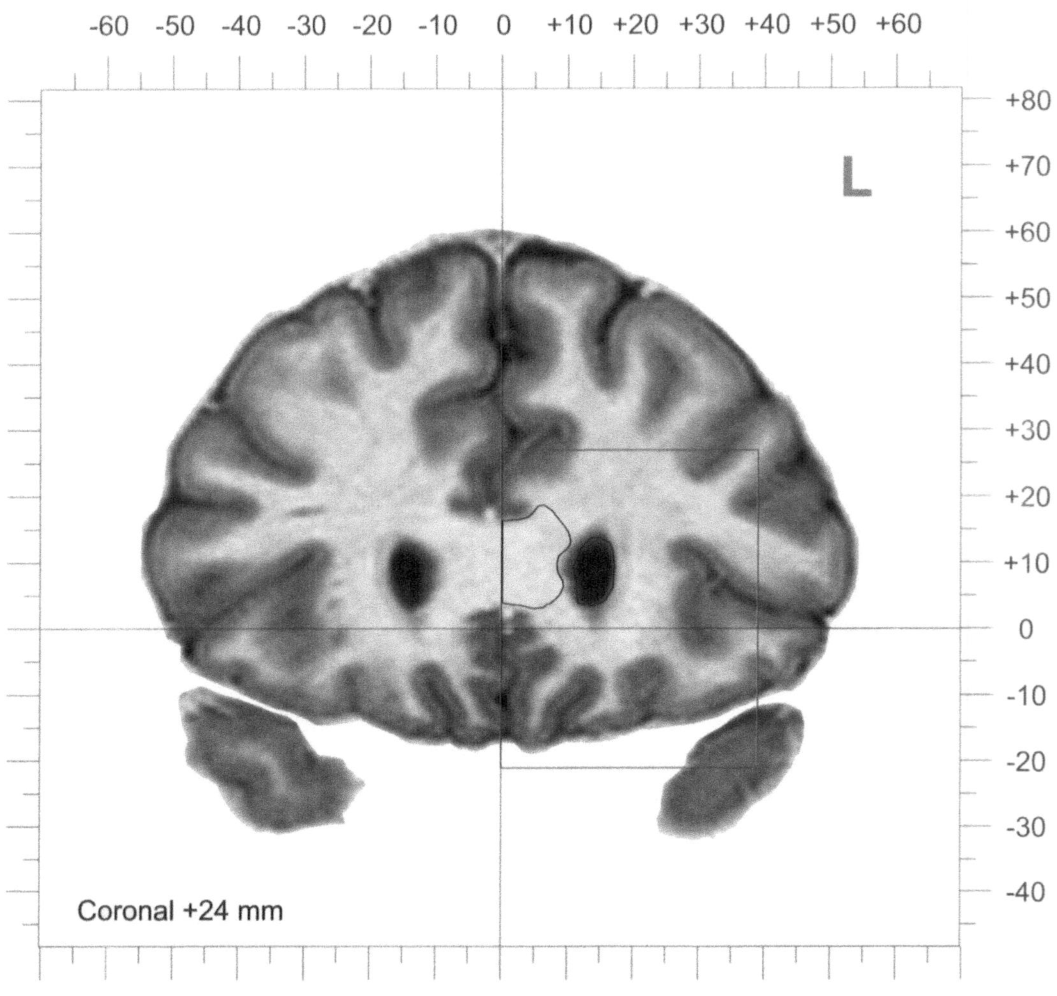


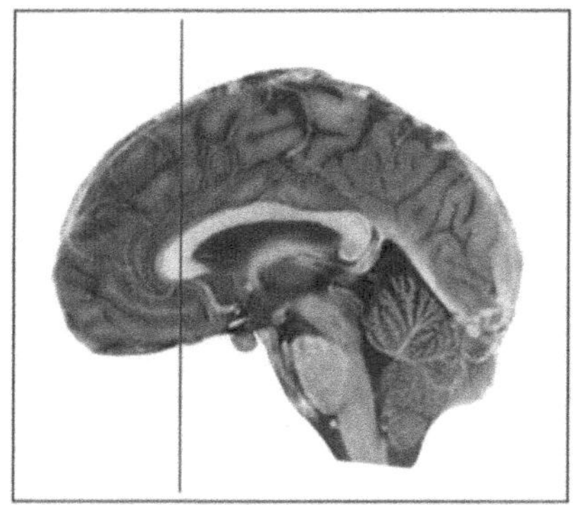

## Plate 19b

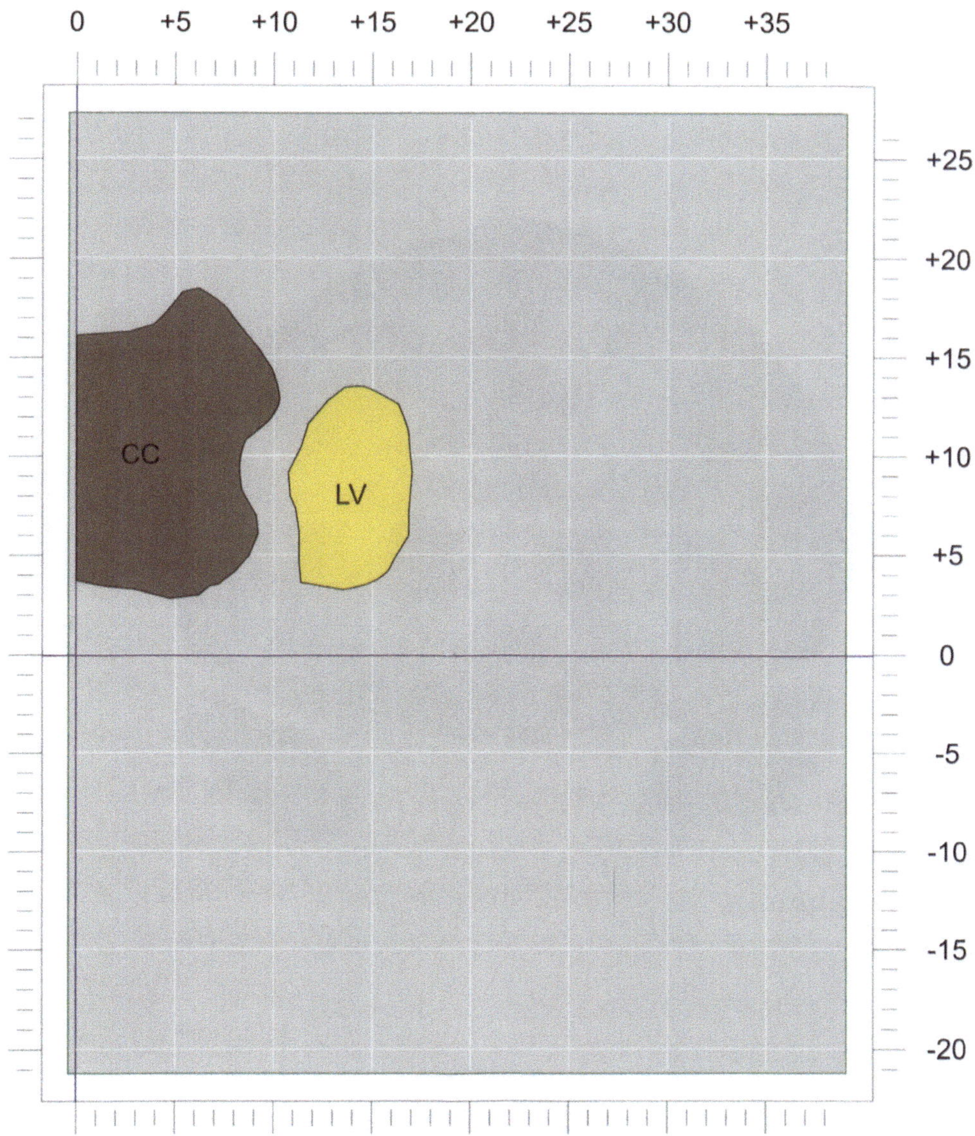


Coronal +24 mm

## Plate 20a

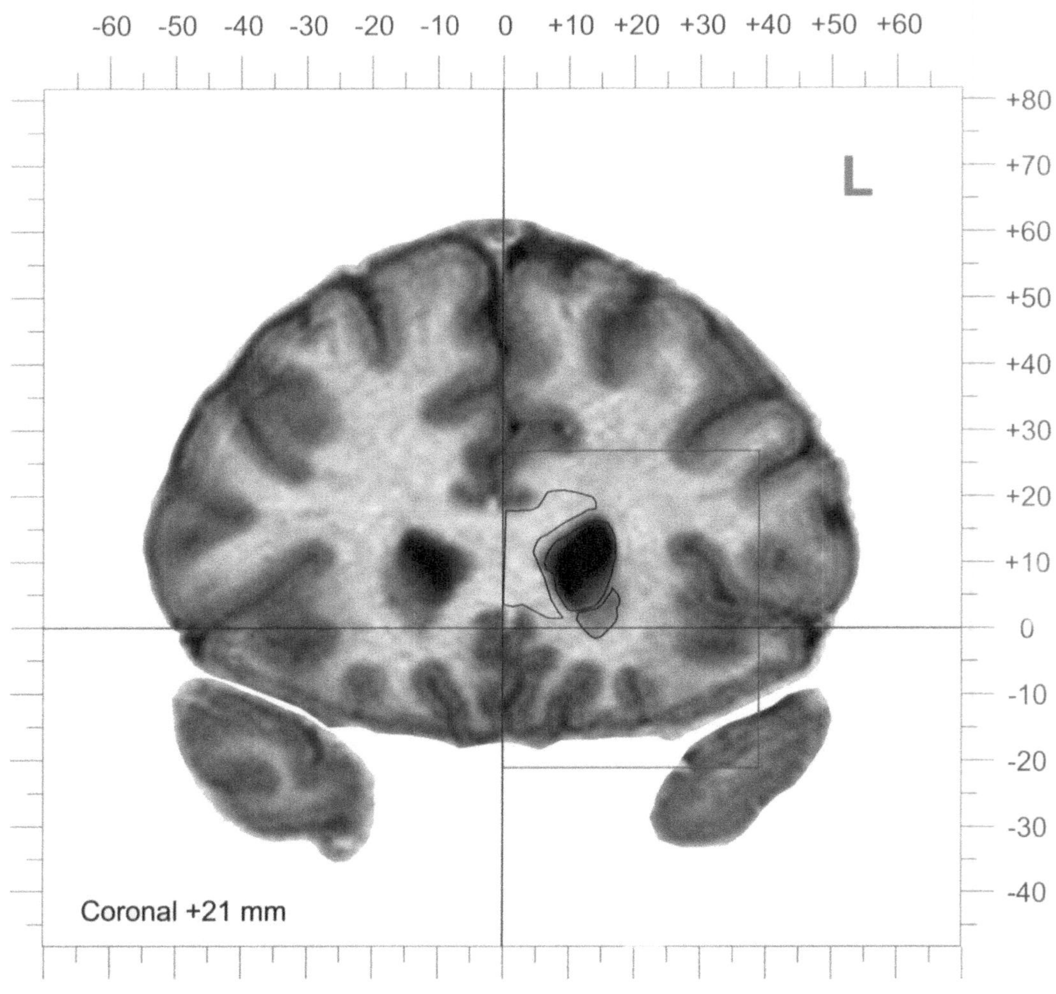


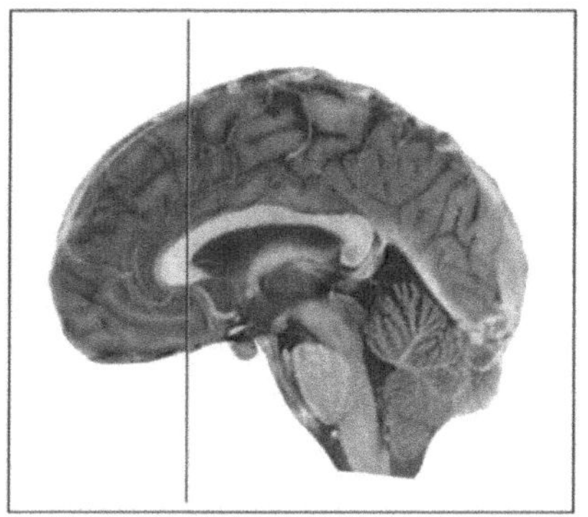

# Plate 20b

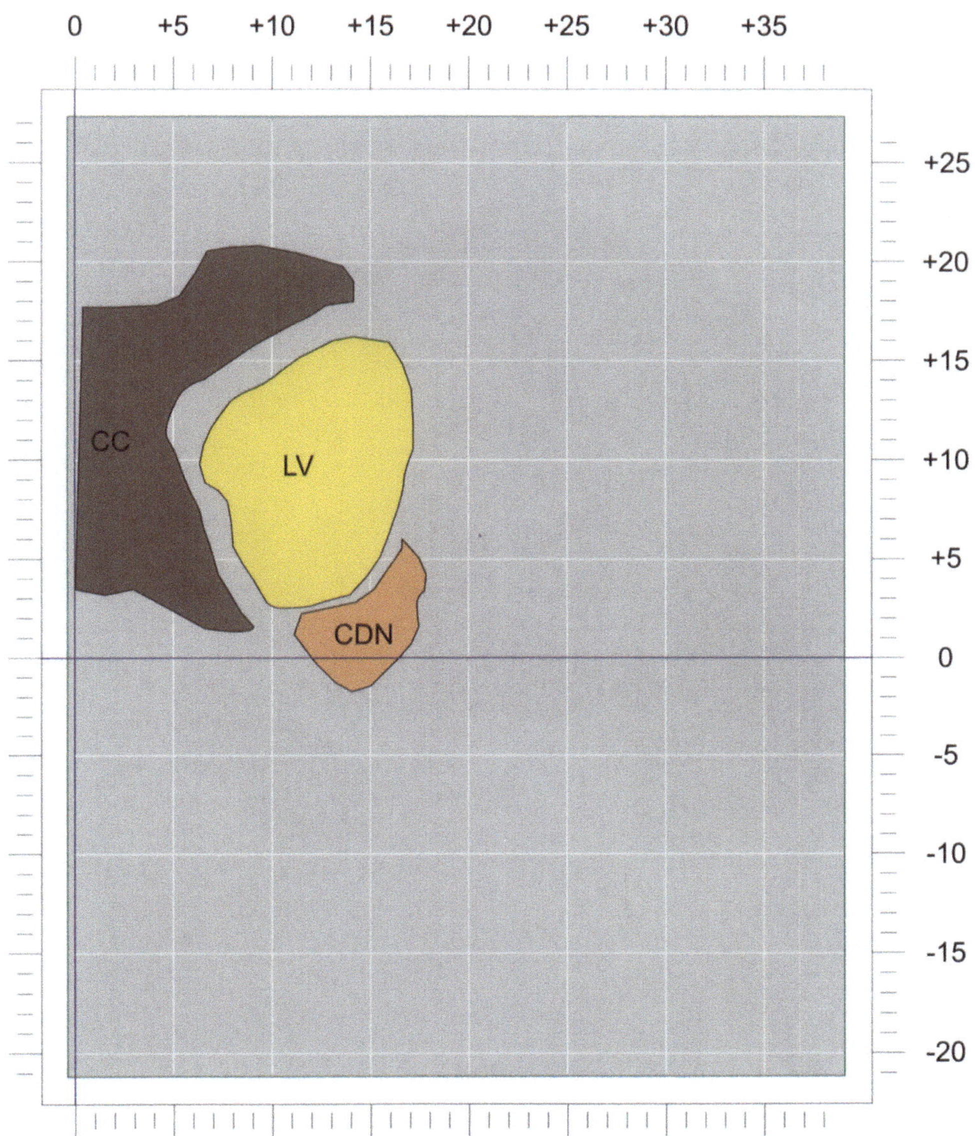


Coronal +21 mm

# Plate 21a

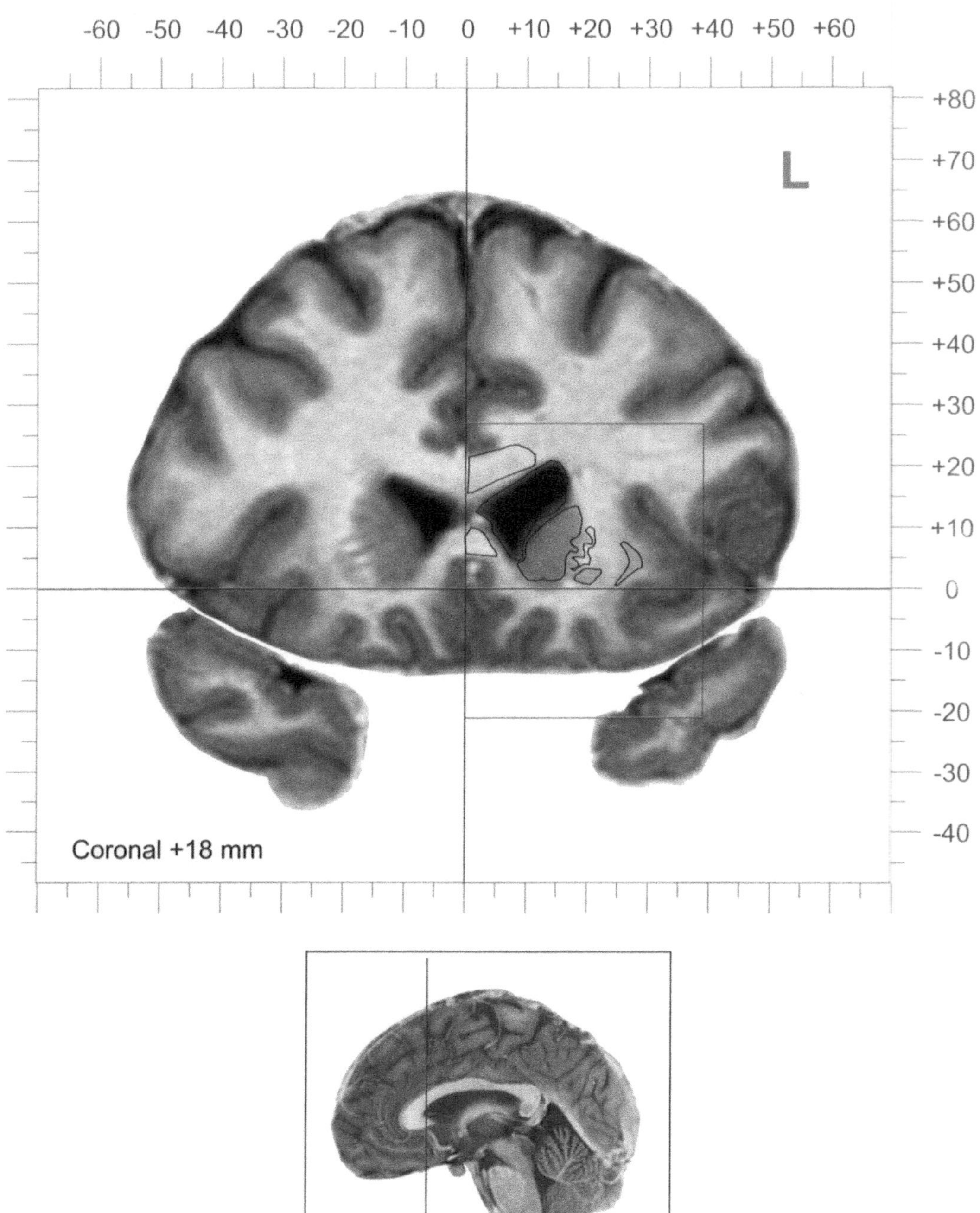

# Plate 21b

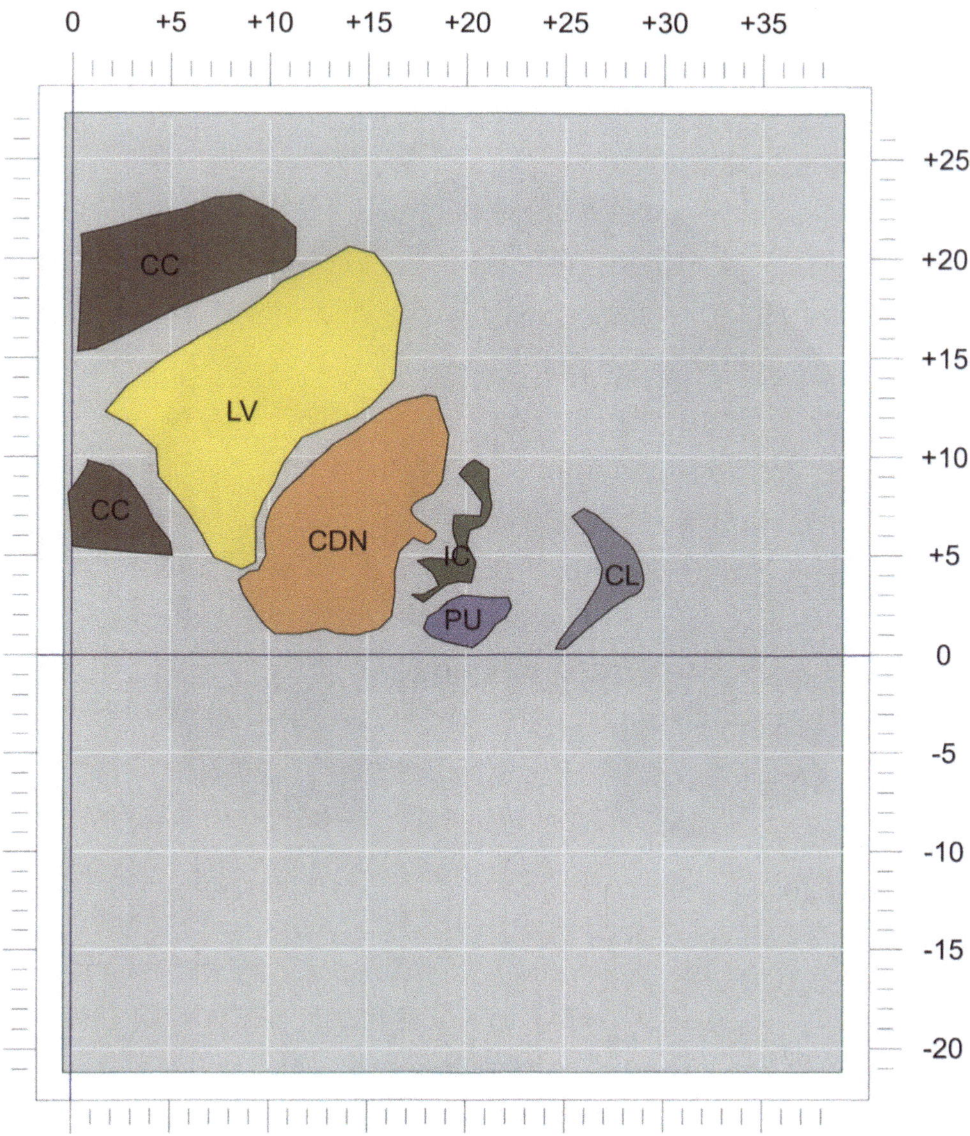


Coronal +18 mm

## Plate 22a

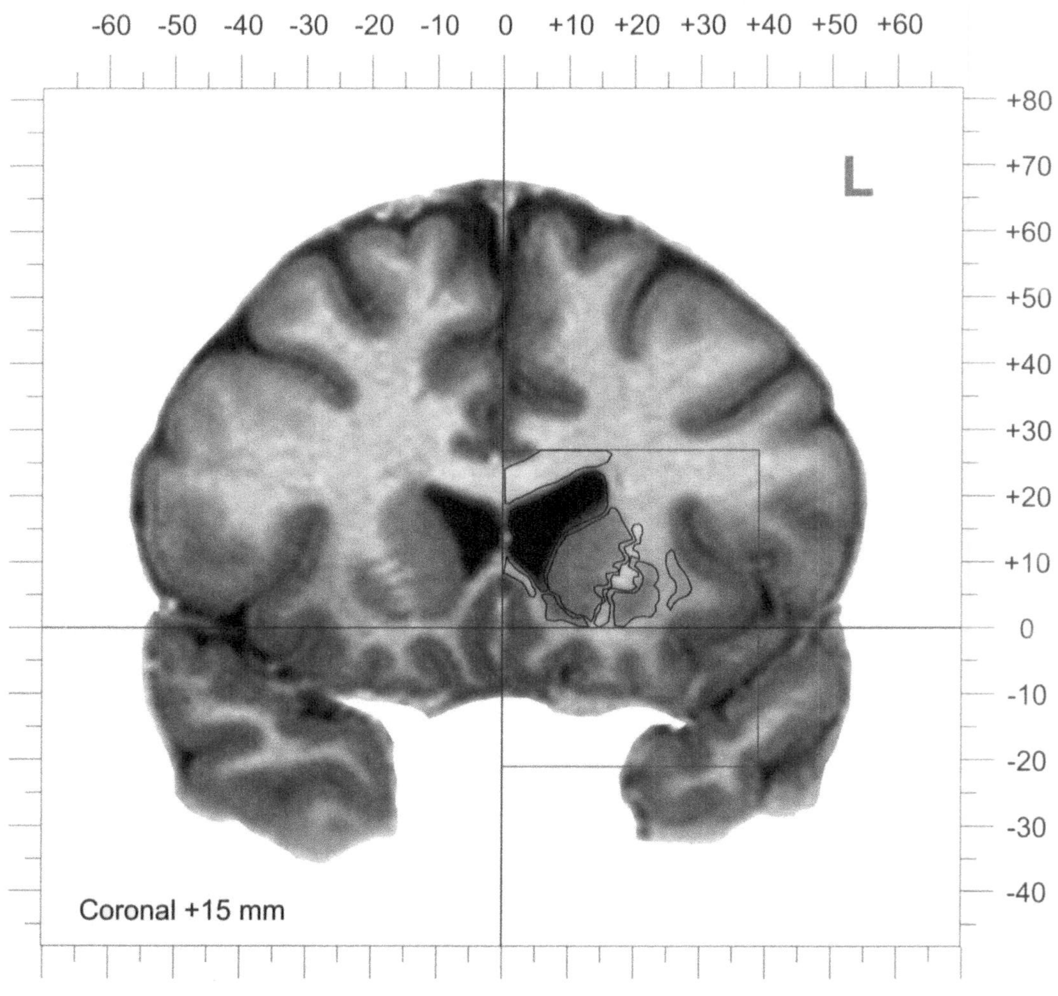


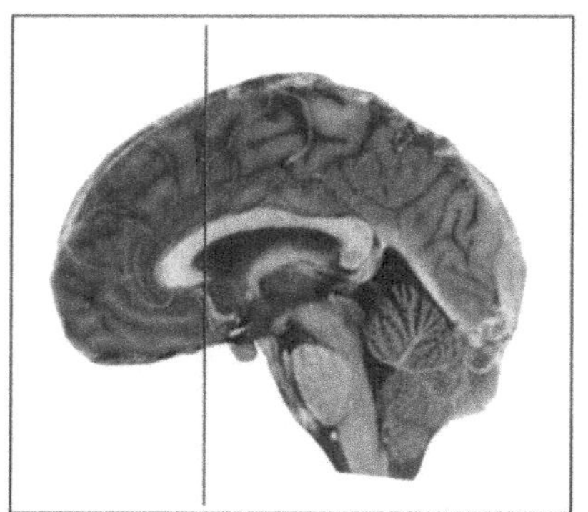

## Plate 22b

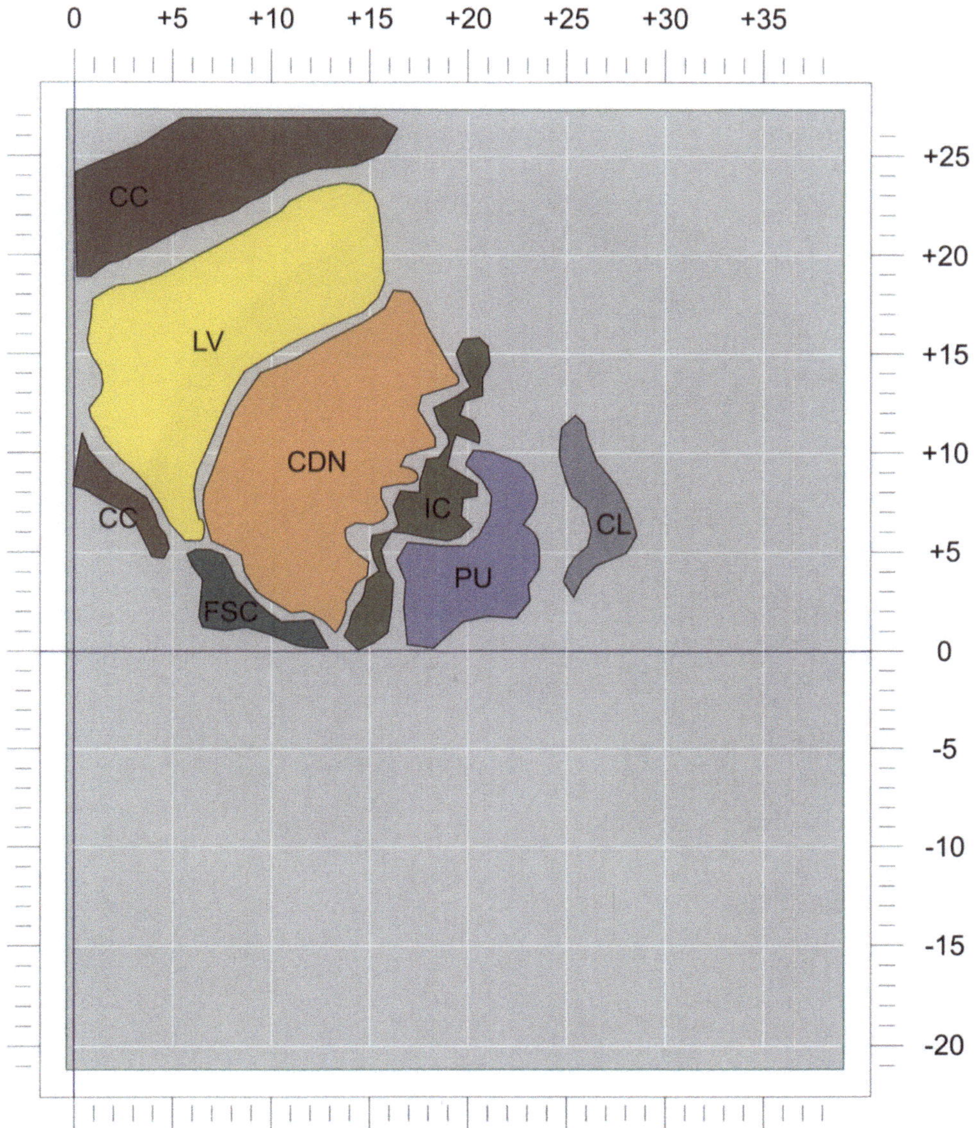


Coronal +15 mm

# Plate 23a

-60
-50
-40
-30
-20
-10
0
+10
+20
+30
+40
+50
+60
+80
+70
+60
+50
+40
+30
+20
+10
0
-10
-20
-30
-40
L
Coronal +12 mm

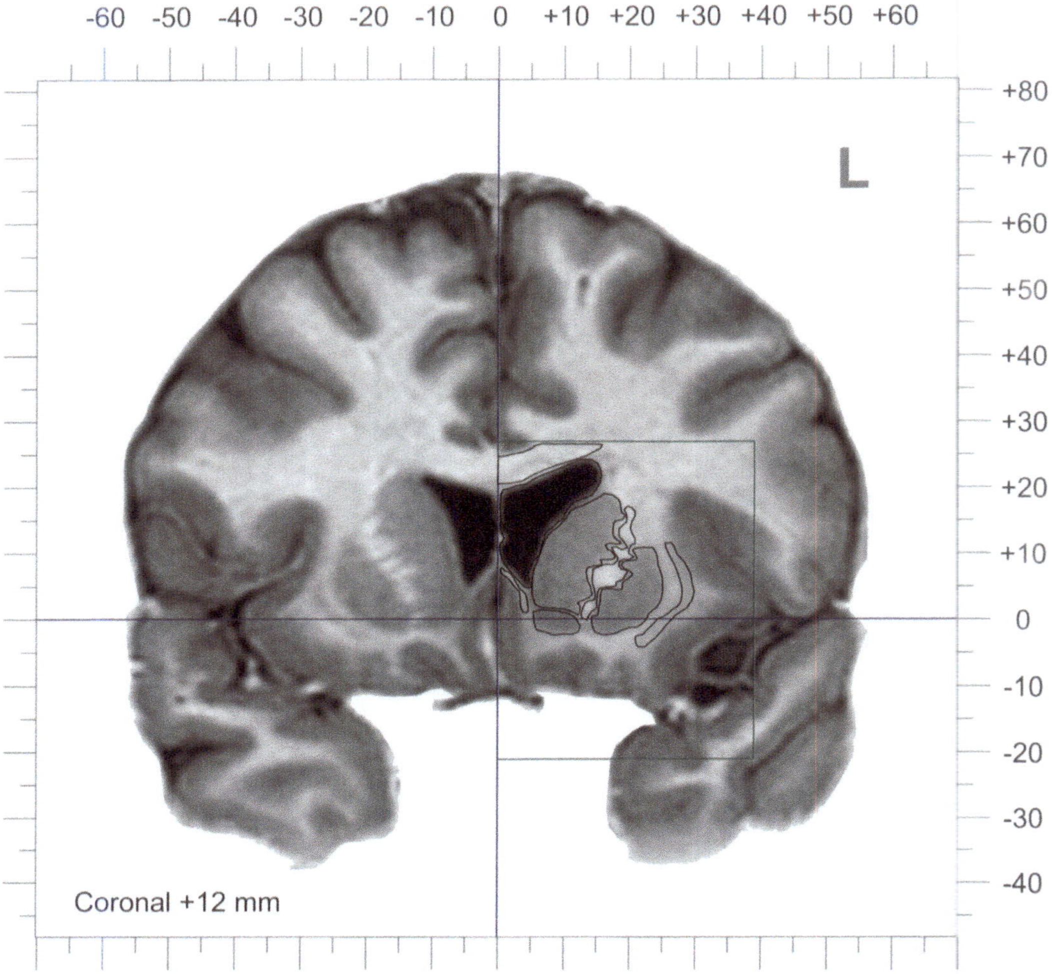

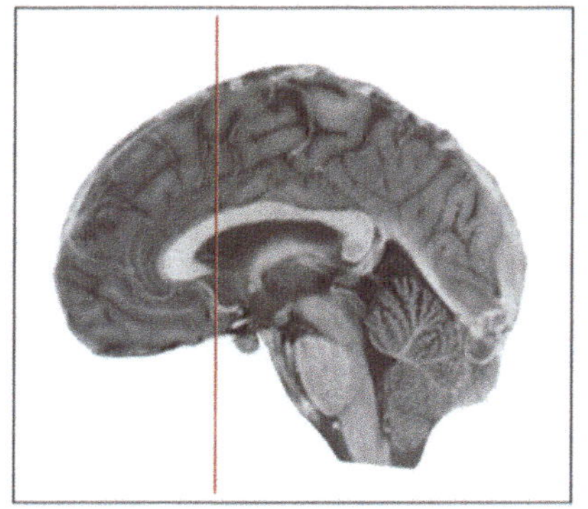

# Plate 23b

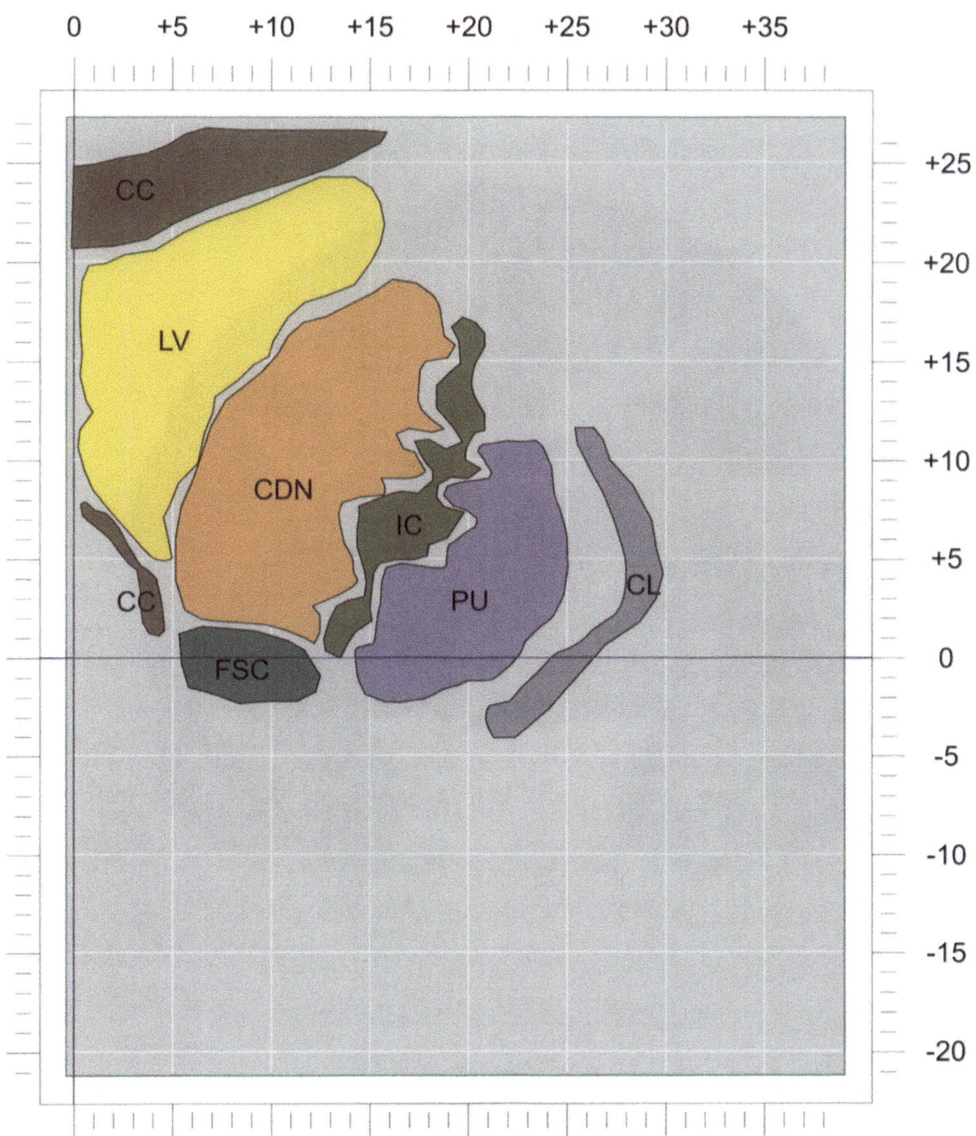



Coronal +12 mm

# Plate 24a

-60 -50 -40 -30 -20 -10 0 +10 +20 +30 +40 +50 +60
+80
+70
L
+60
+50
+40
+30
+20
+10
0
-10
-20
-30
-40

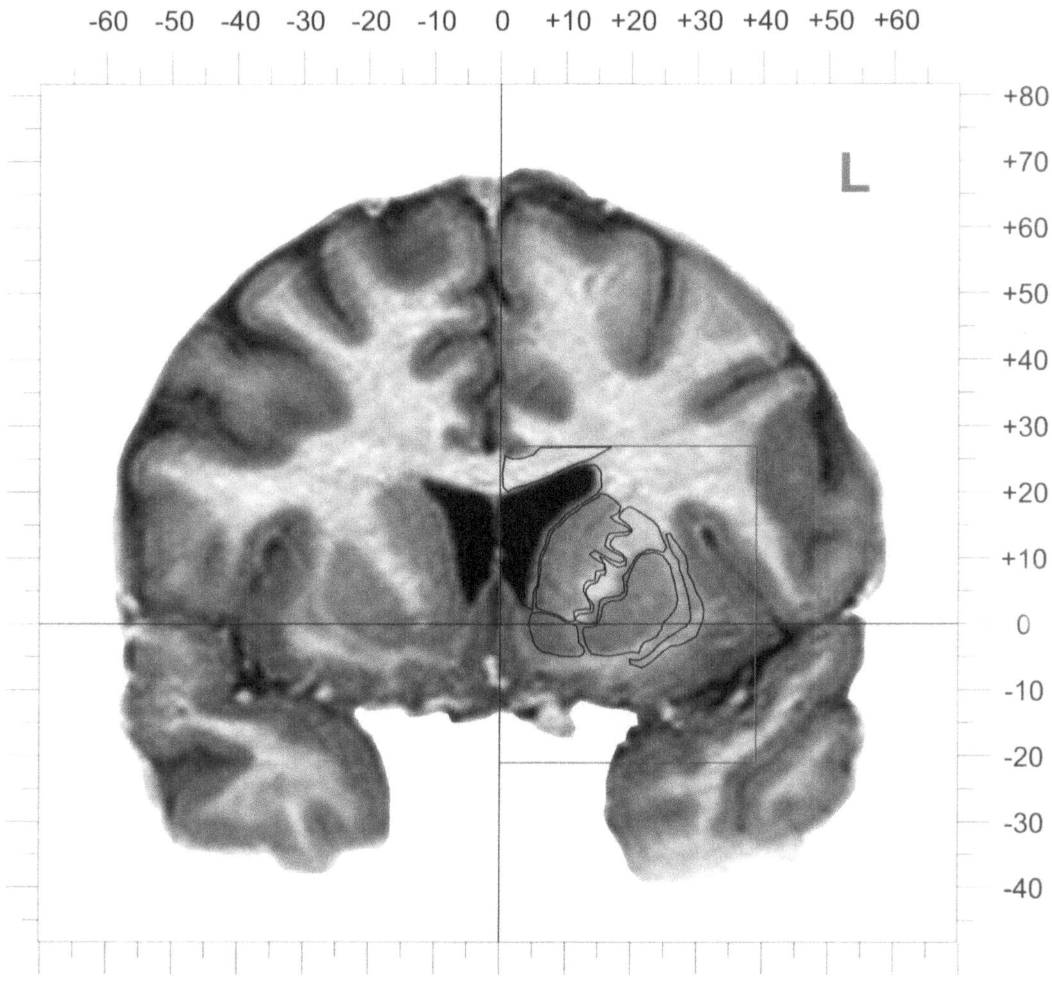

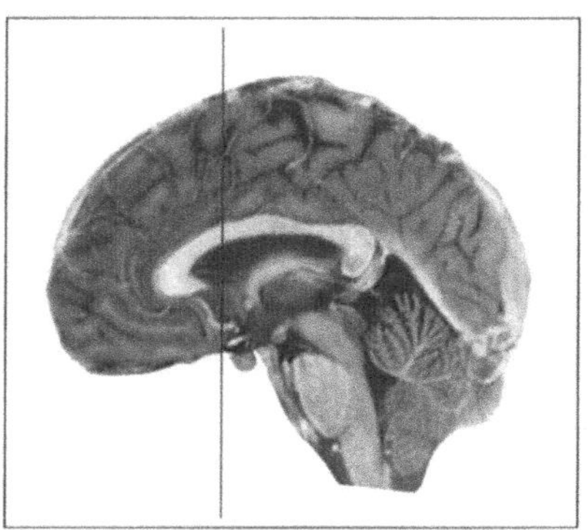

## Plate 24b

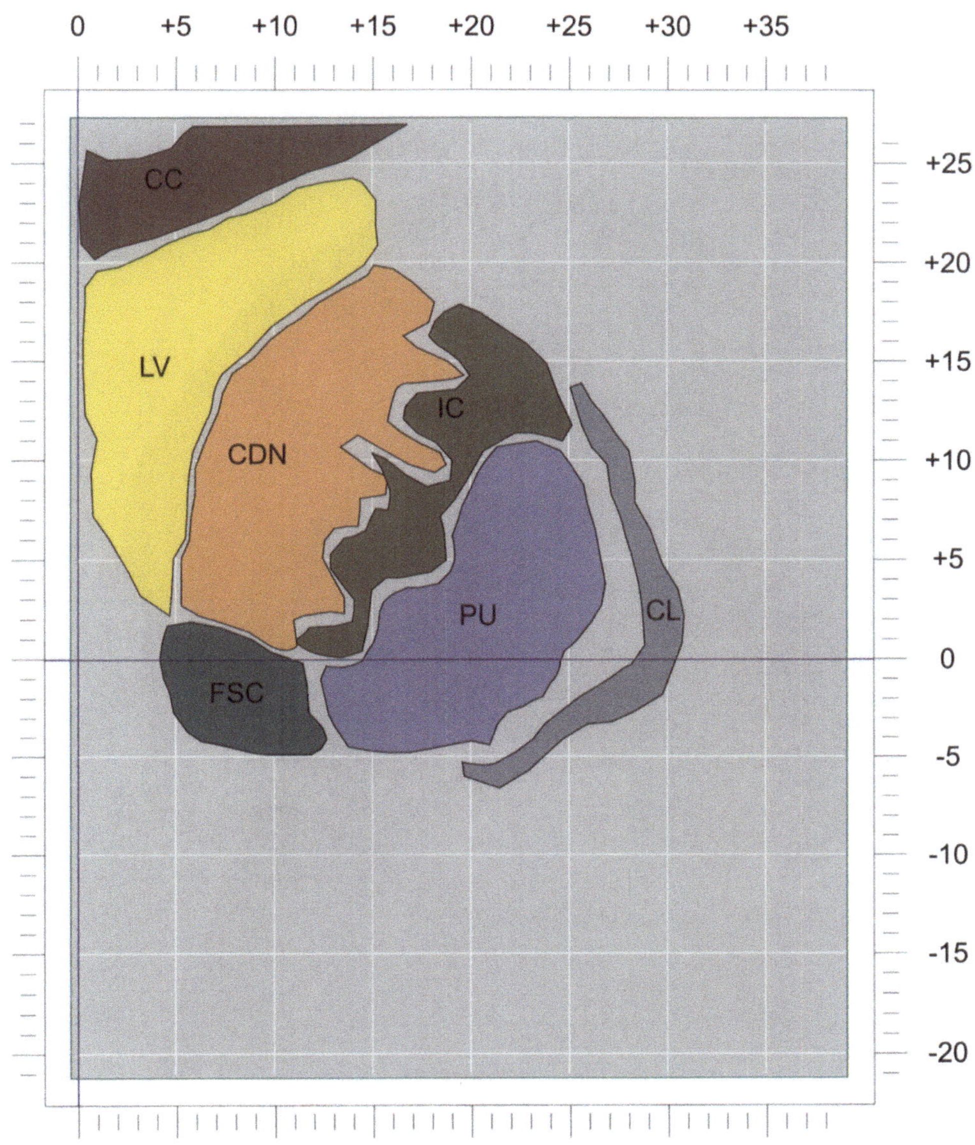


Coronal +9 mm

## Plate 25a

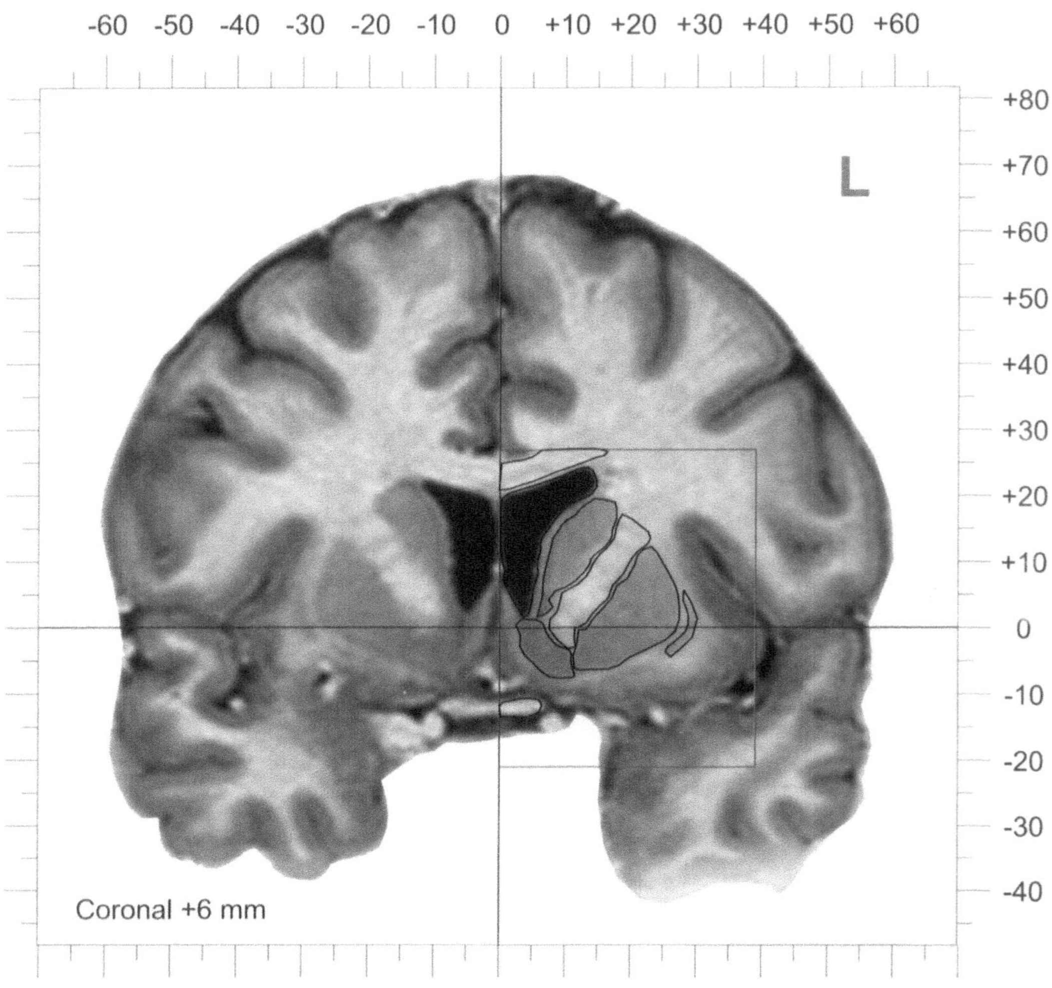


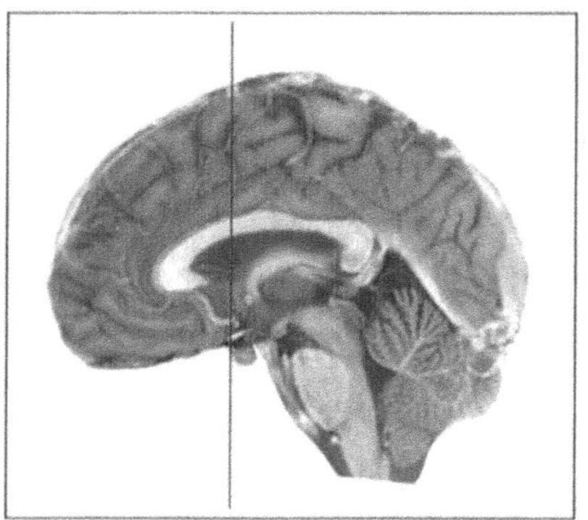

## Plate 25b

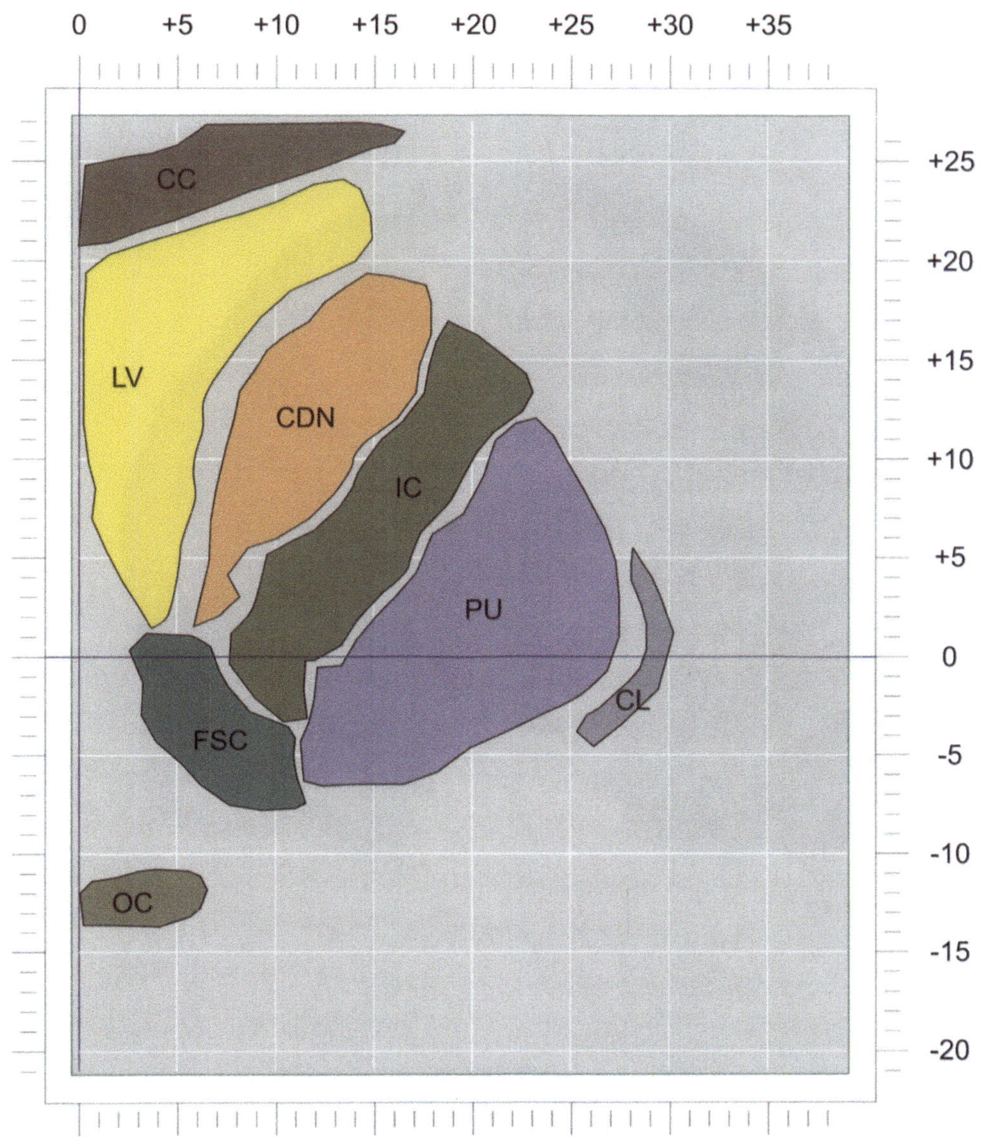


Coronal +6 mm

# Plate 26a

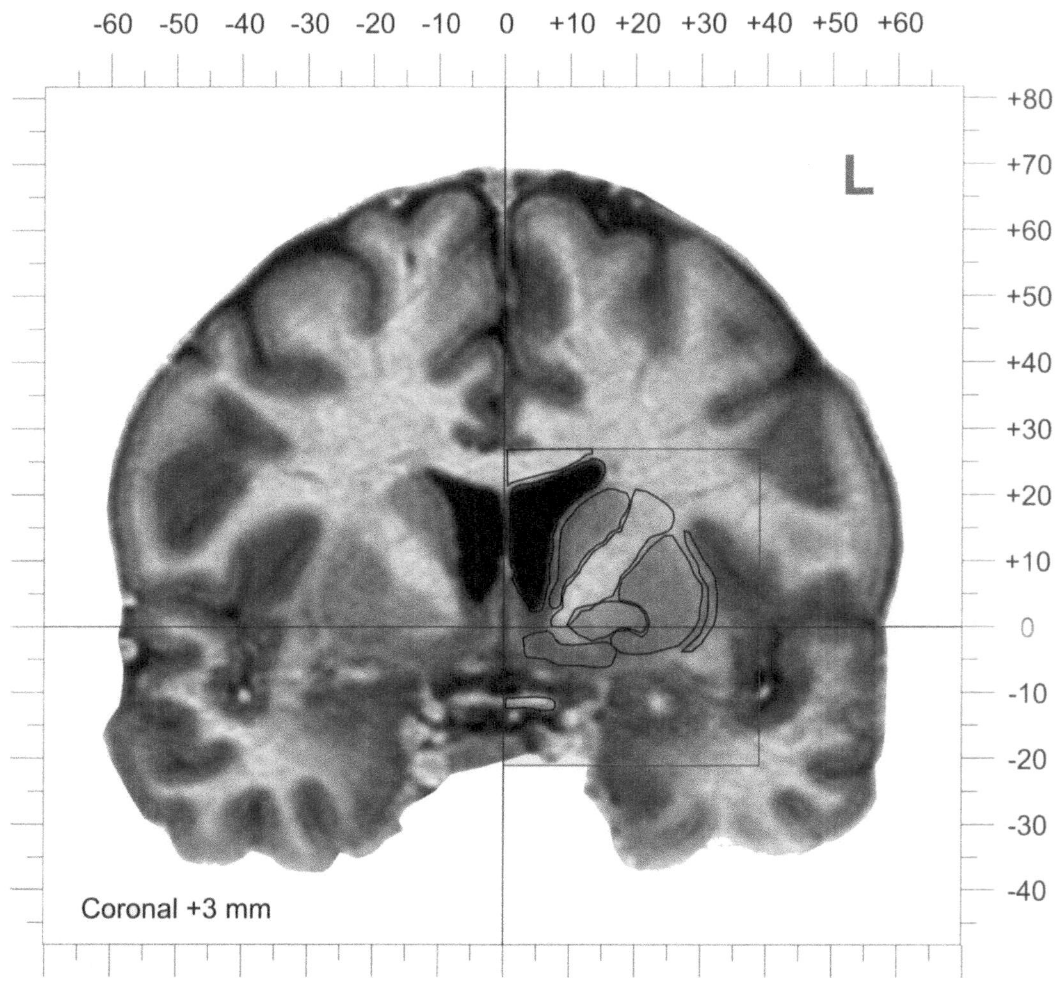



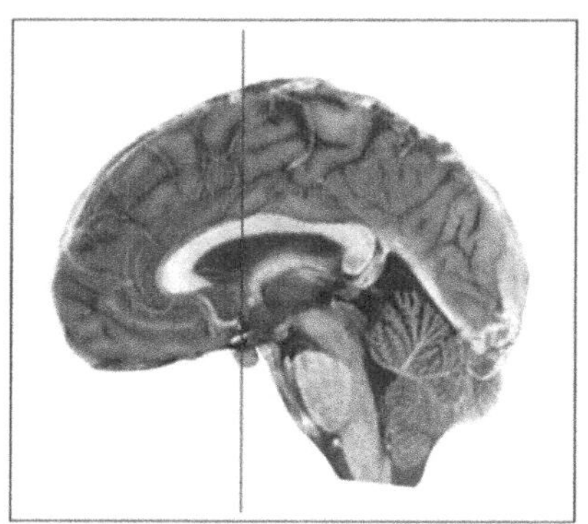

# Plate 26b

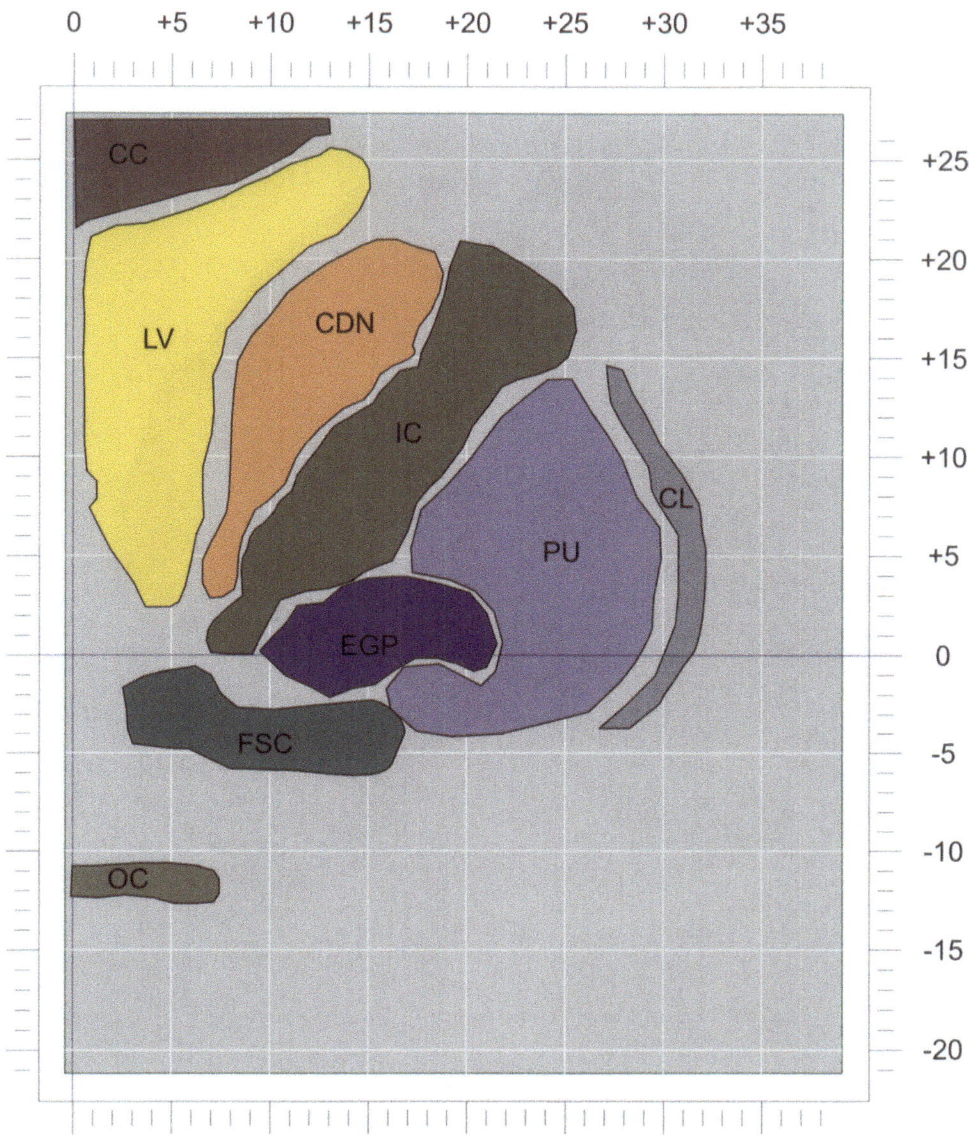


Coronal +3 mm

## Plate 27a

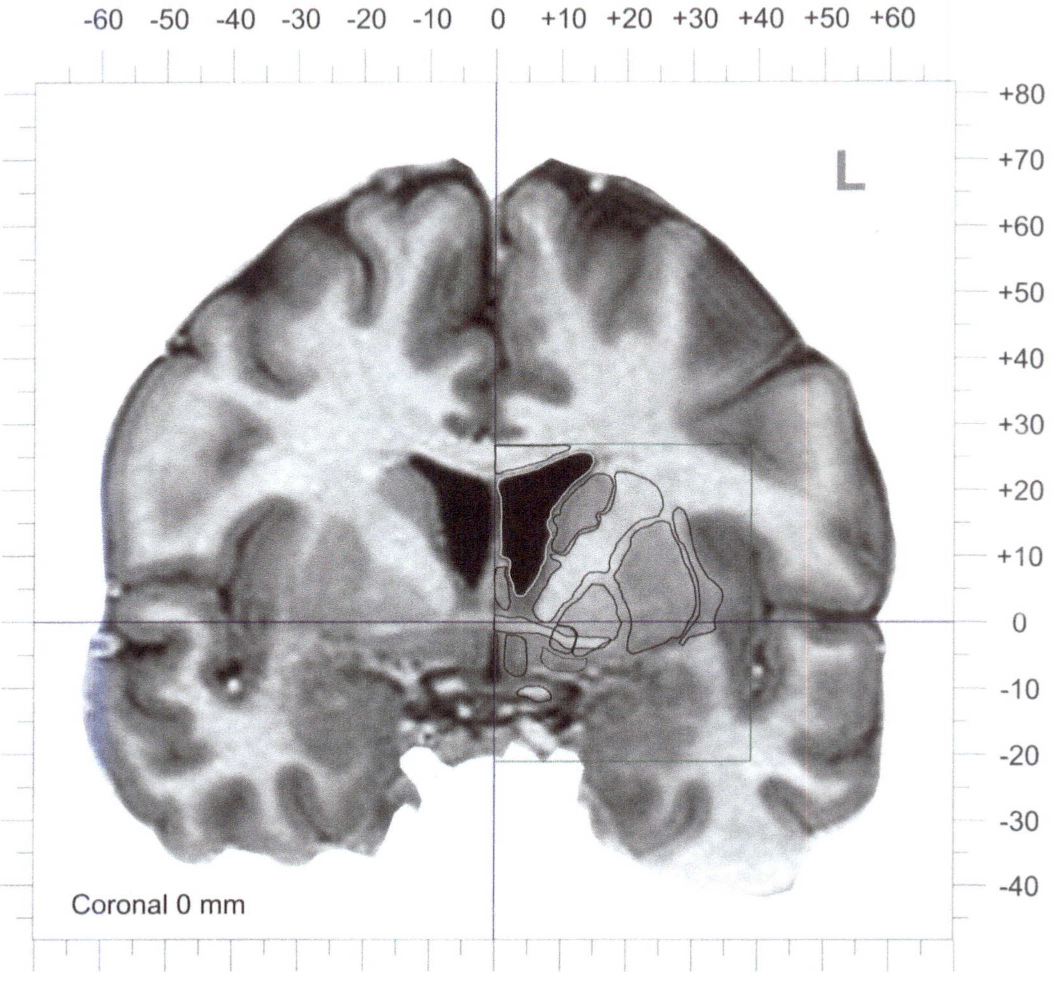


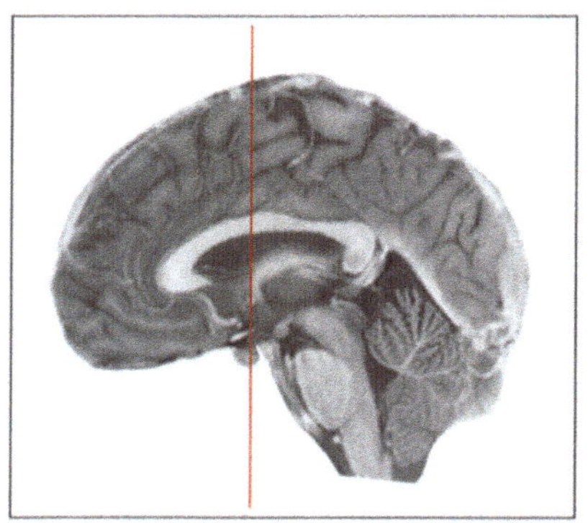

## Plate 27b

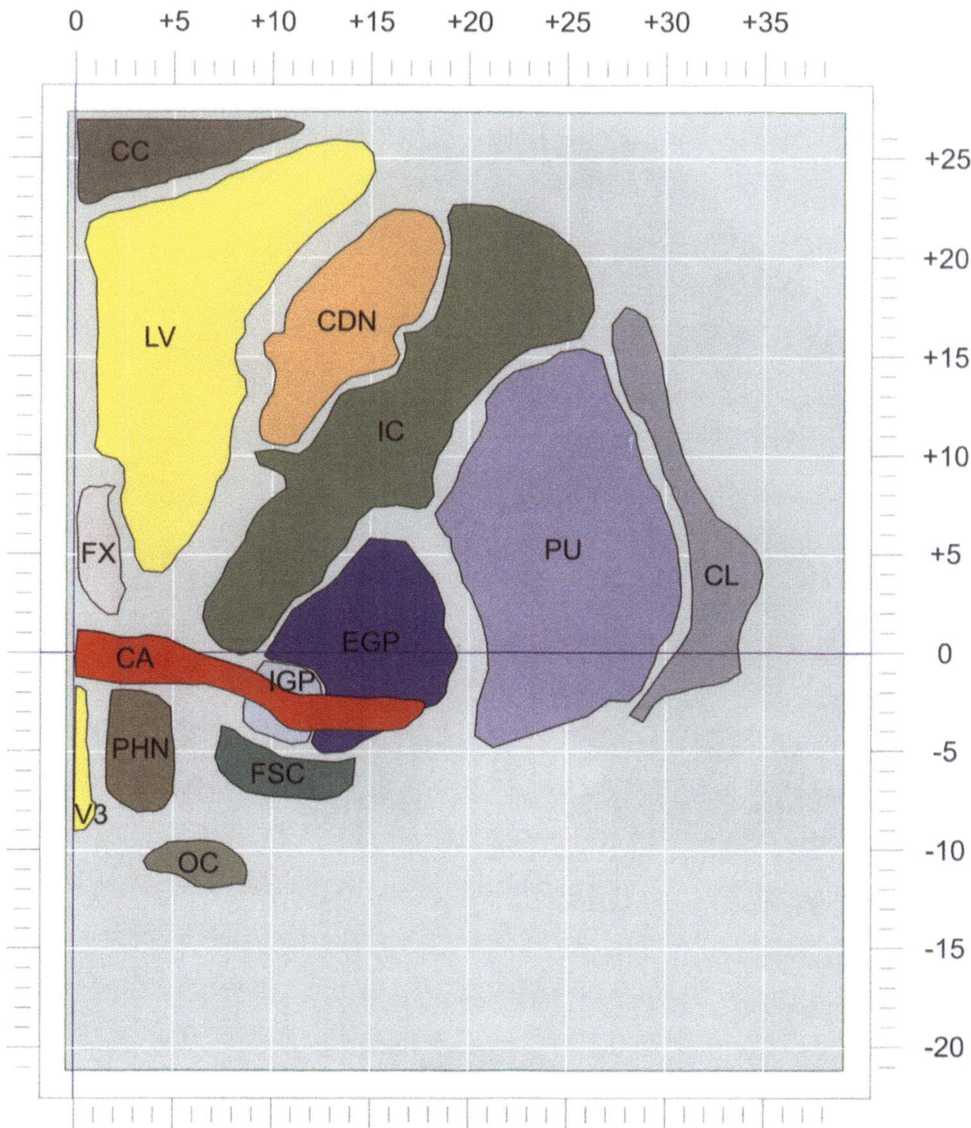


Coronal 0 mm

# Plate 28a

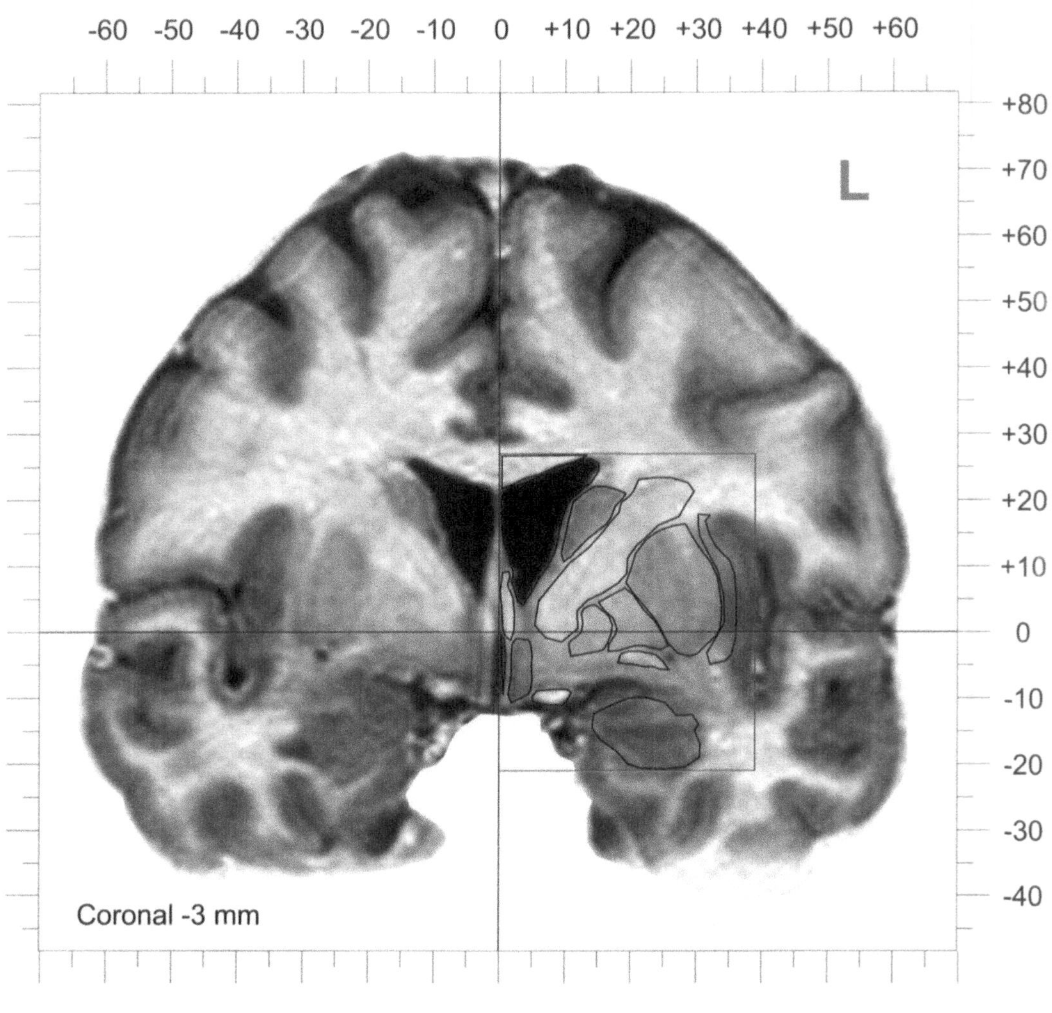


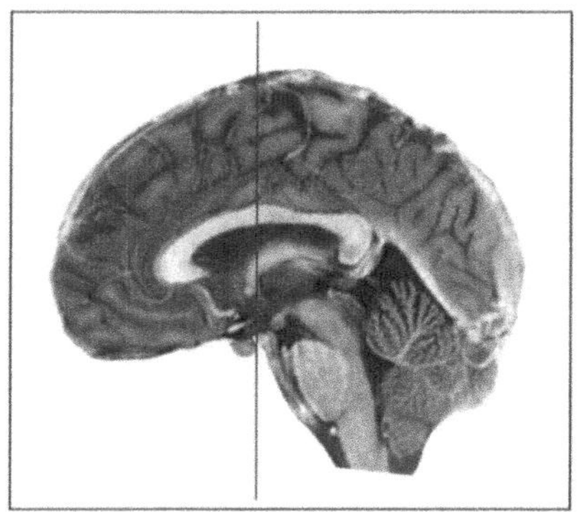

## Plate 28b

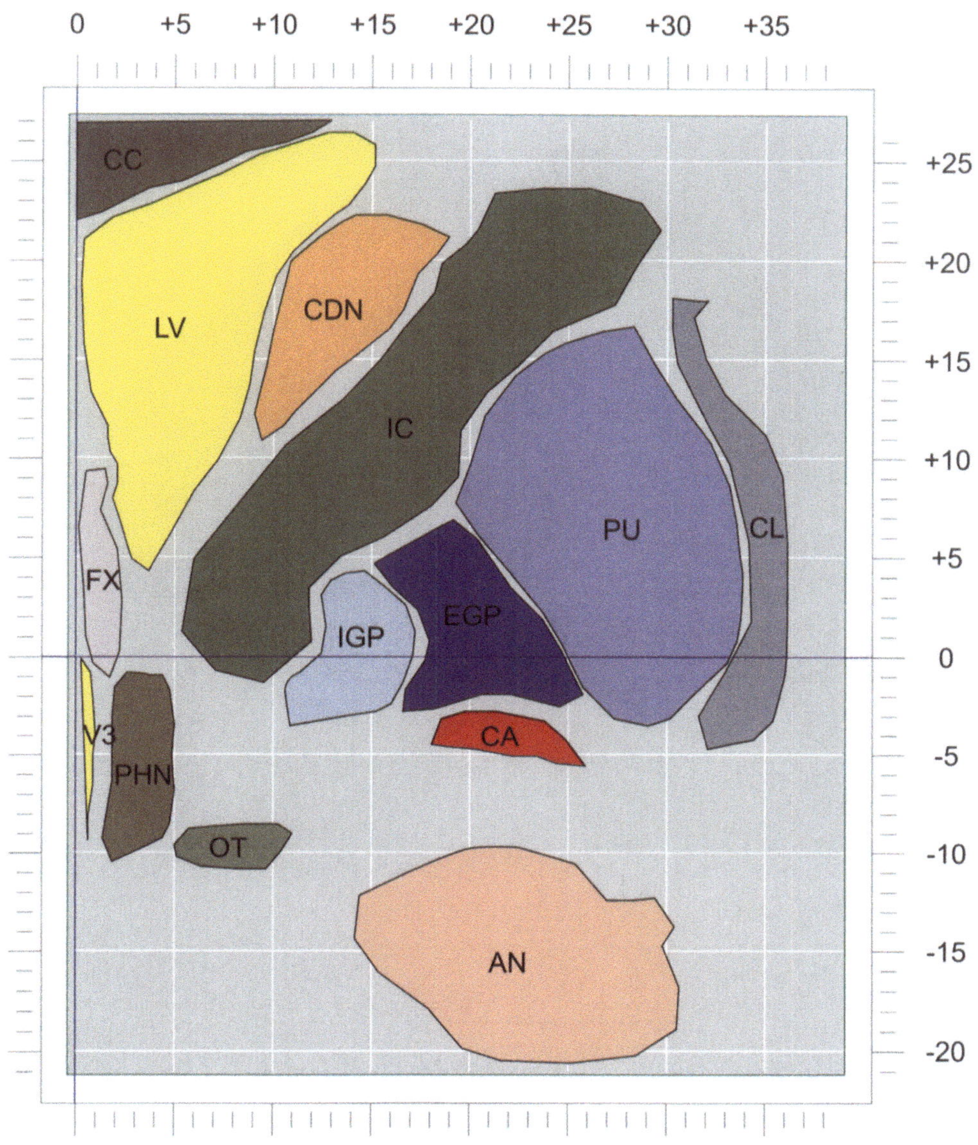


Coronal -3 mm

## Plate 29a

-60 -50 -40 -30 -20 -10 0 +10 +20 +30 +40 +50 +60
+80
+70
+60
+50
+40
+30
+20
+10
0
-10
-20
-30
-40
L
Coronal -6 mm

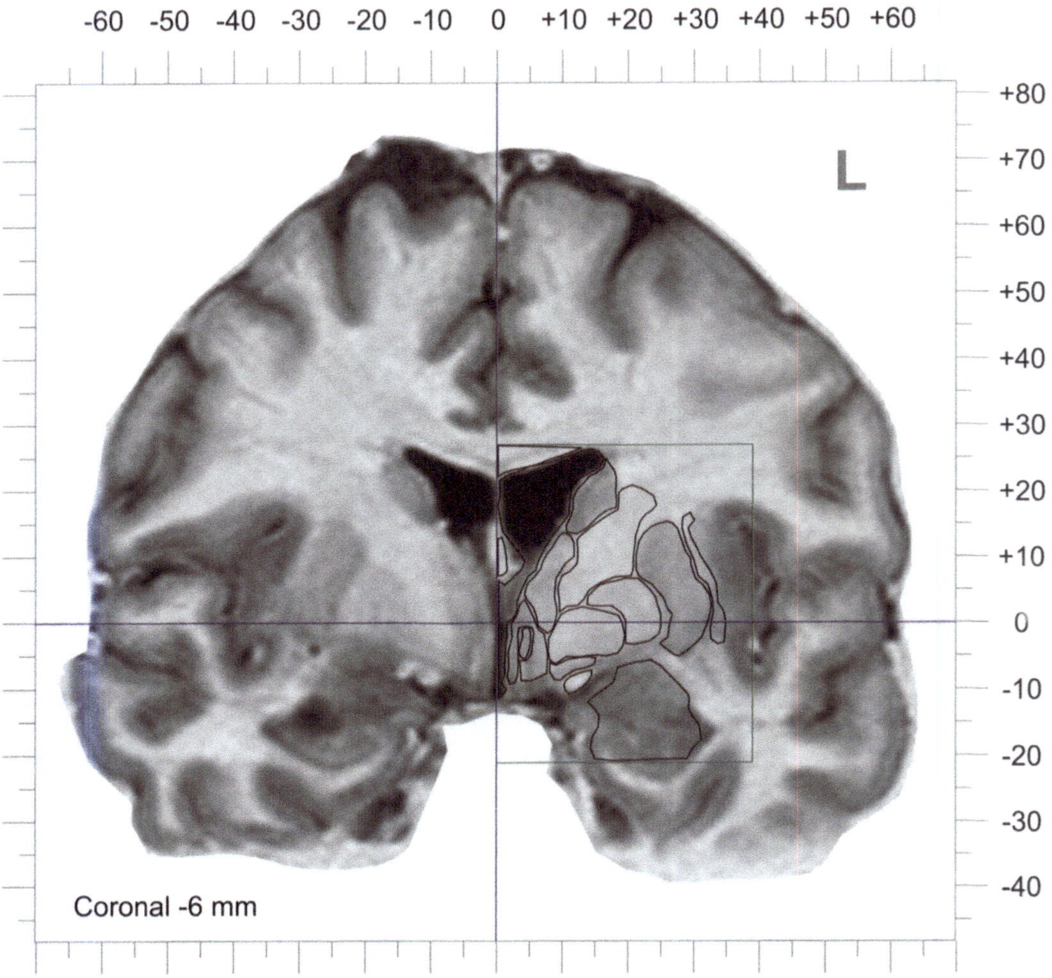

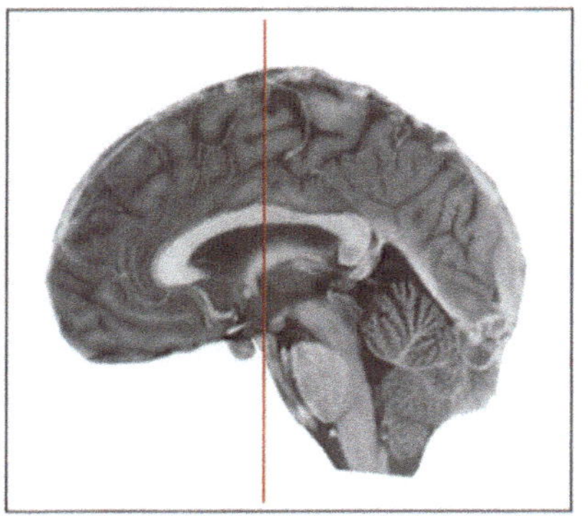

## Plate 29b

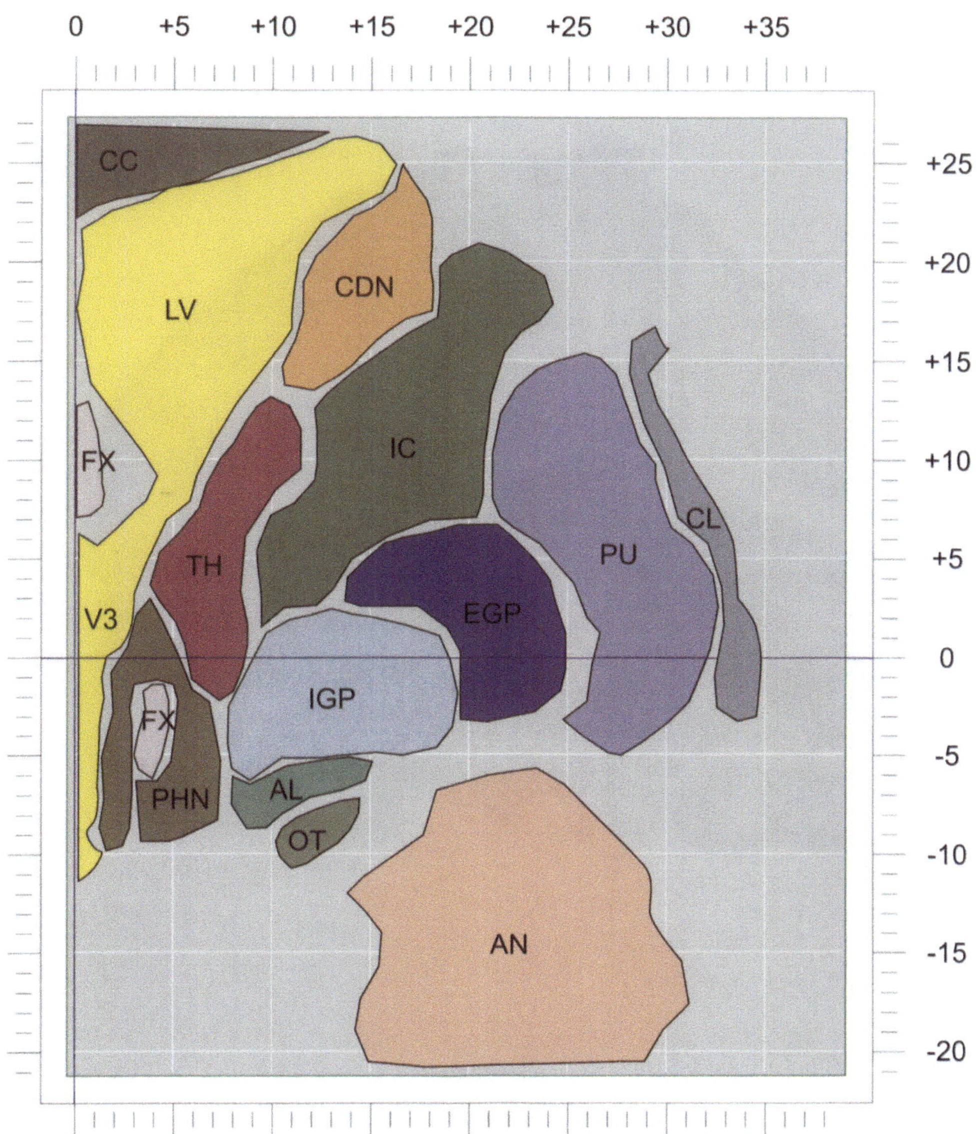


Coronal -6 mm

## Plate 30a

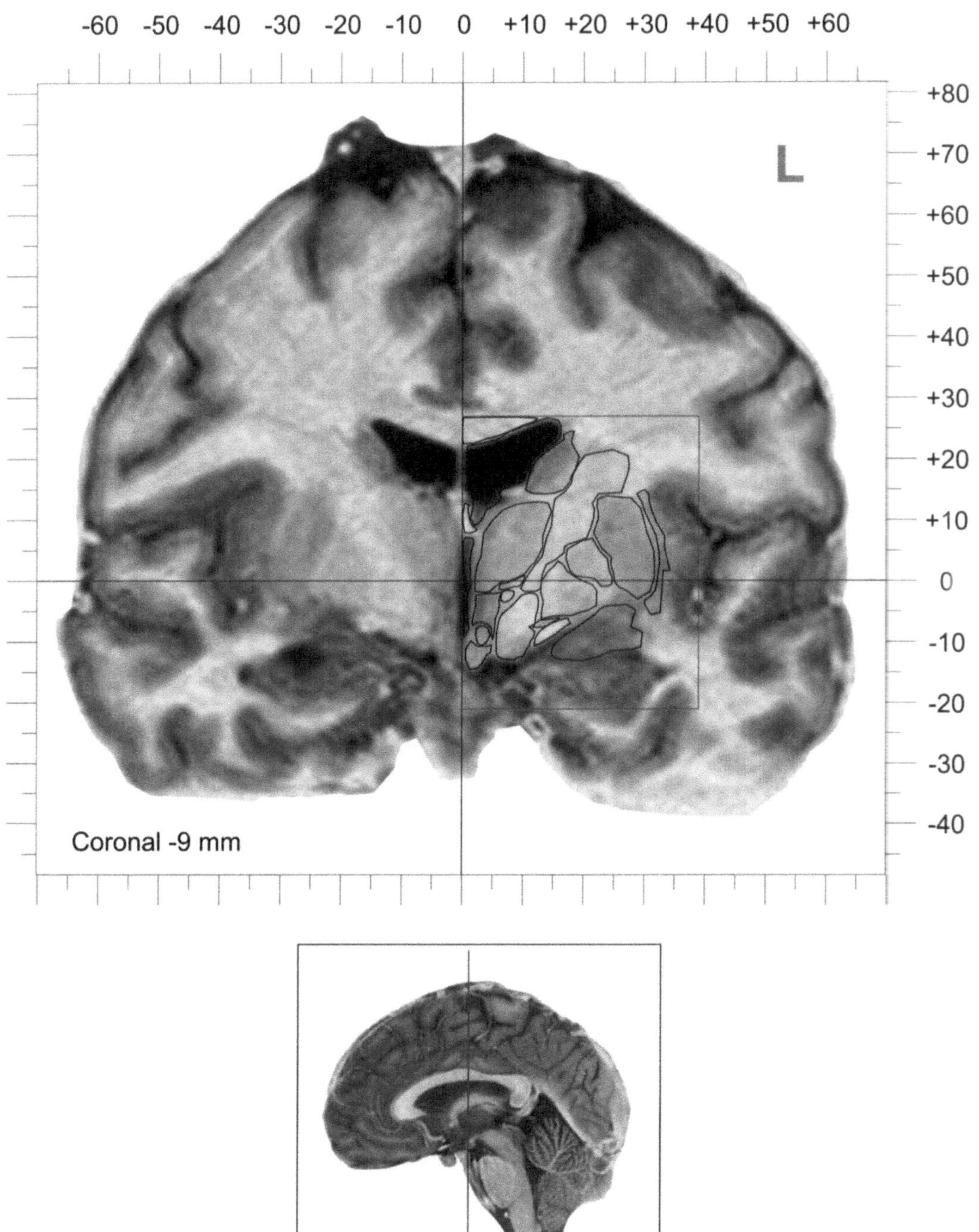

## Plate 30b

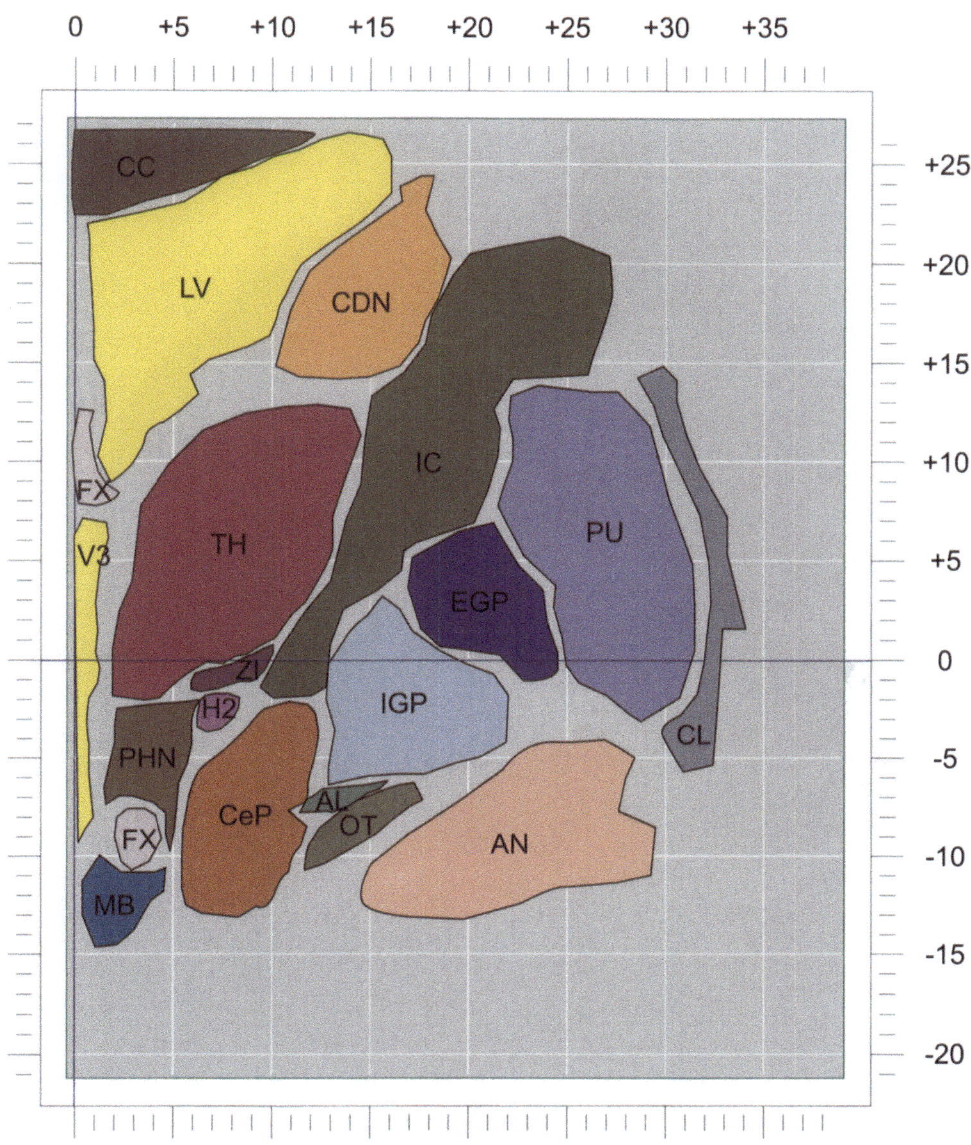


Coronal -9 mm

## Plate 31a

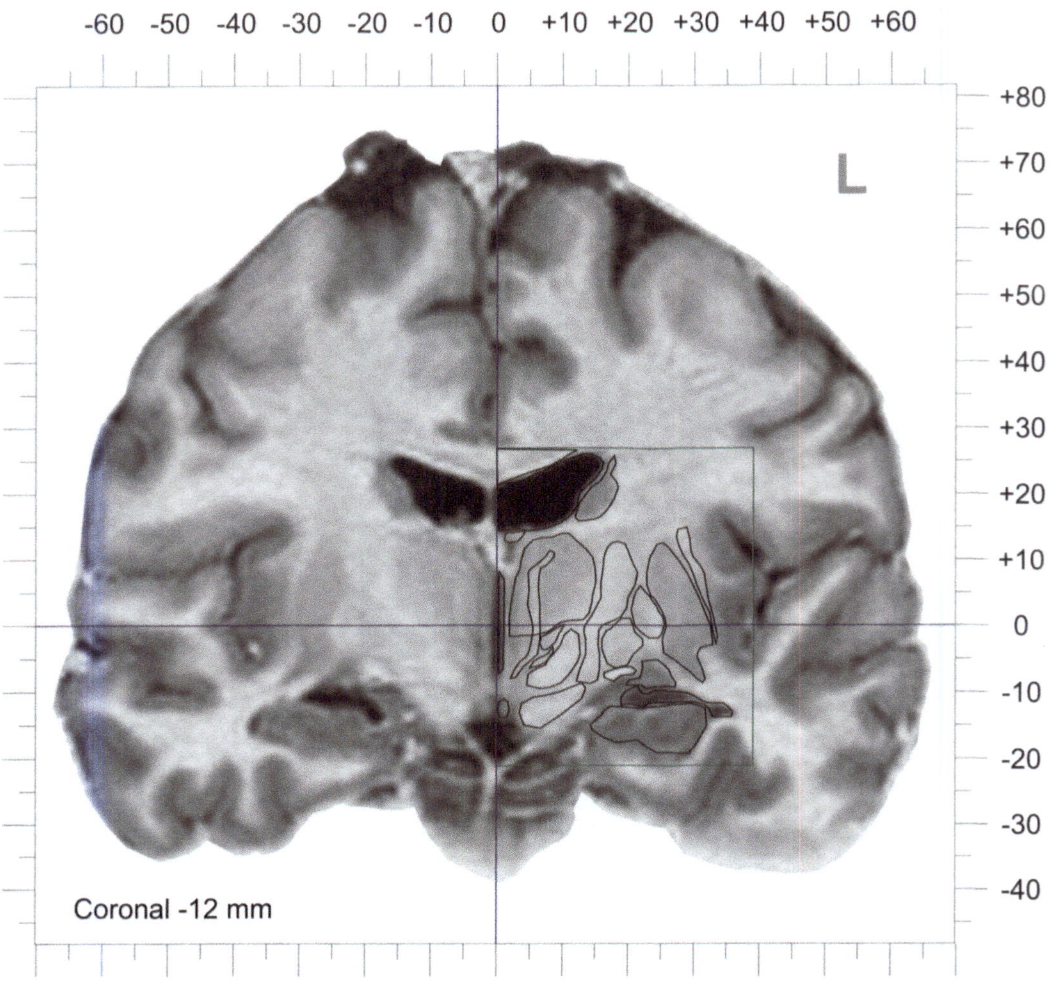


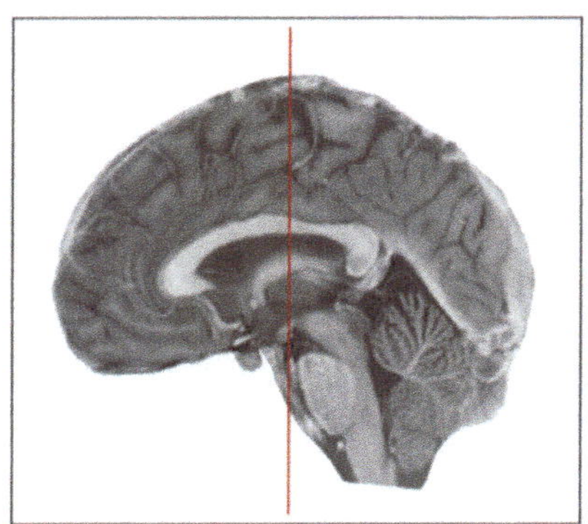

# Plate 31b

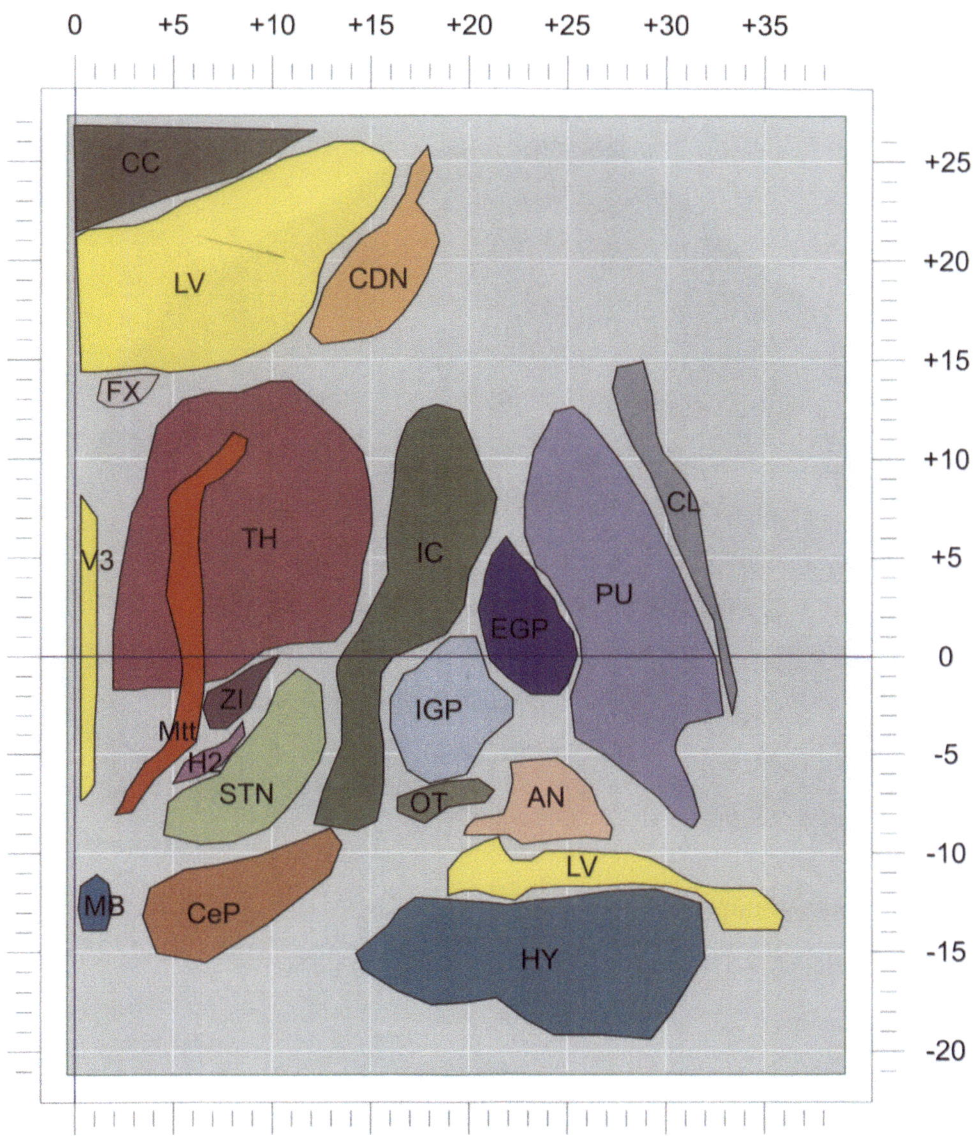


Coronal -12 mm

## Plate 32a

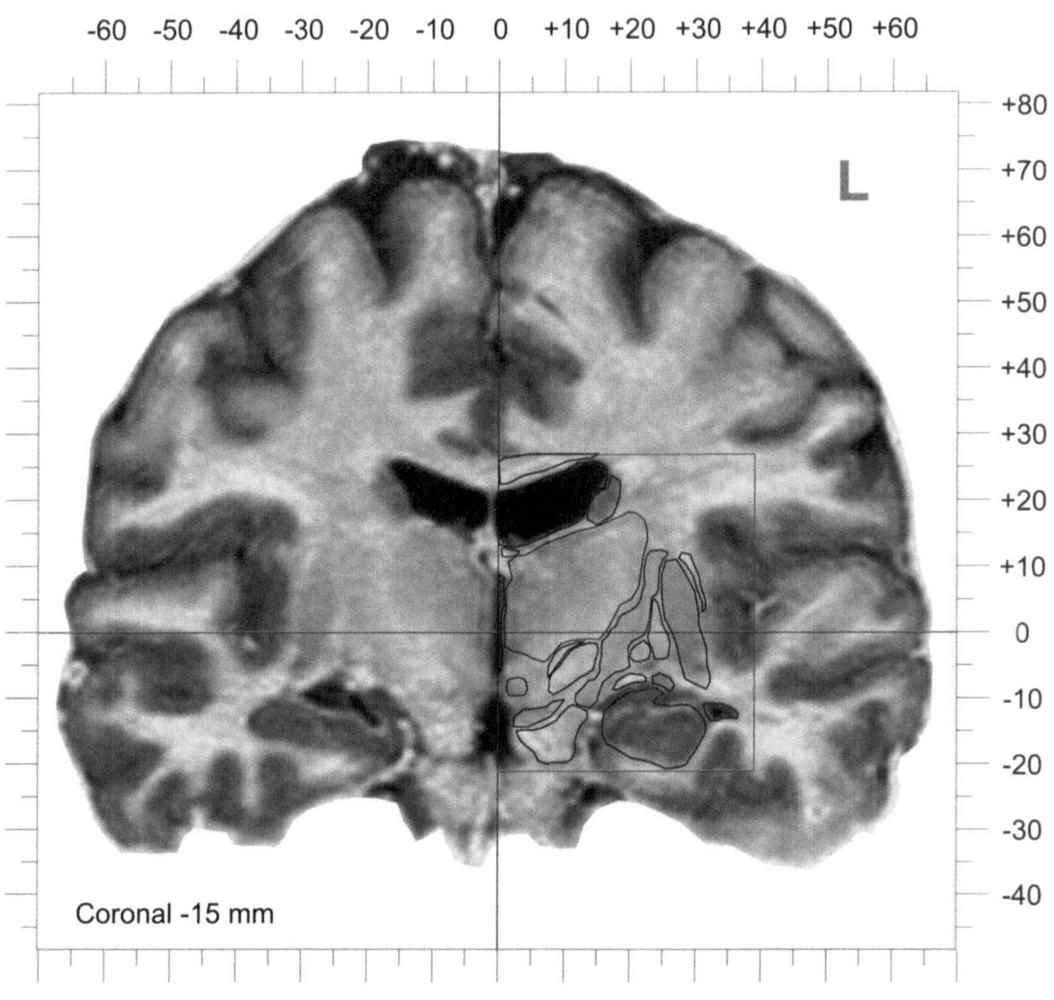


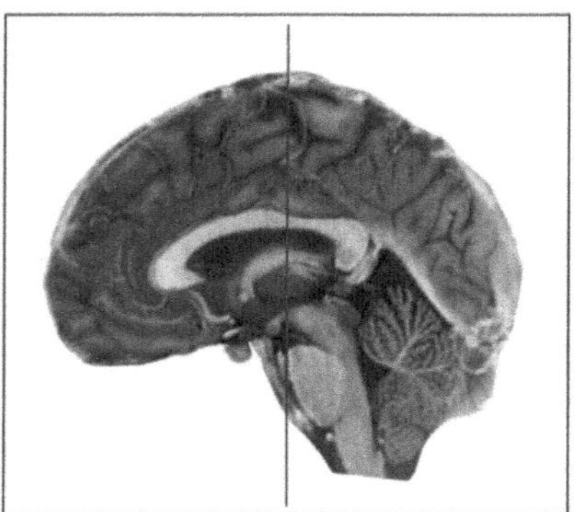

# Plate 32b

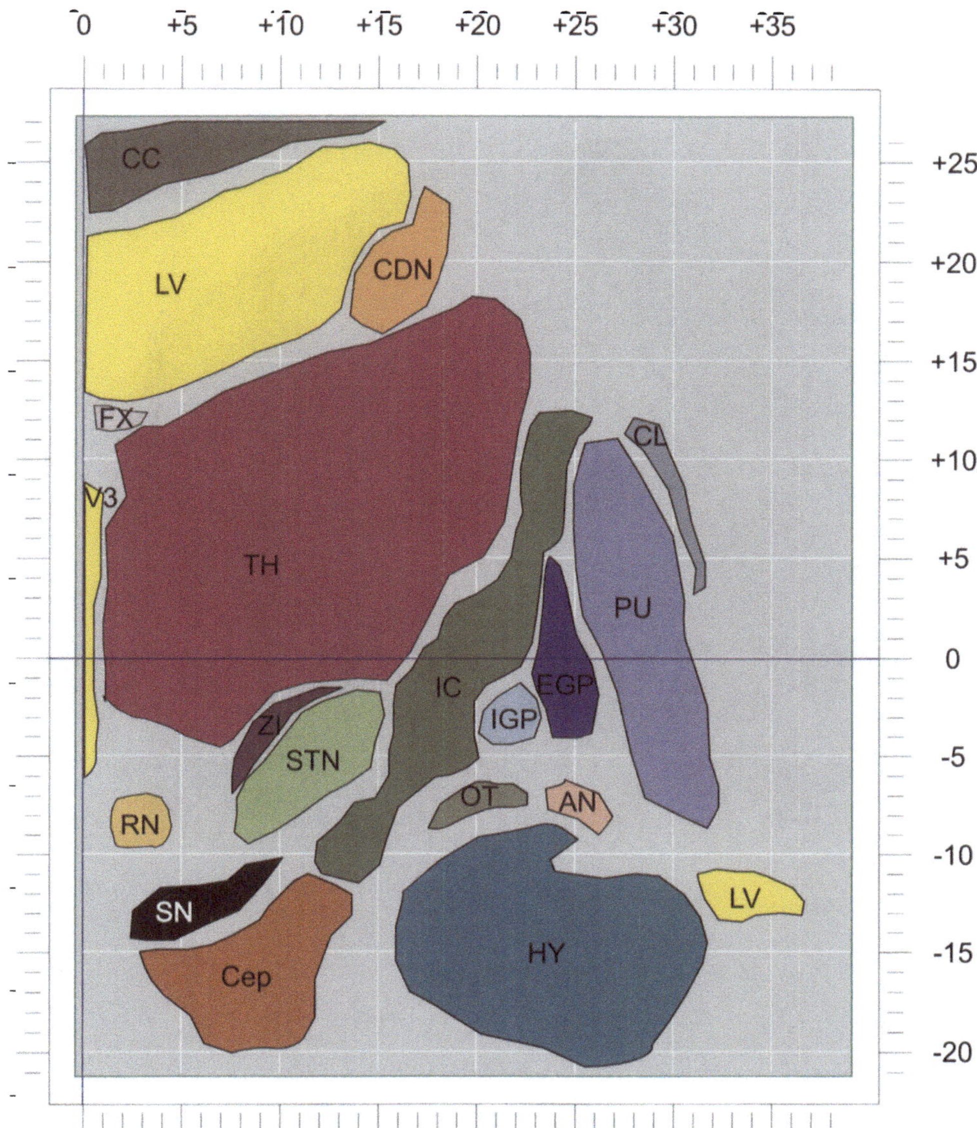


Coronal -15 mm

Coronal -15 mm

## Plate 33a

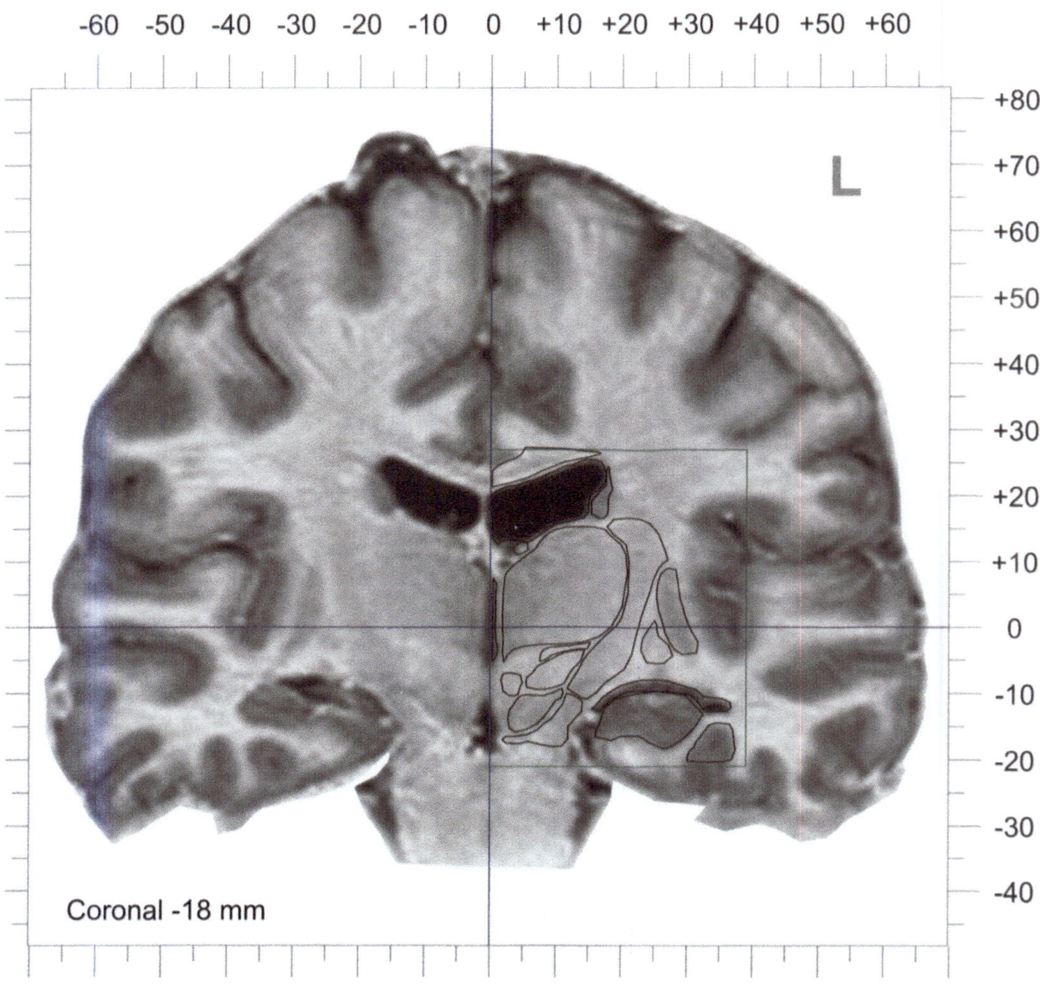


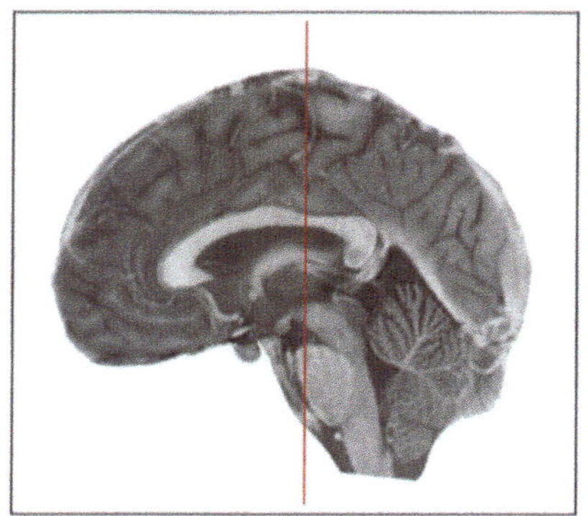

# Plate 33b

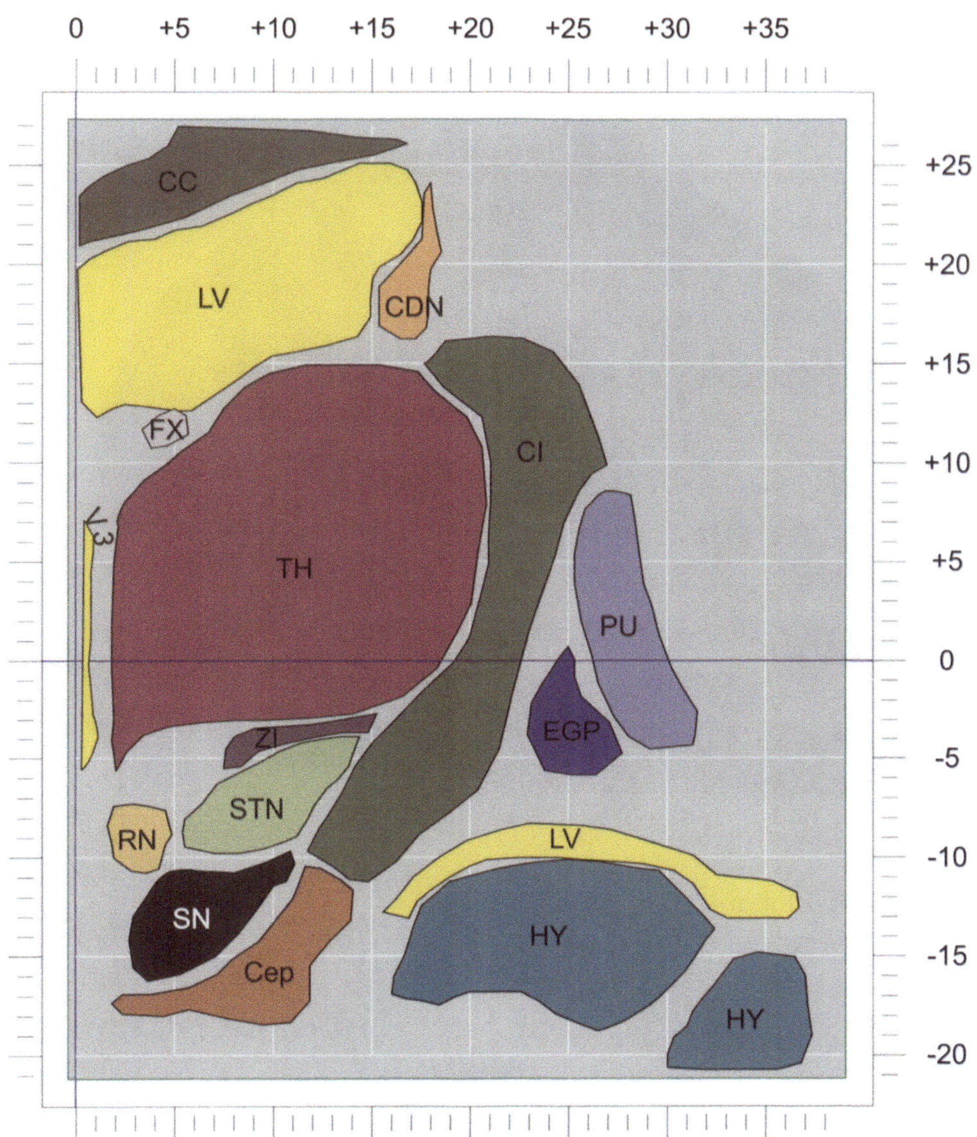



Coronal -18 mm

## Plate 34a

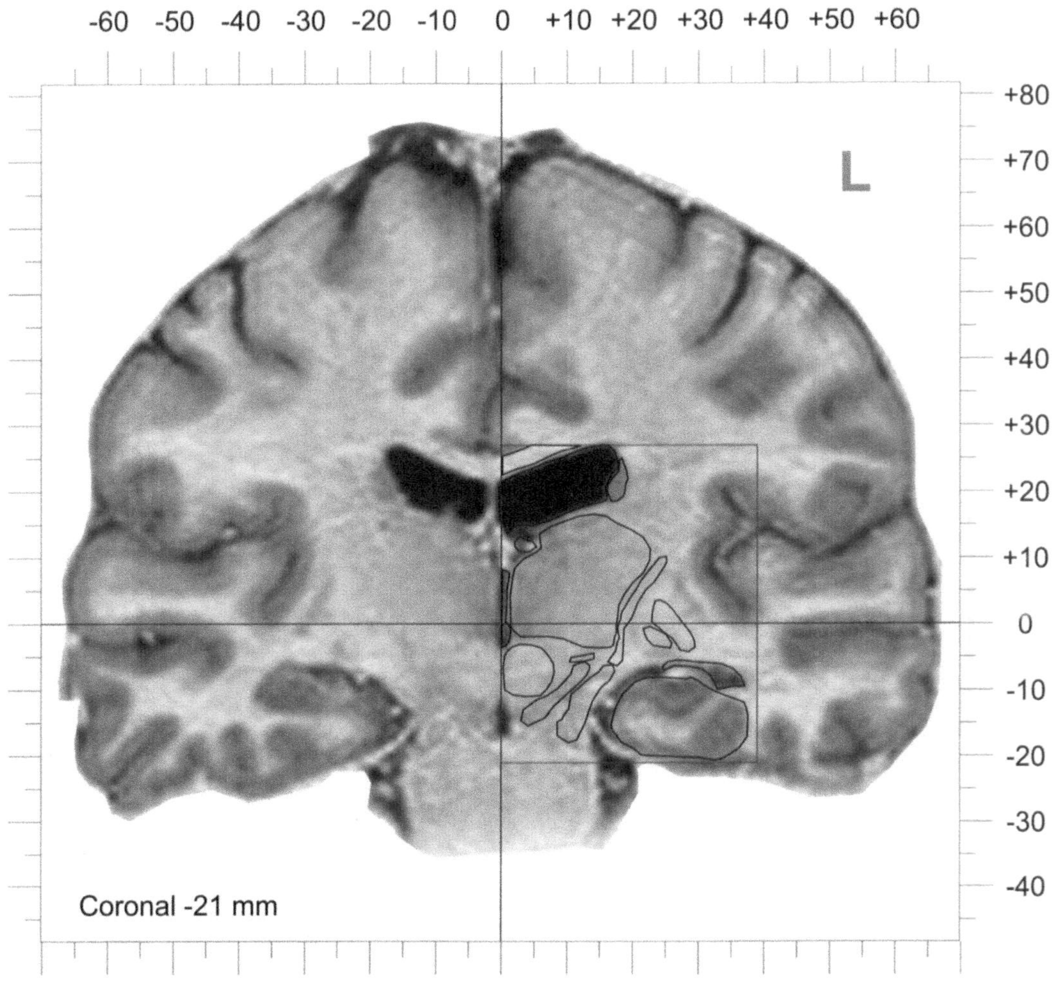


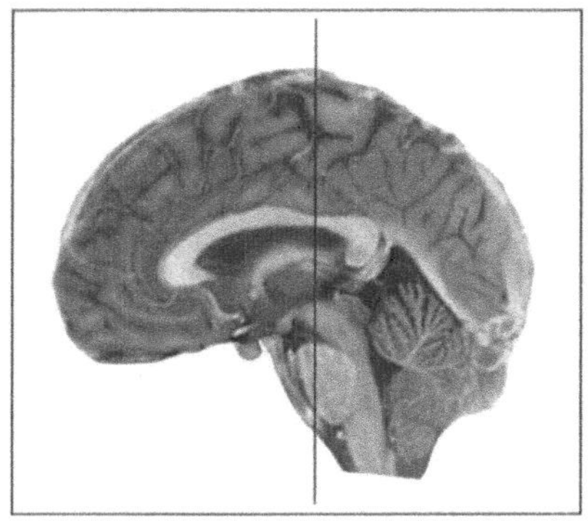

# Plate 34b

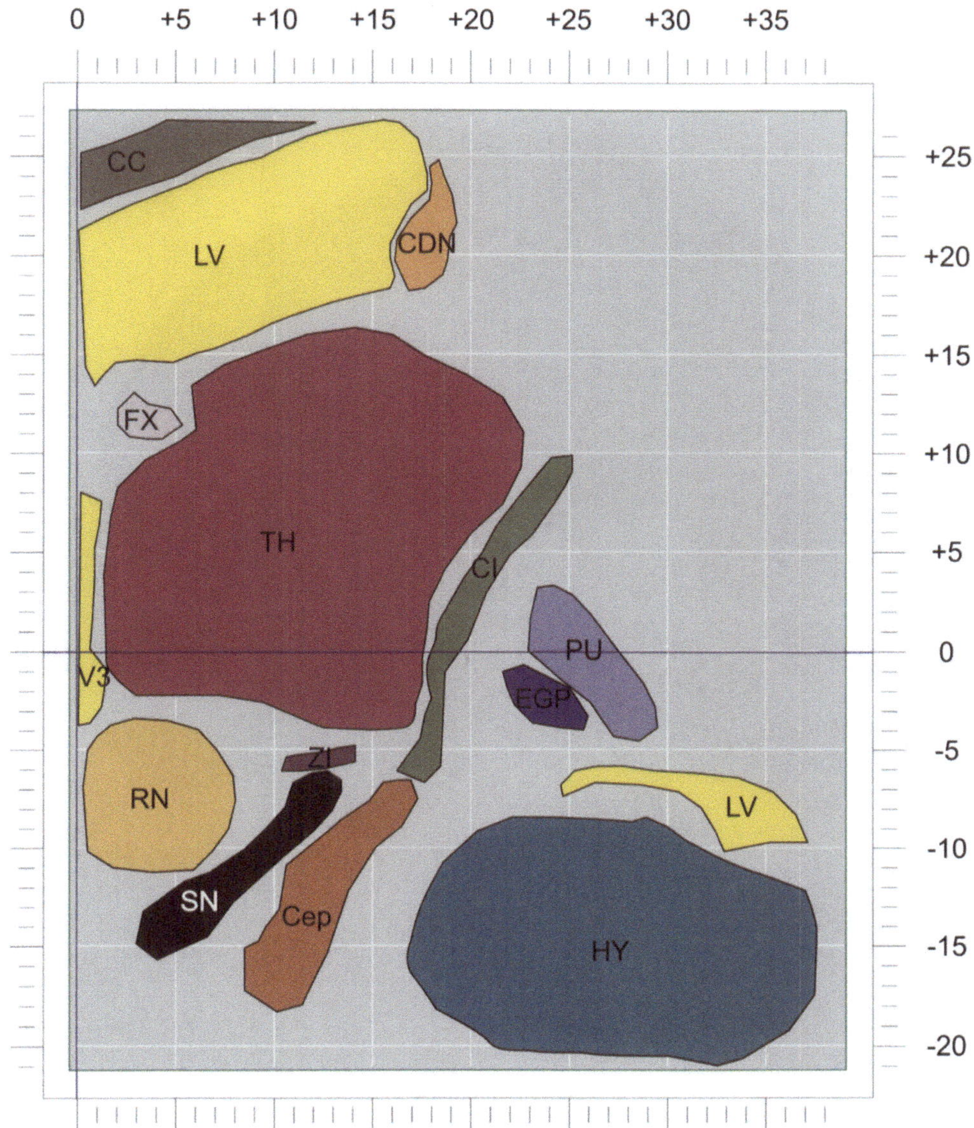


Coronal -21 mm

## Plate 35a

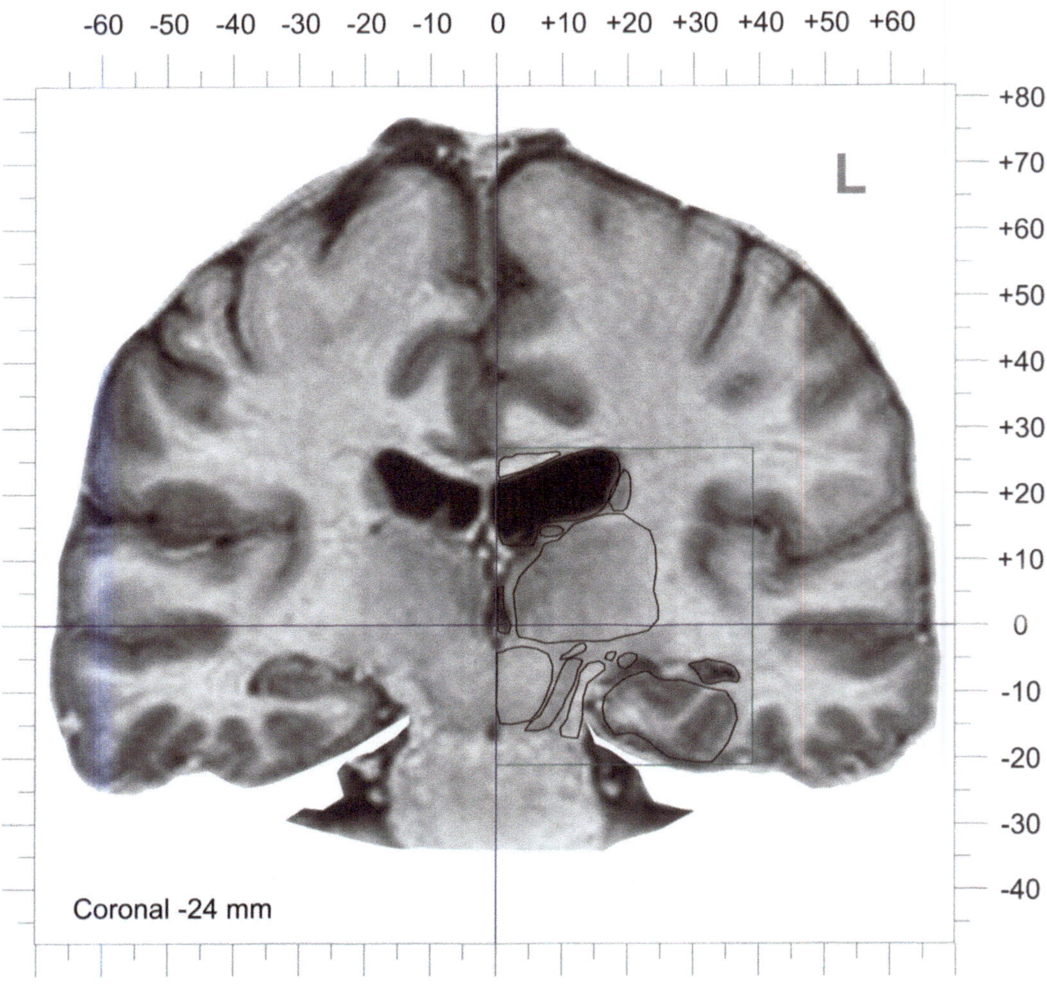


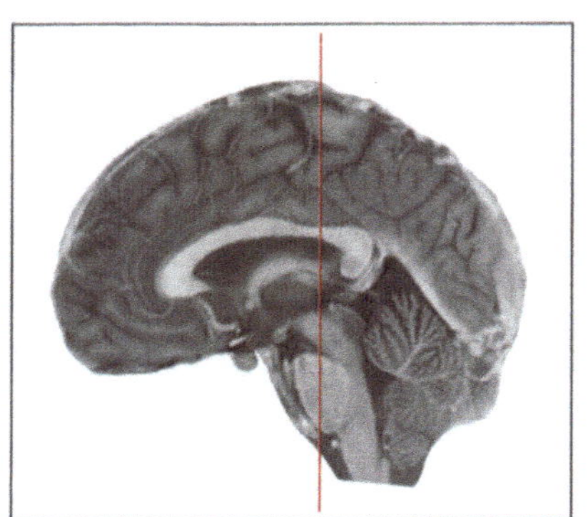

## Plate 35b

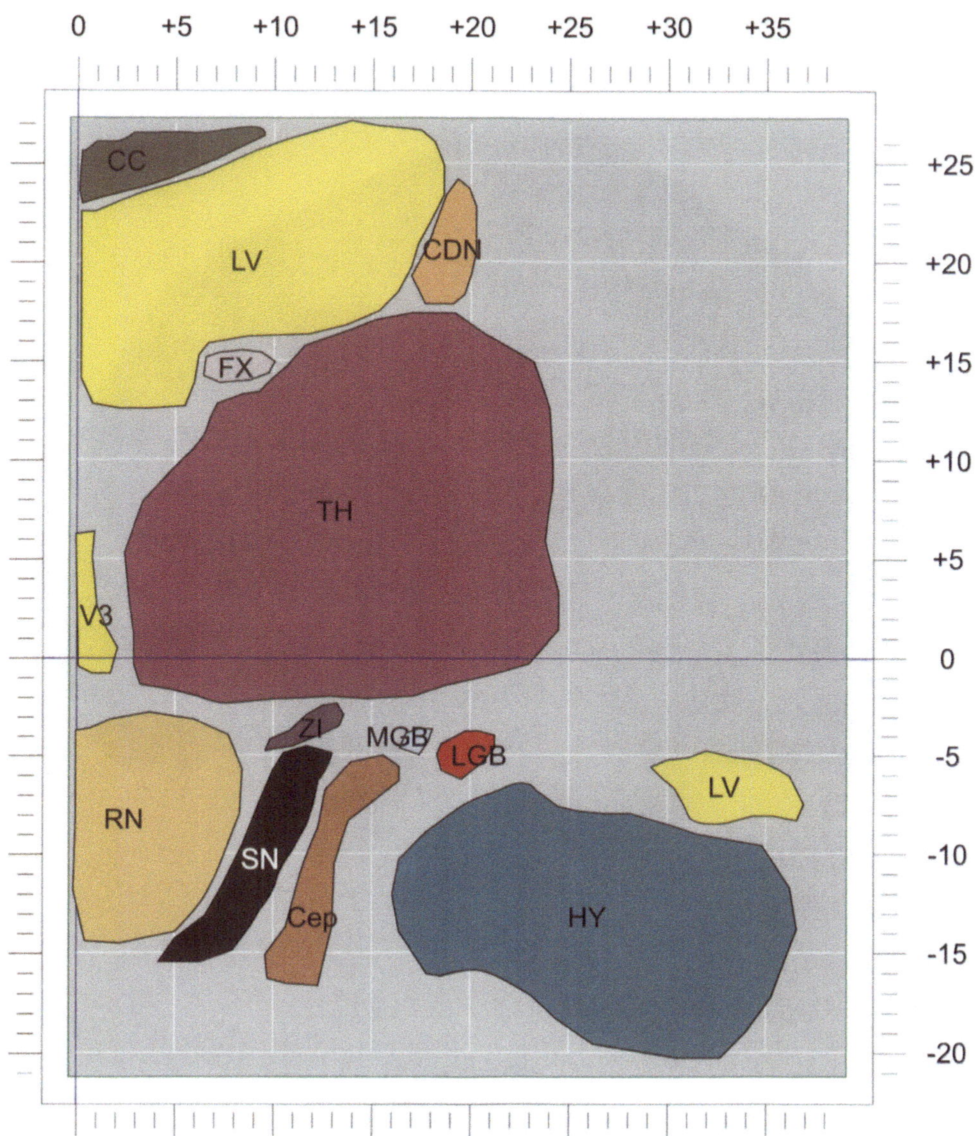


Coronal -24 mm

## Plate 36a

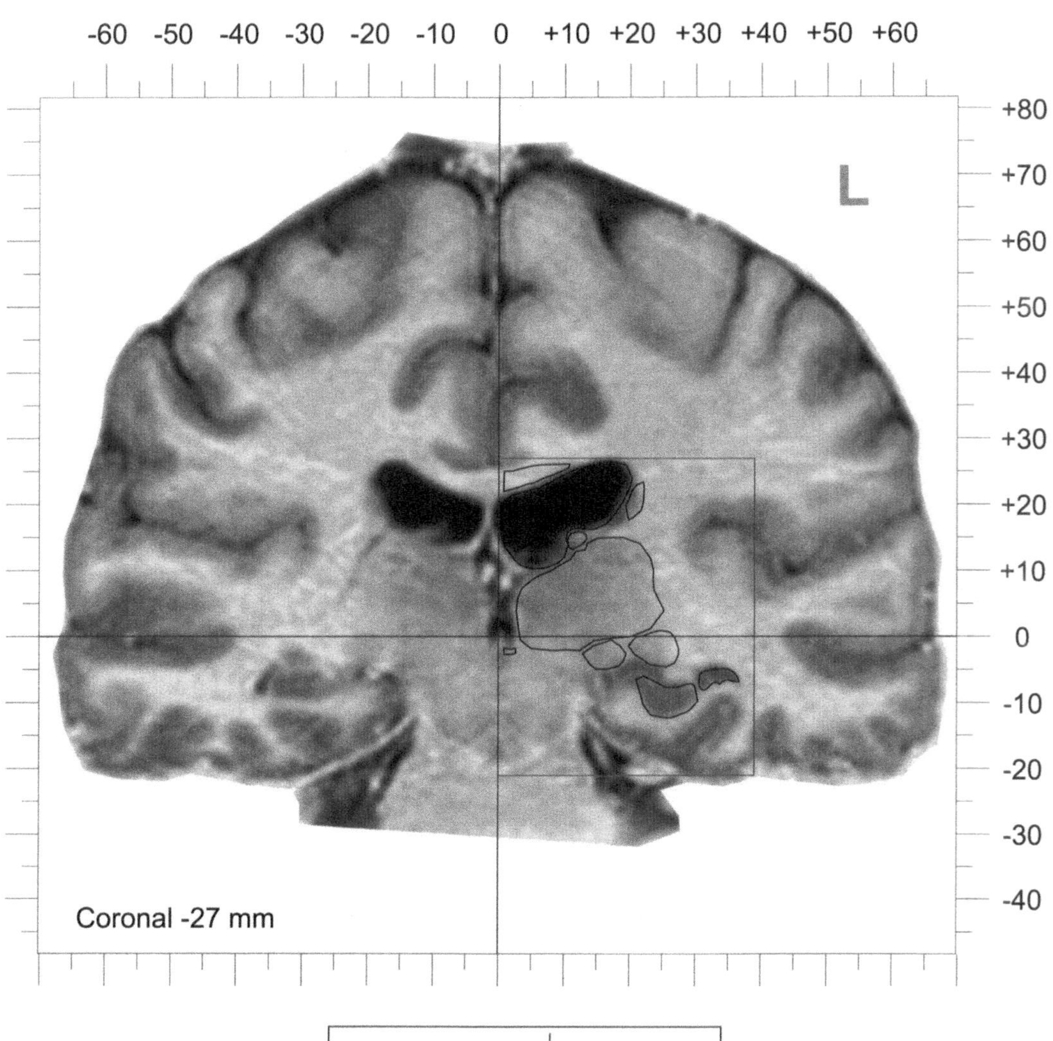


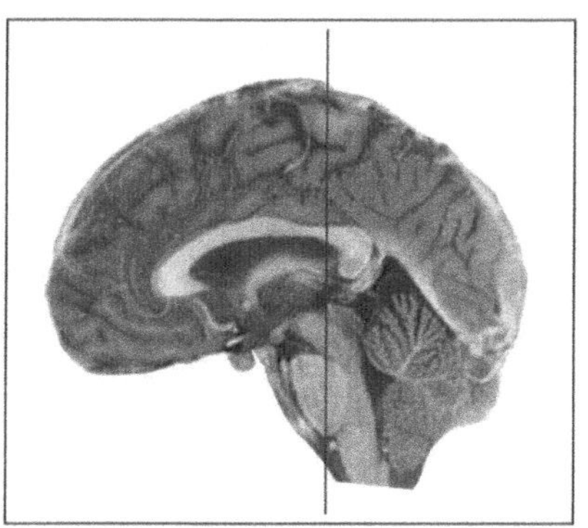

## Plate 36b

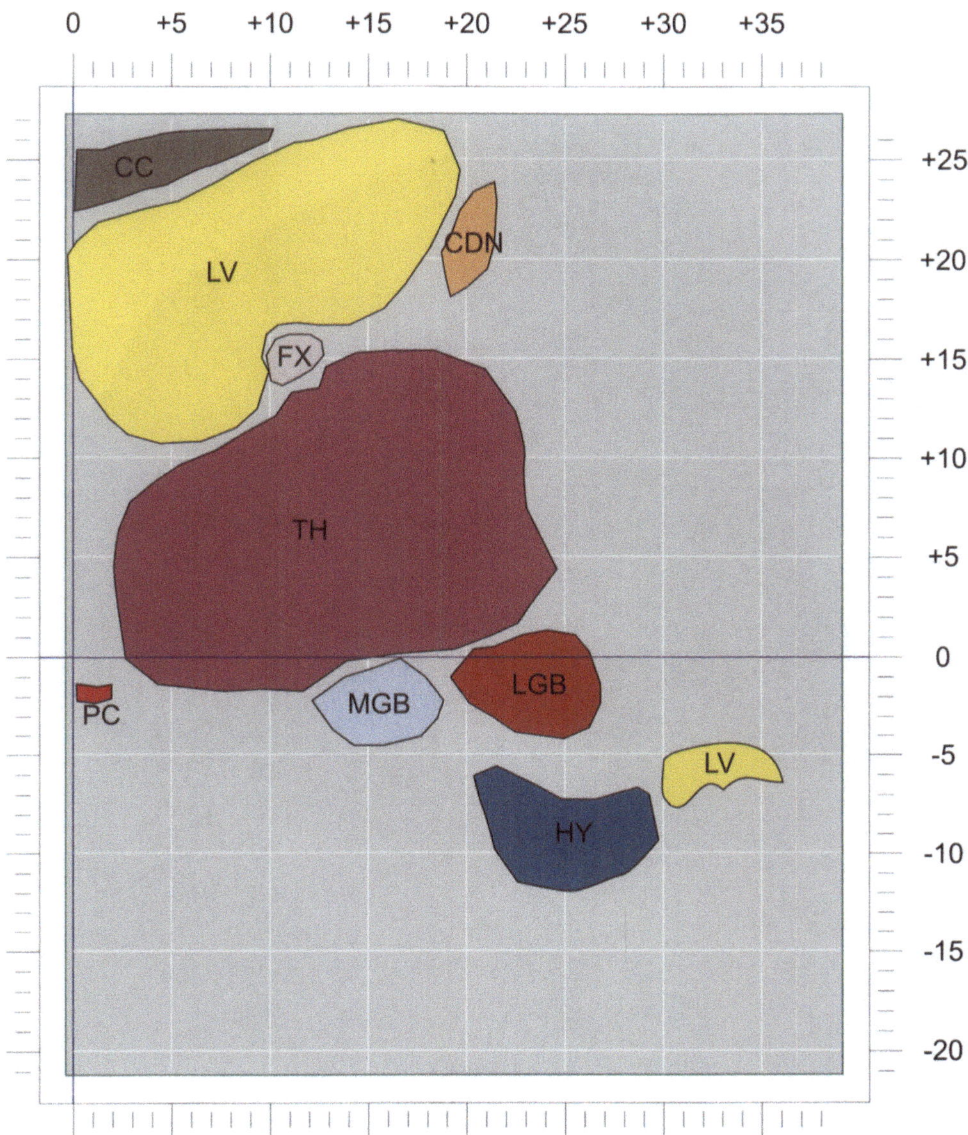


Coronal -27 mm

## Plate 37a

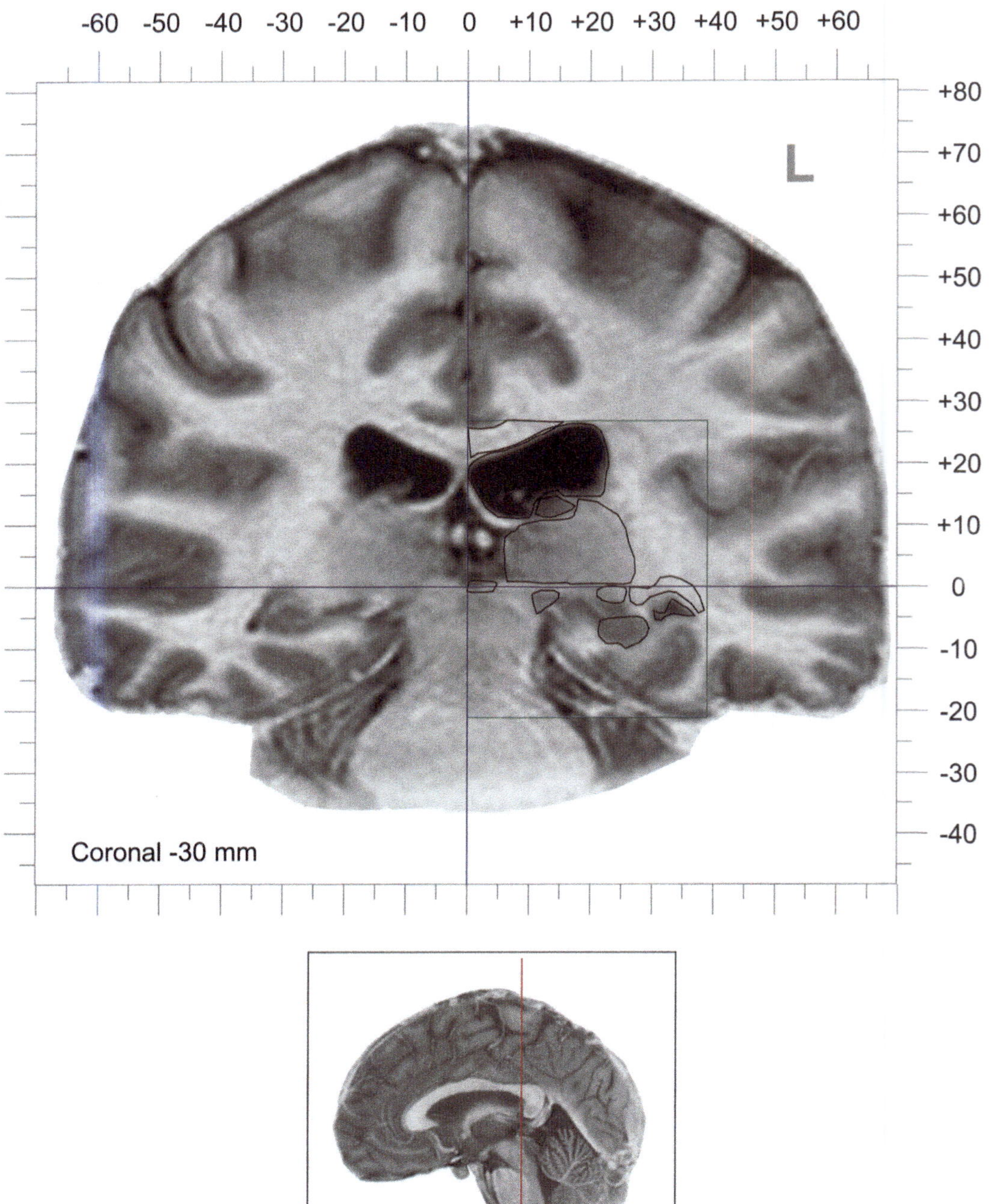

# Plate 37b

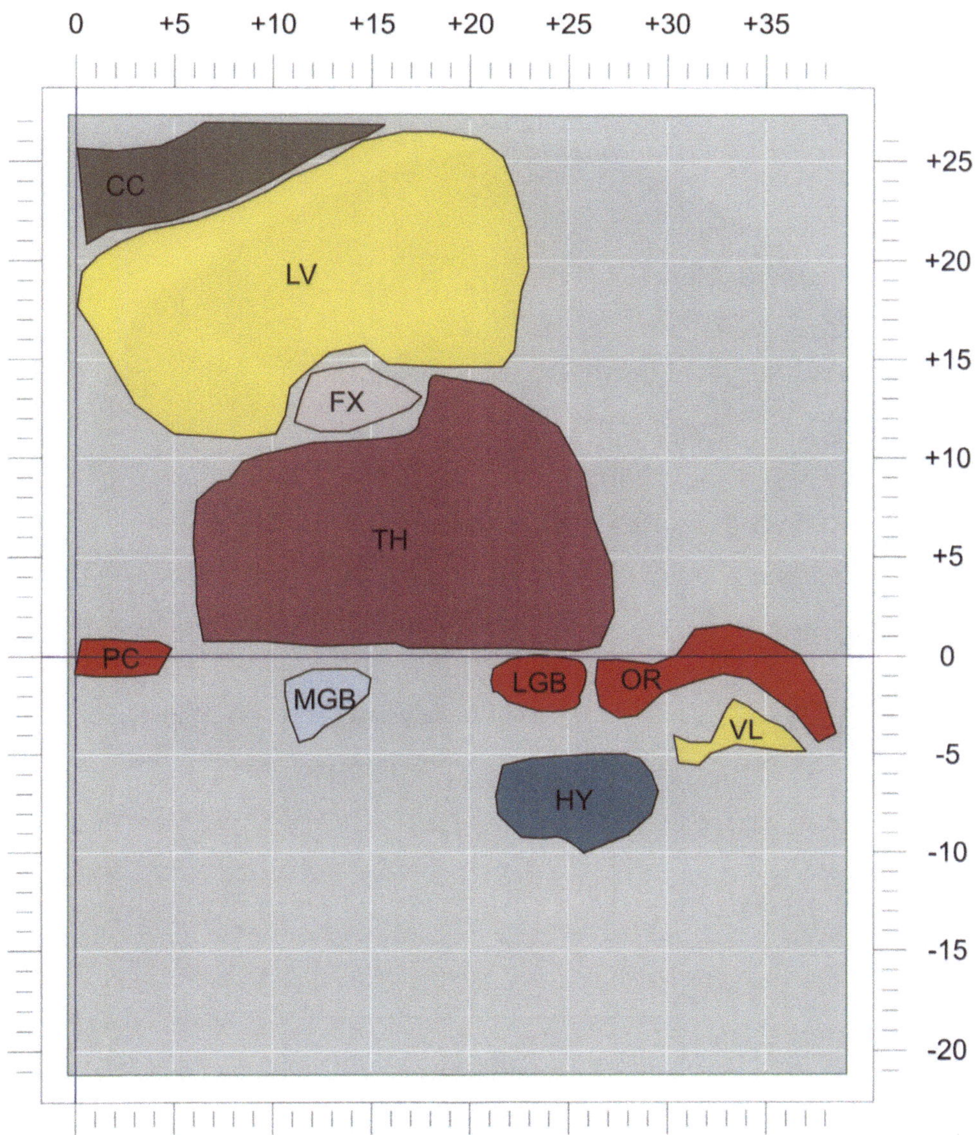


Coronal -30 mm

## Plate 38a

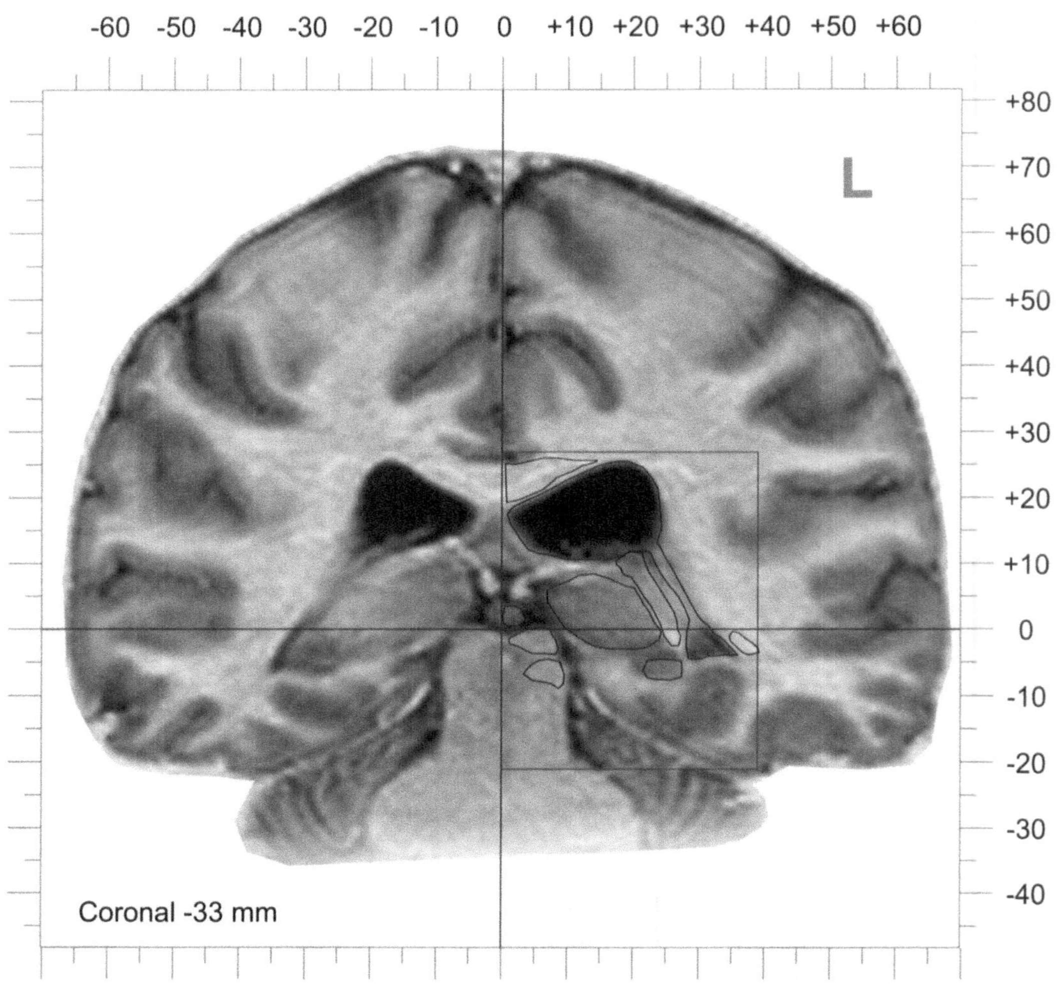


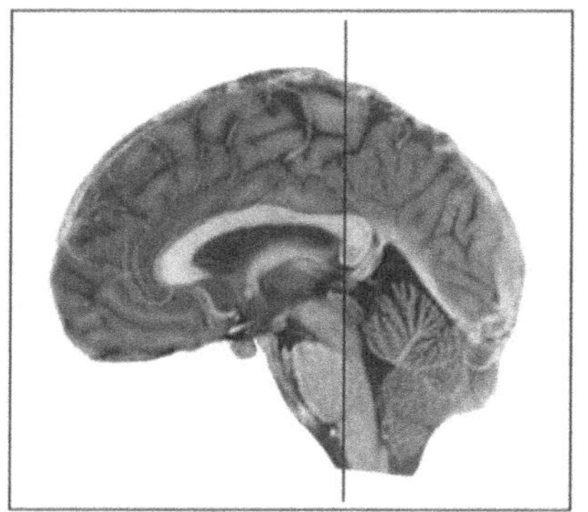

## Plate 38b

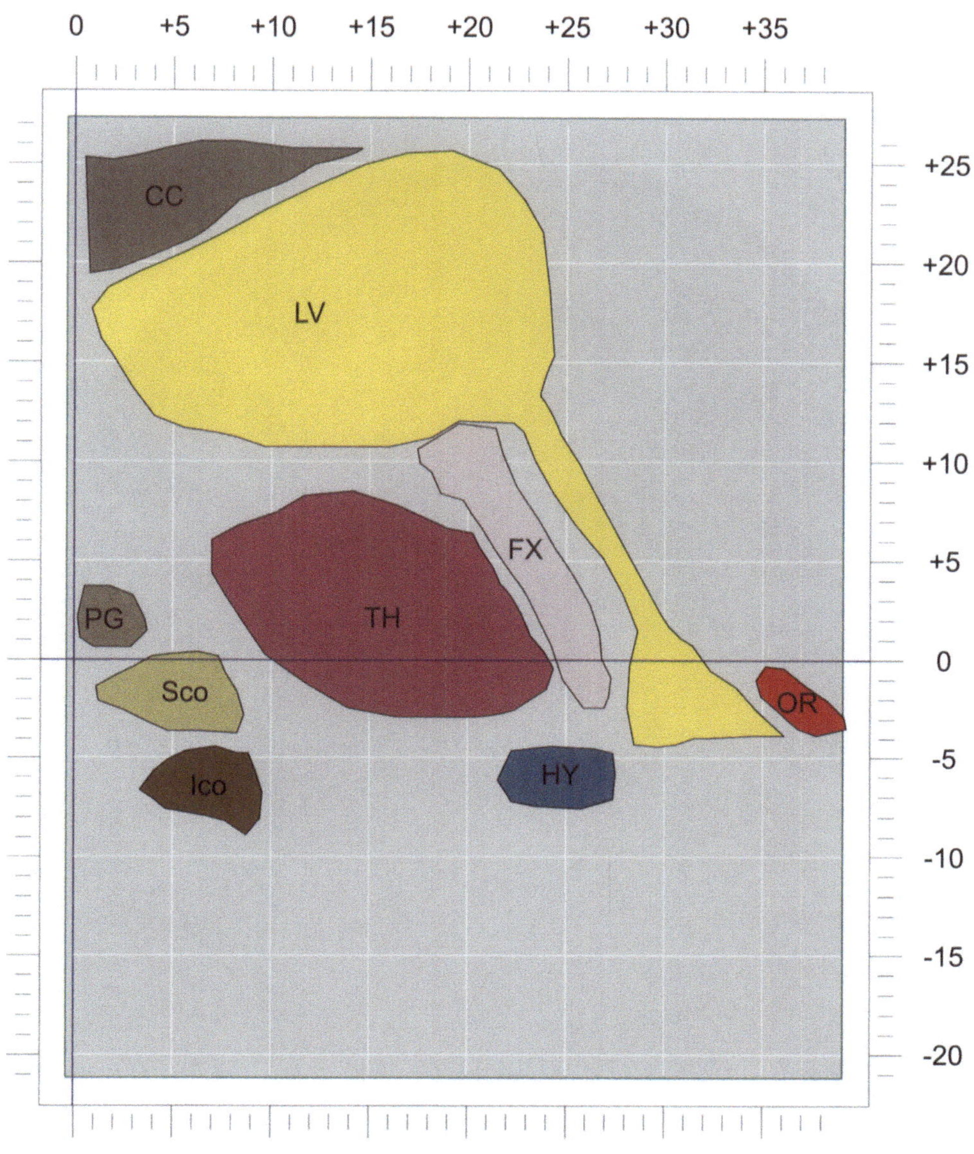


Coronal -33 mm

## Plate 39a

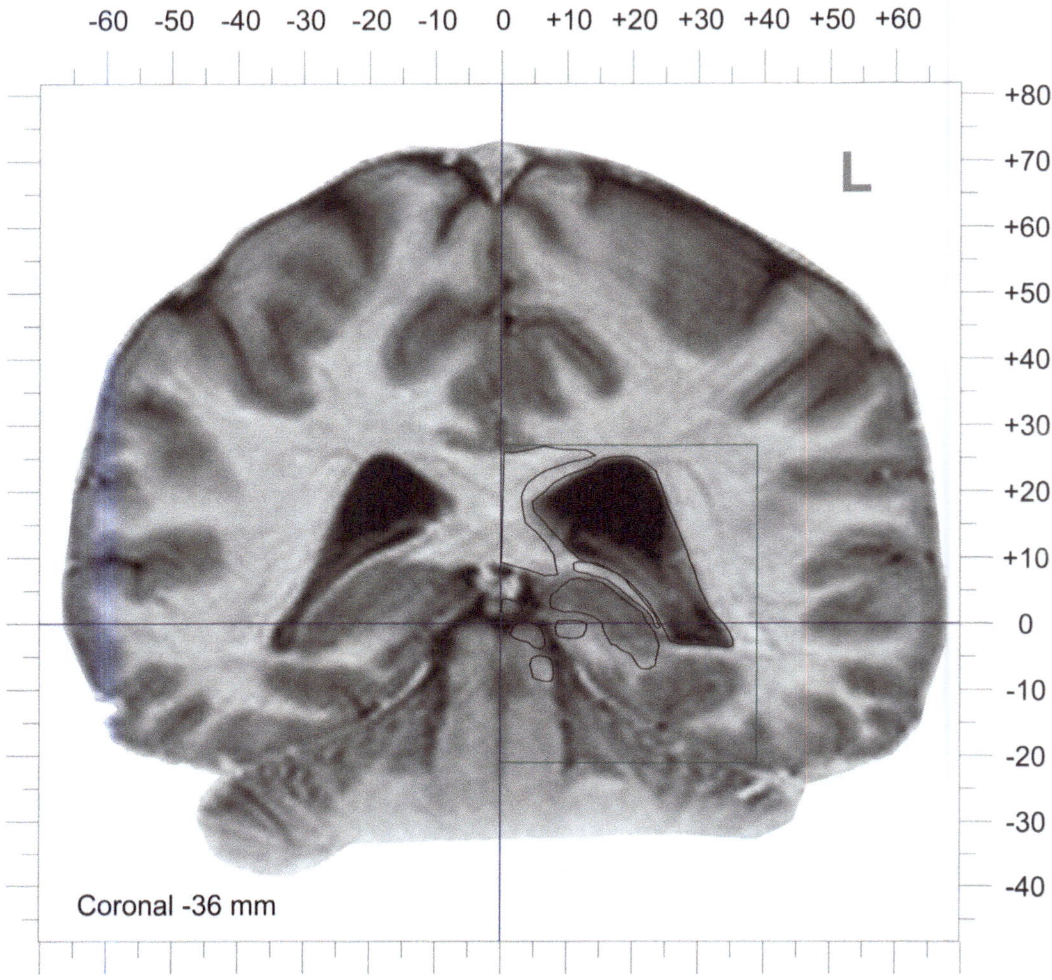


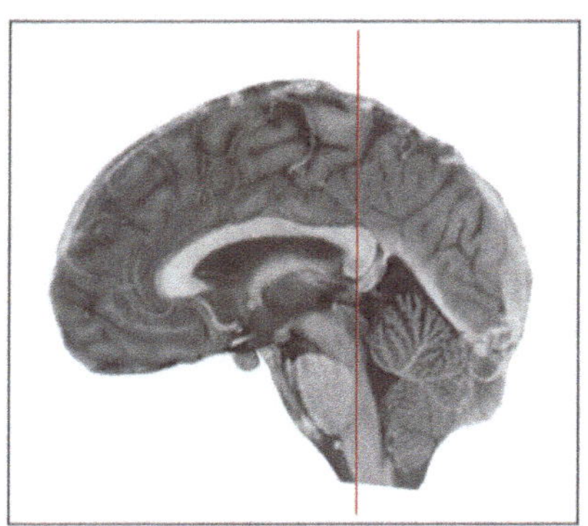

## Plate 39b

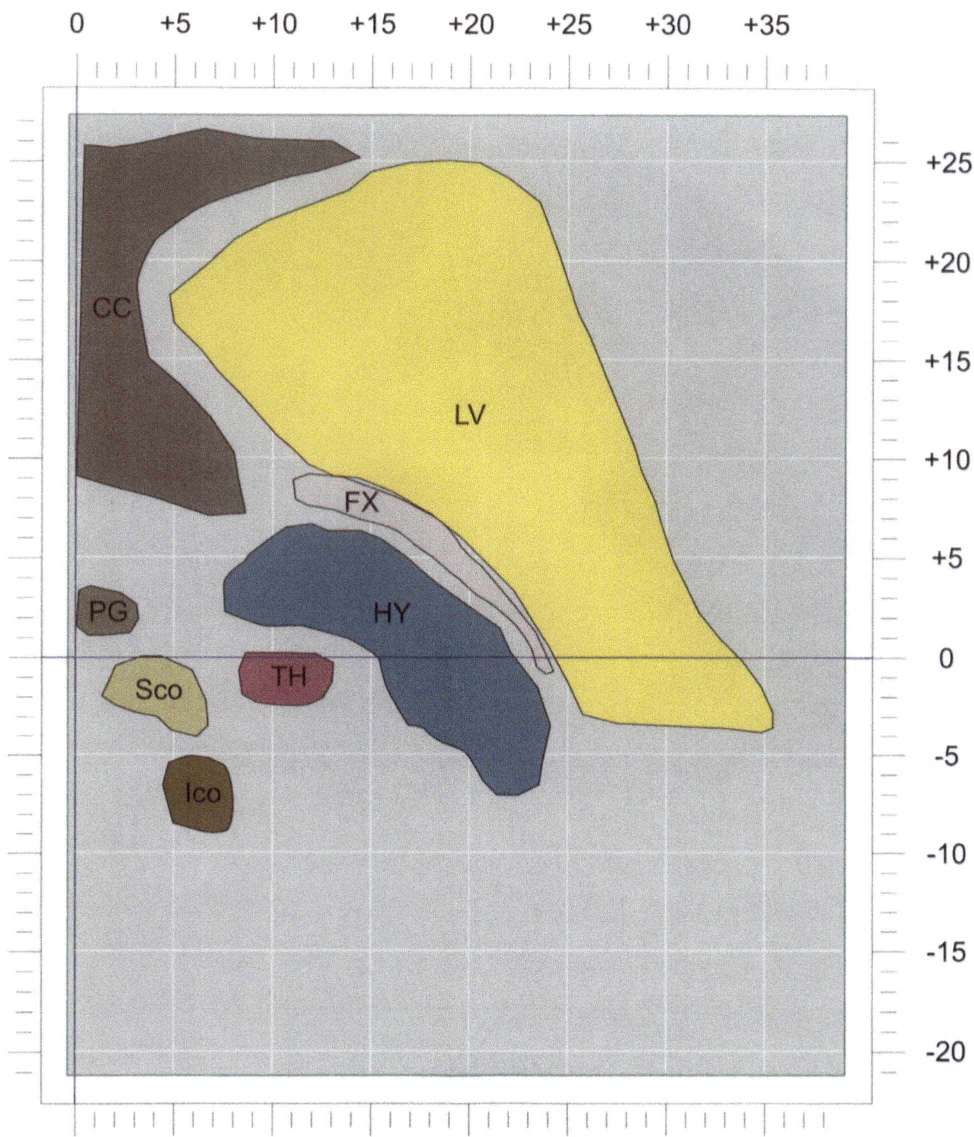


Coronal -36 mm

## Plate 40a

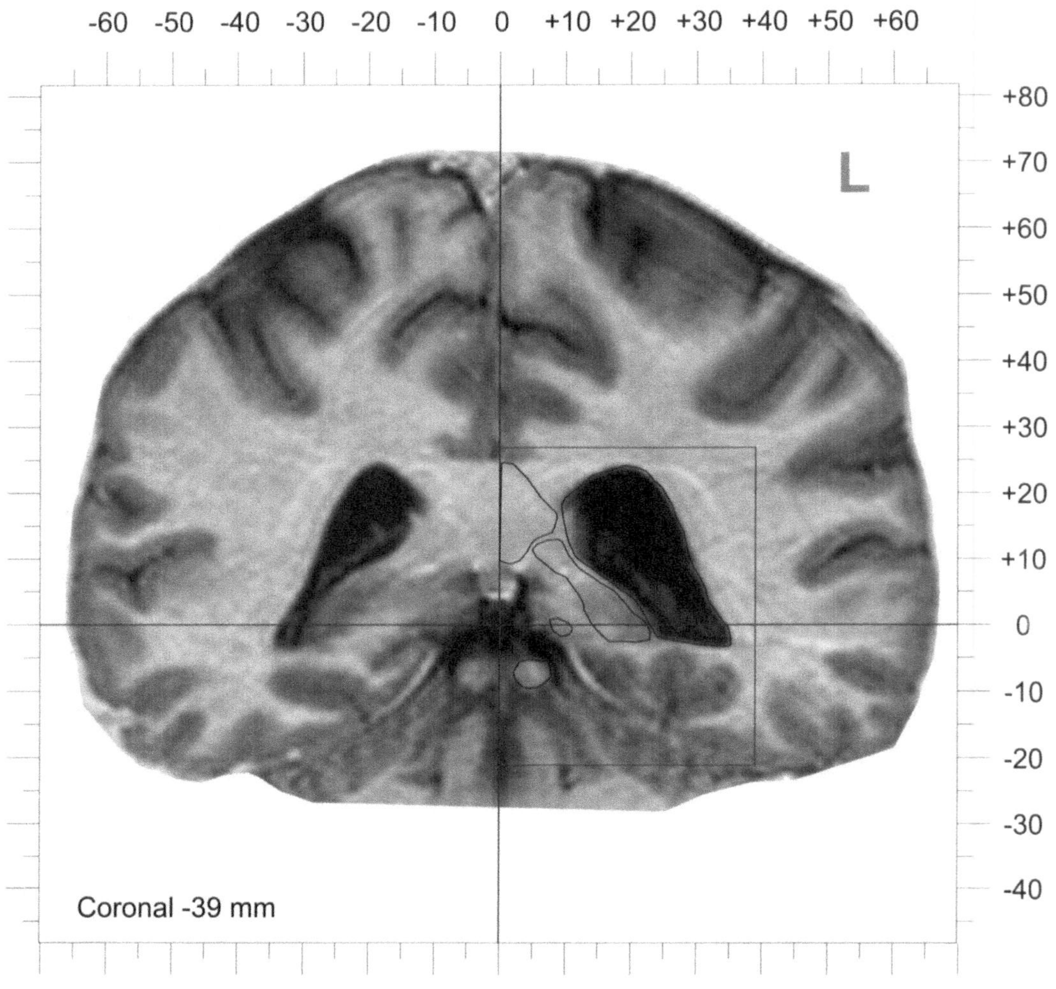


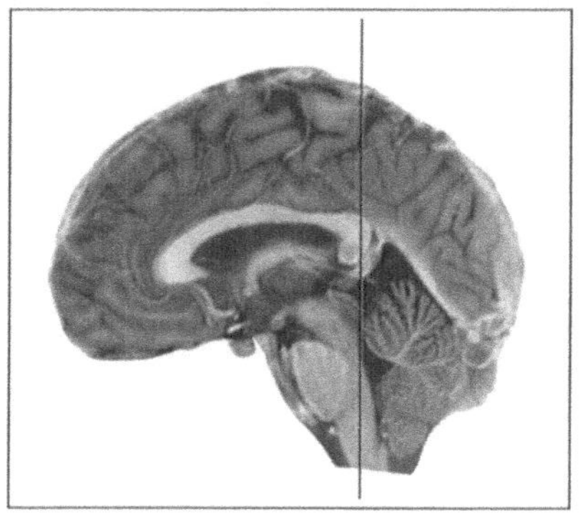

# Plate 40b

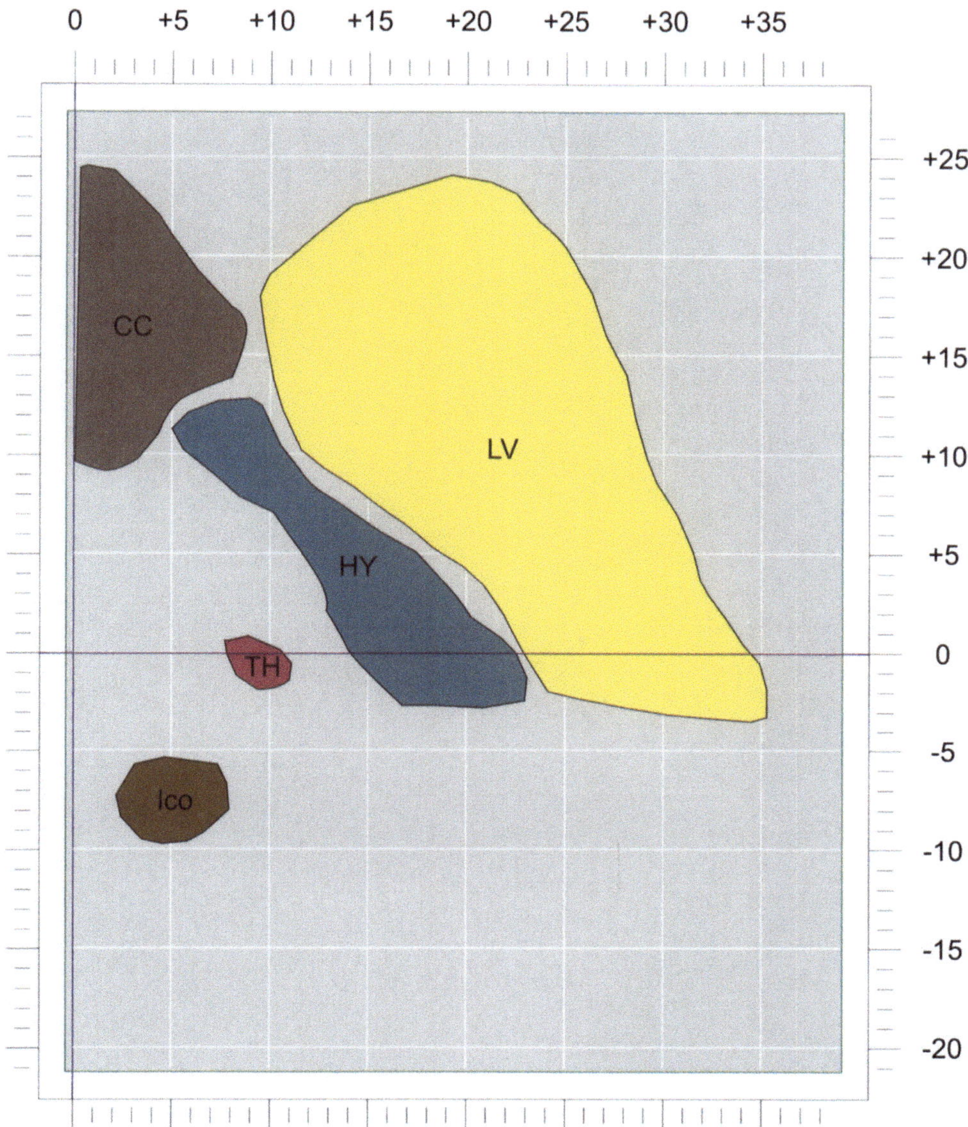


Coronal -39 mm

# Sagittal Sections

Plates 41-54

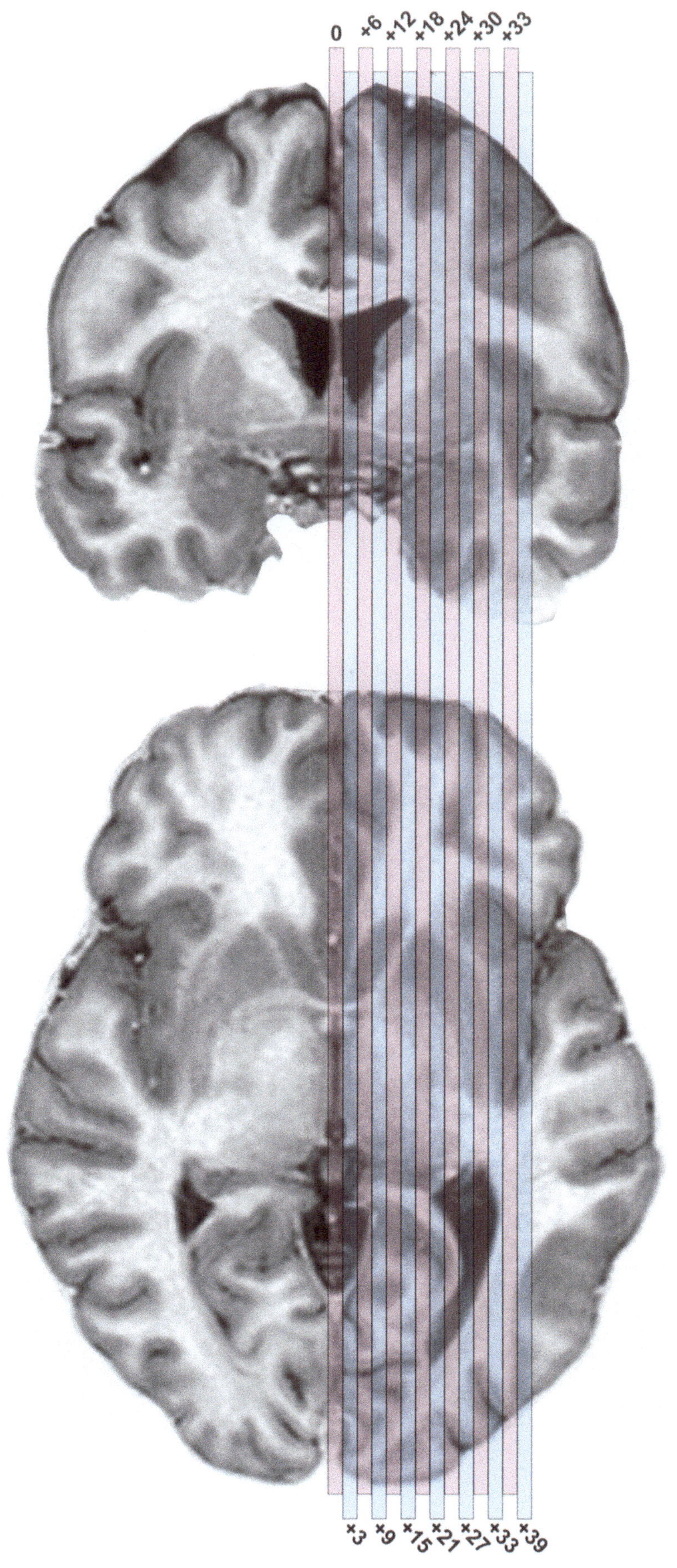
0 +6 +12 +18 +24 +30 +33
+3 +9 +15 +21 +27 +33 +39

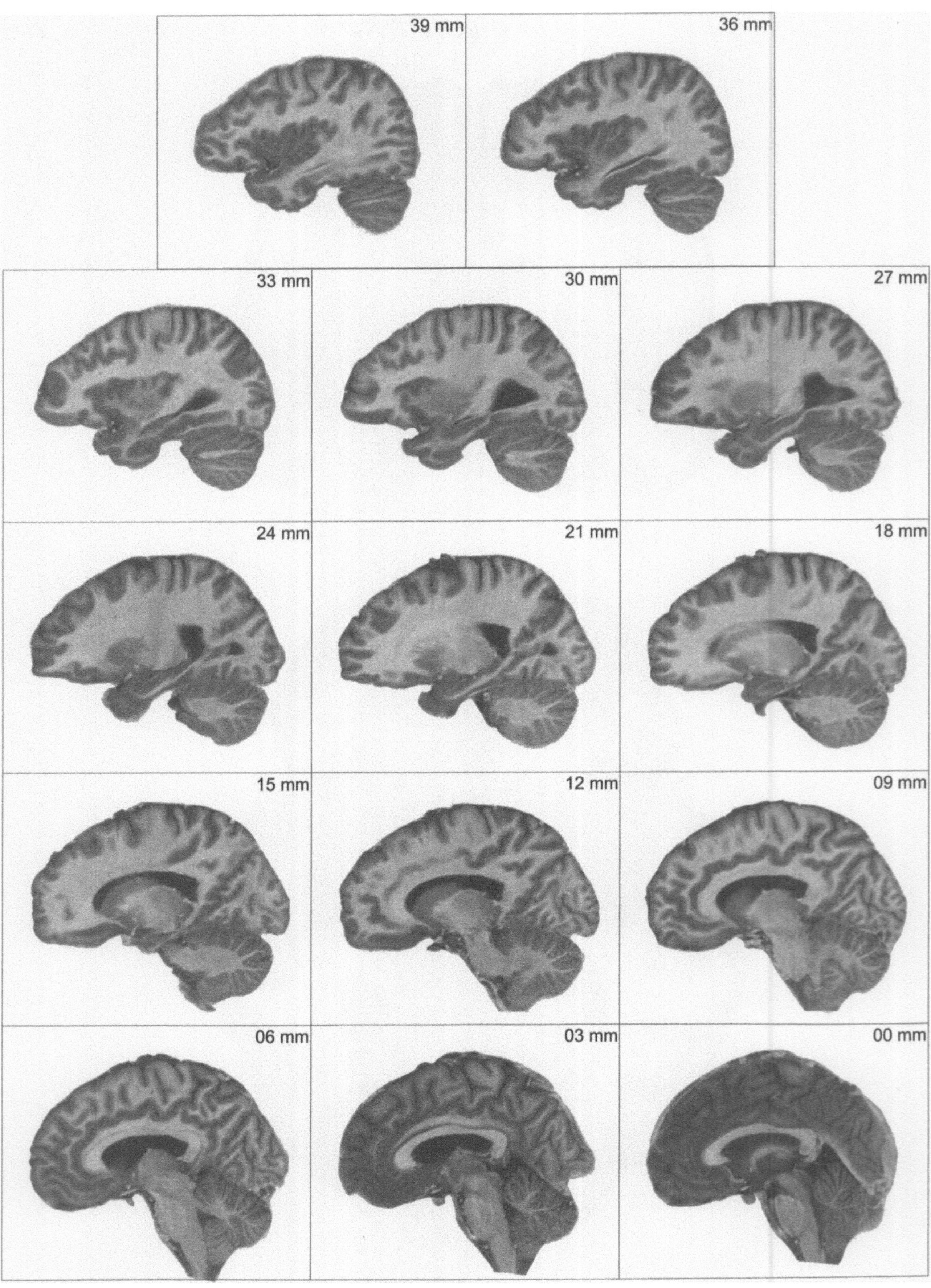


39 mm
36 mm
33 mm
30 mm
27 mm
24 mm
21 mm
18 mm
15 mm
12 mm
09 mm
06 mm
03 mm
00 mm

# Abbreviation – Nomenclature – Color Codes

| | | | | | | | | |
|---|---|---|---|---|---|---|---|---|
| **AC** | Anterior Commissure | | **Ico** | Inferior colliculus | | **PU** | Putamen | |
| **AL** | Ansa Lenticularis | | **IGP** | Int. Globus Pallidum | | **RN** | Red Nucleus | |
| **AN** | Amigdaloid Nucleus | | **LGB** | Lat. Geniculate Body | | **TH** | Thalamus | |
| **CC** | Corpus Callosum | | **LV** | Lateral Ventricles | | **Sco** | Superior Colliculus | |
| **CDN** | Caudate Nucleus | | **MB** | Mammillary Body | | **SN** | Substantia Nigra | |
| **Cep** | Cerebral peduncle | | **MGB** | Med. Genic. Body | | **STN** | Subthalamic Nucleus | |
| **CL** | Claustrum | | **MTT** | Mammillo thal. tract | | **V3** | Third ventricle | |
| **DE** | Diencephalon | | **OC** | Optic Chiasm | | **ZI** | Zona Incerta | |
| **EGP** | Ext.globus pallidum | | **OR** | Optic Radiation | | | | |
| **FSC** | Fundus striati, caudati | | **OT** | Optic Tract | | | | |
| **FX** | Fornix | | **PC** | Post. Commissure | | | | |
| **H2** | H2 Forel's field | | **PG** | Pineal Gland | | | | |
| **HY** | Hyppocampus | | **PHN** | Paraventricular Hypothalamic Nuclei | | | | |
| **IC** | Internal Capsula | | | | | | | |

# Plate 41a

+70 +60 +50 +40 +30 +20 +10 0 -10 -20 -30 -40 -50 -60 -70 -80 -90 -100
+90
+80
+70
+60
+50
+40
+30
+20
+10
0
-10
-20
-30
-40
-50
-60
Sagittal +39 mm

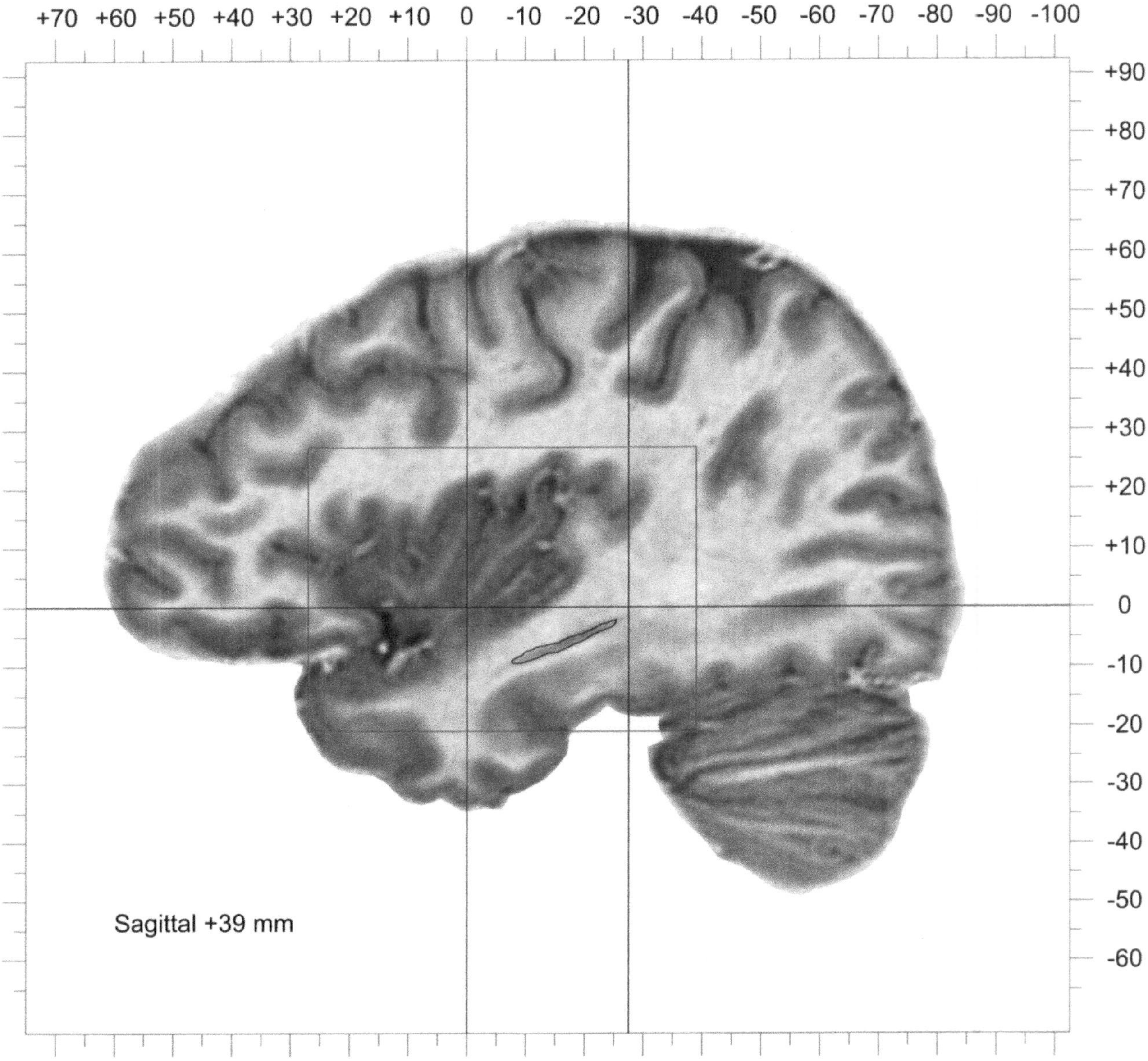

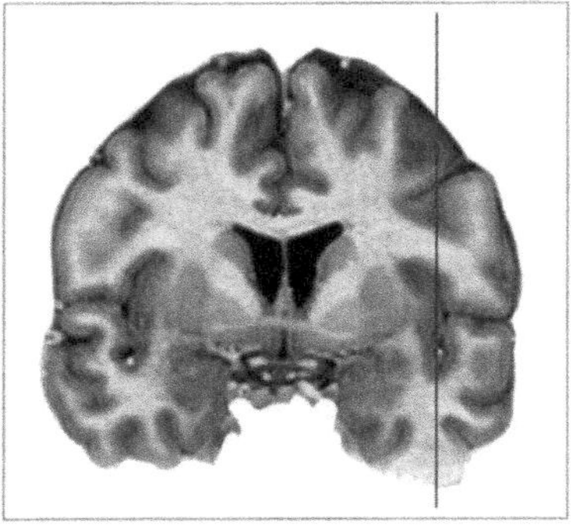

# Plate 41b

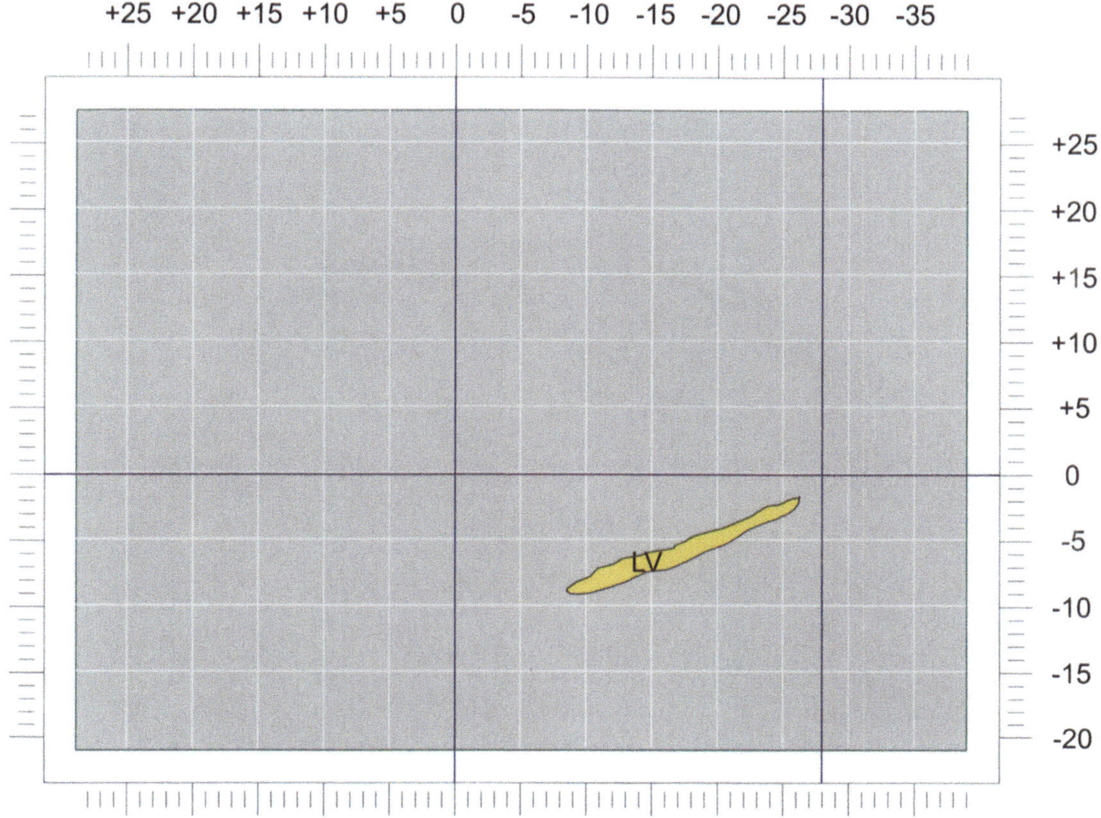


Sagittal 39 mm

# Plate 42a

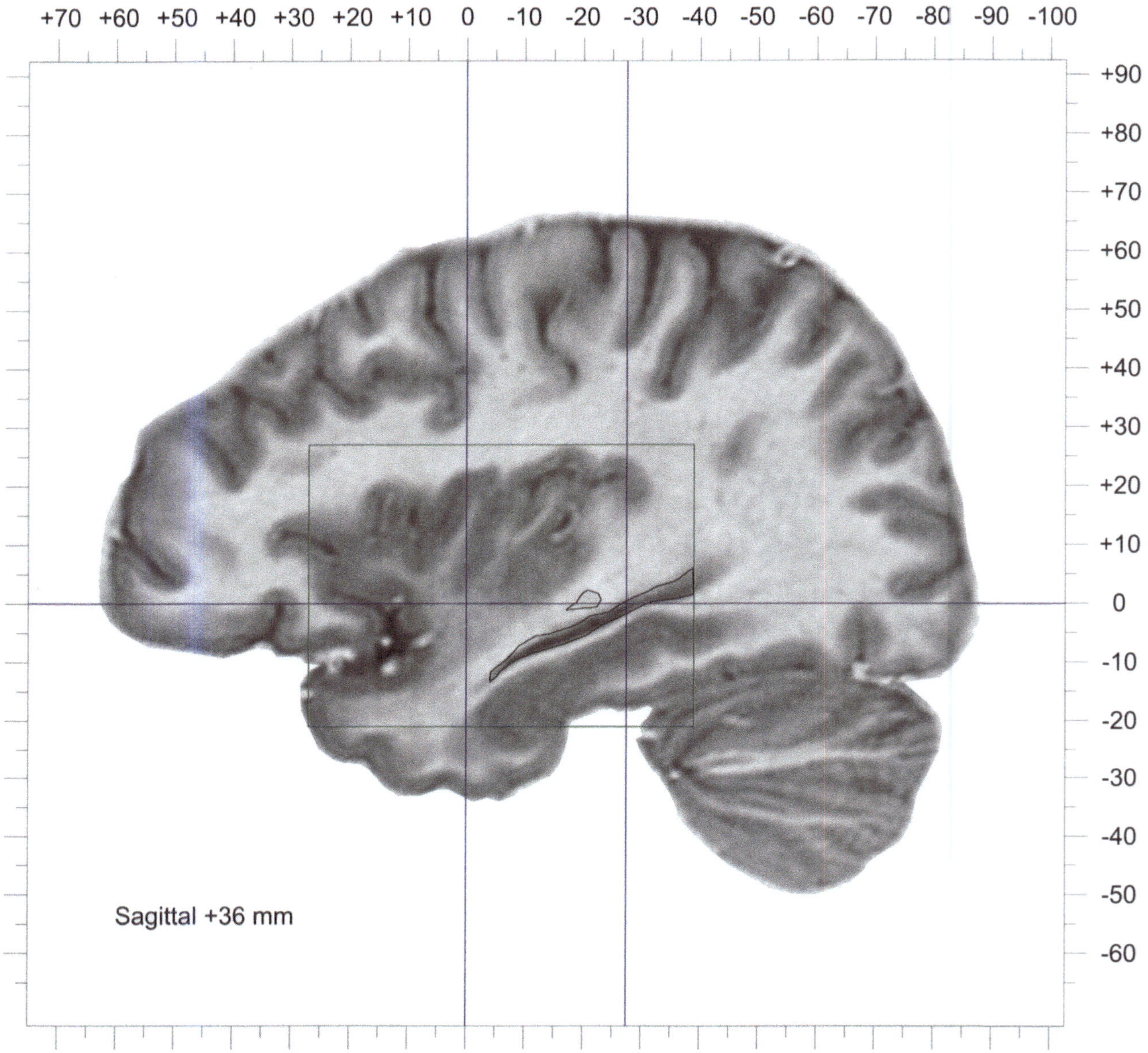

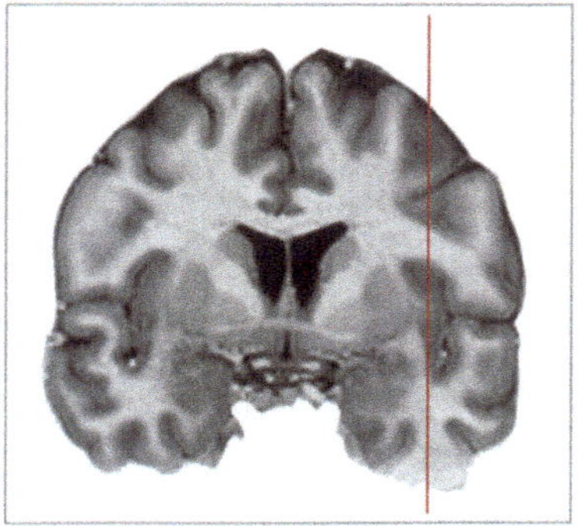

## Plate 42b

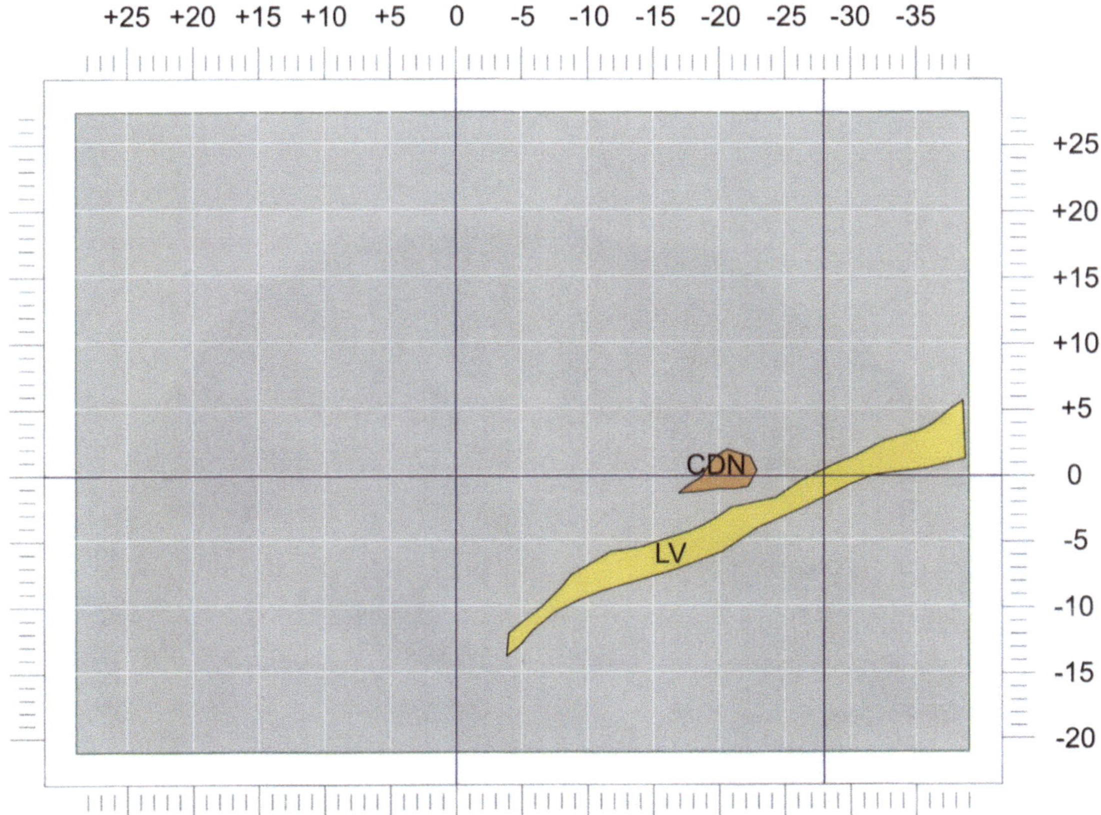


Sagittal 36 mm

## Plate 43a

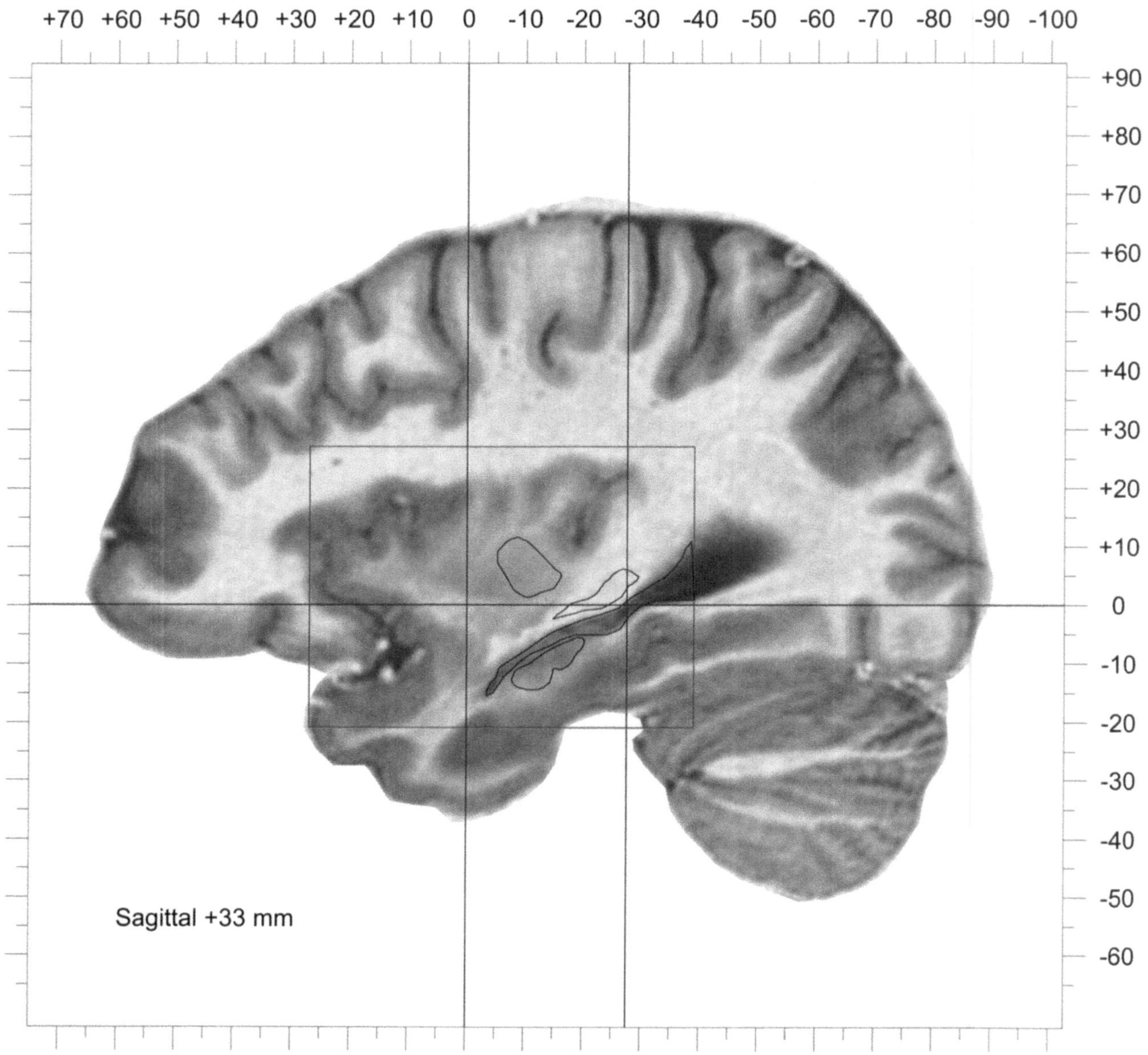

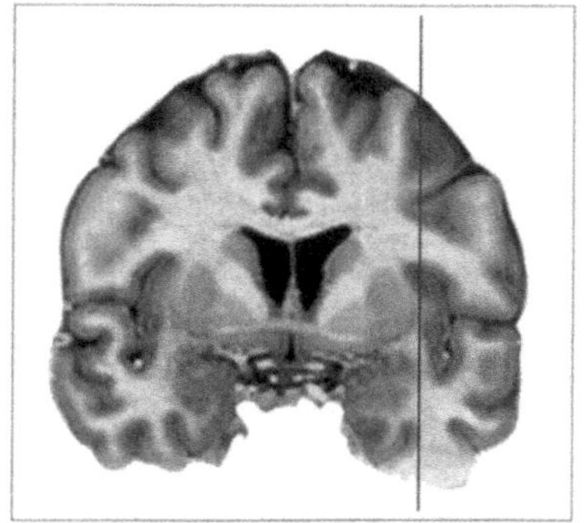

## Plate 43b

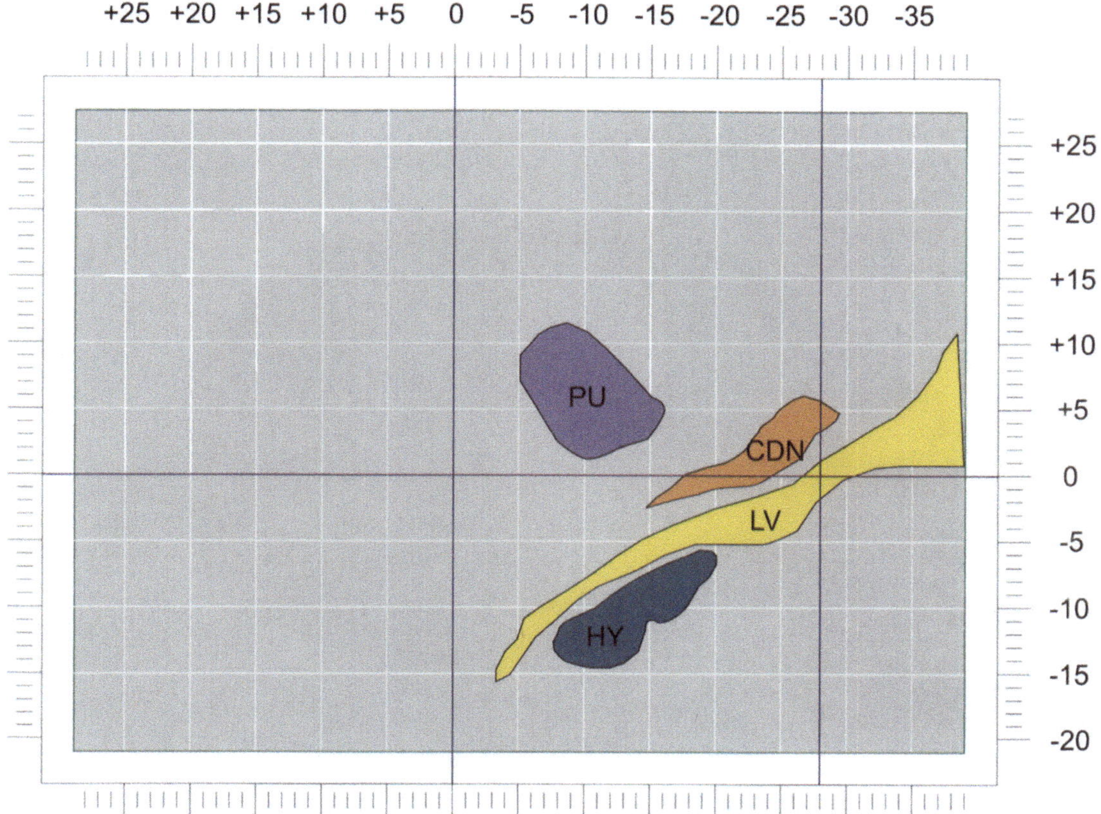


Sagittal 33 mm

## Plate 44a

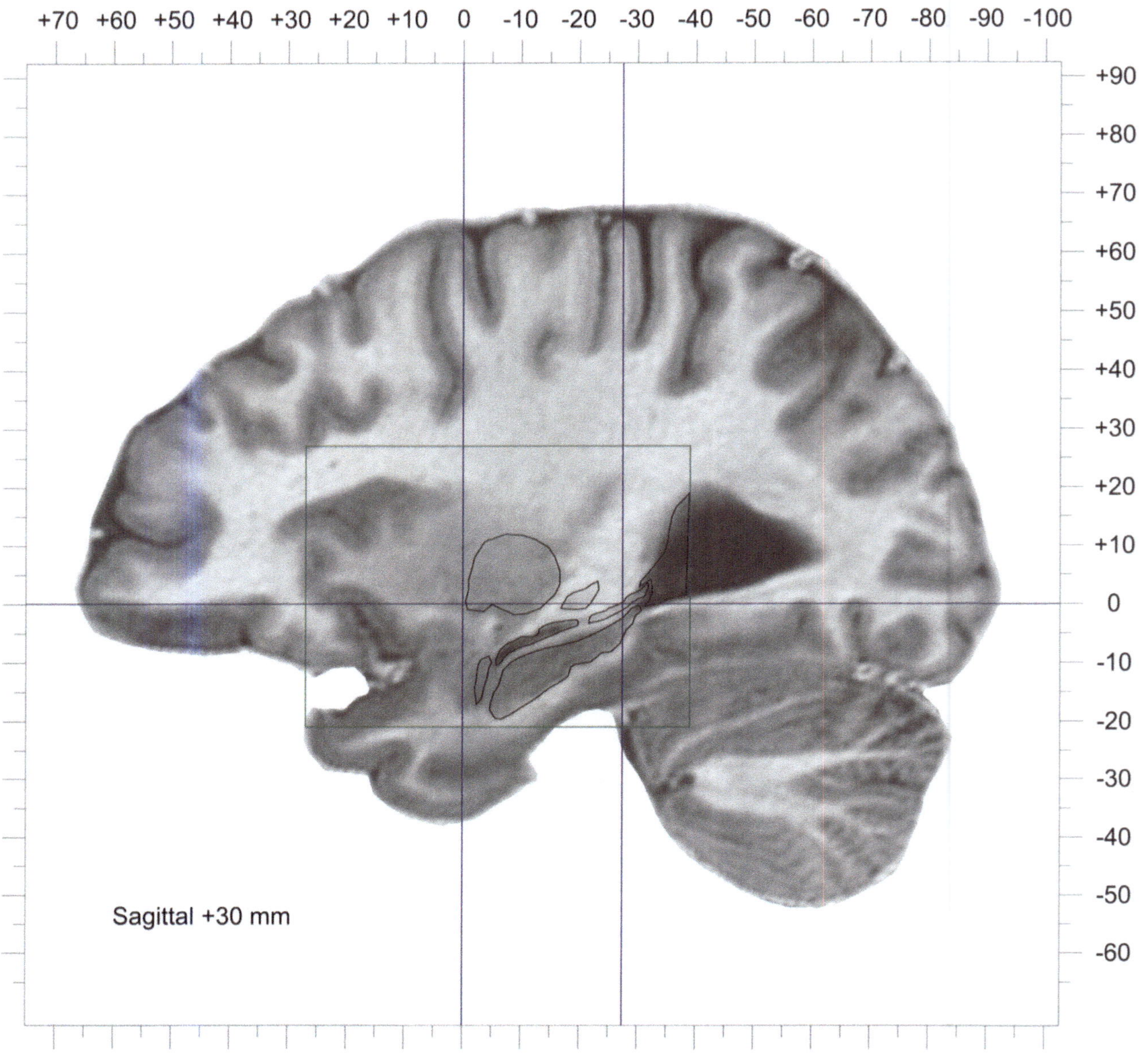

+70  +60  +50  +40  +30  +20  +10   0   -10  -20  -30  -40  -50  -60  -70  -80  -90  -100

+90
+80
+70
+60
+50
+40
+30
+20
+10
0
-10
-20
-30
-40
-50
-60

Sagittal +30 mm

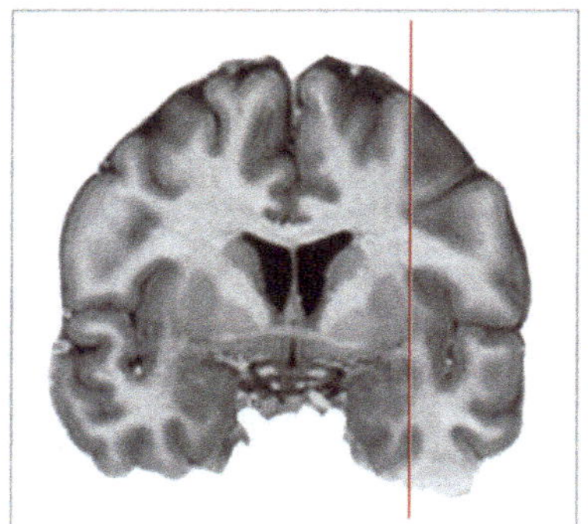

## Plate 44b

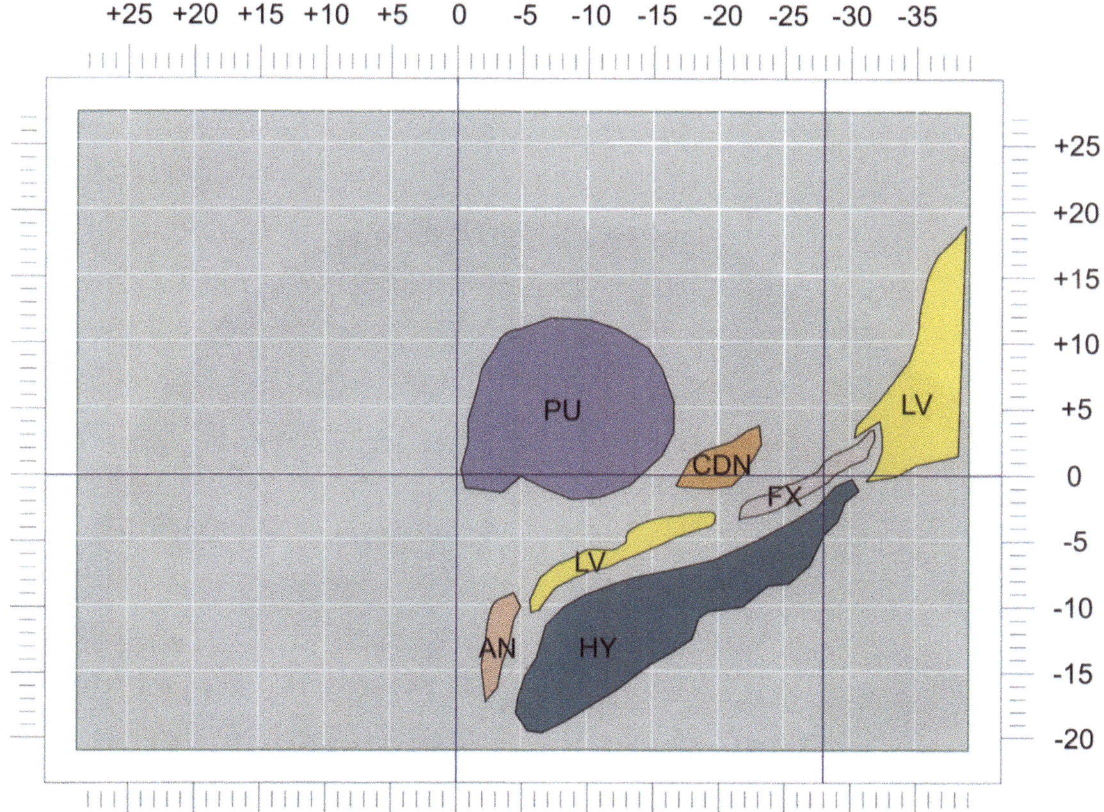


Sagittal 30 mm

## Plate 45a

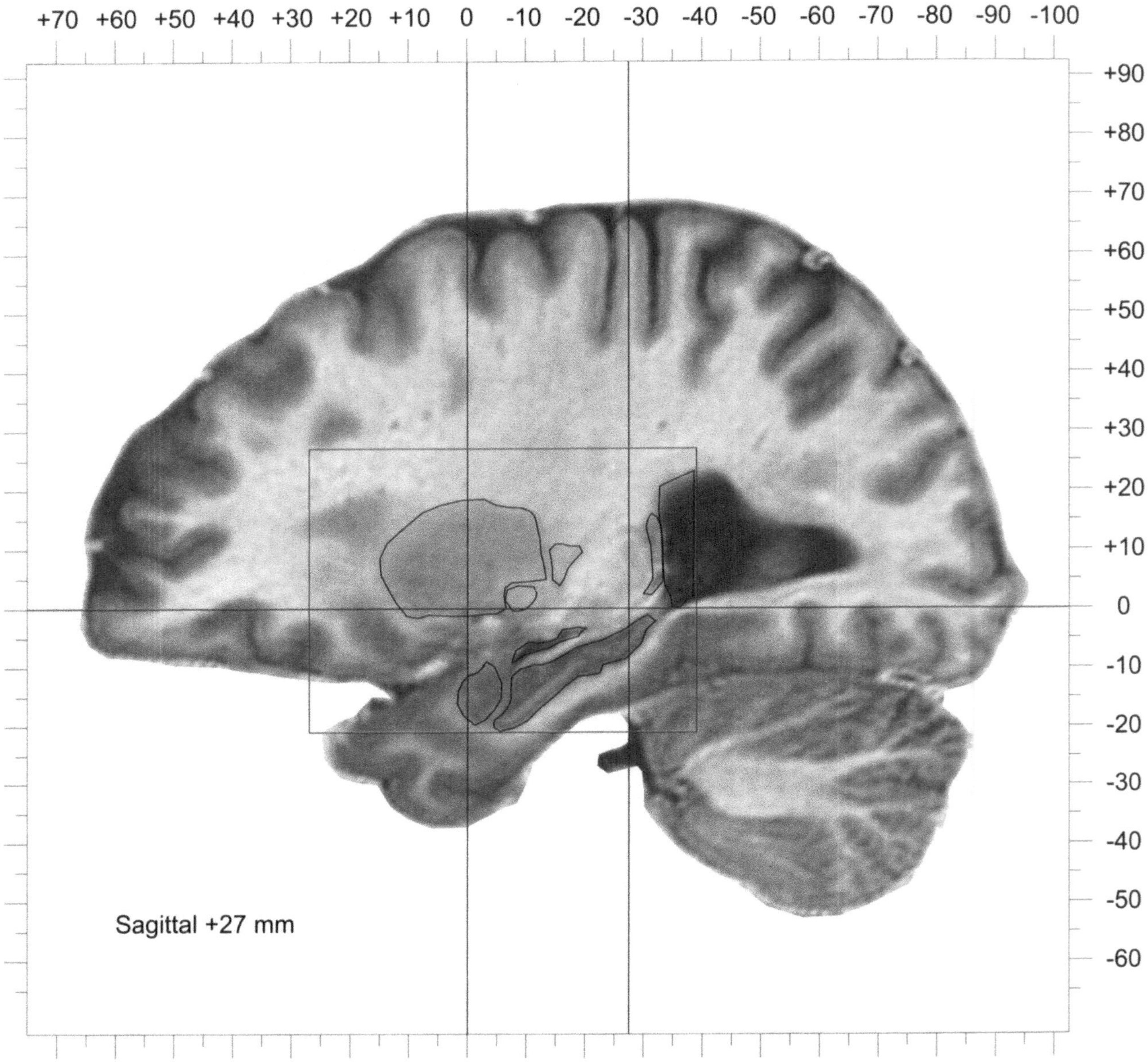

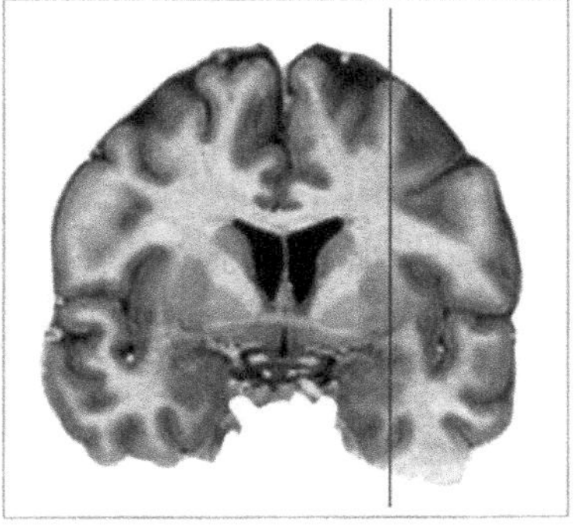

## Plate 45b

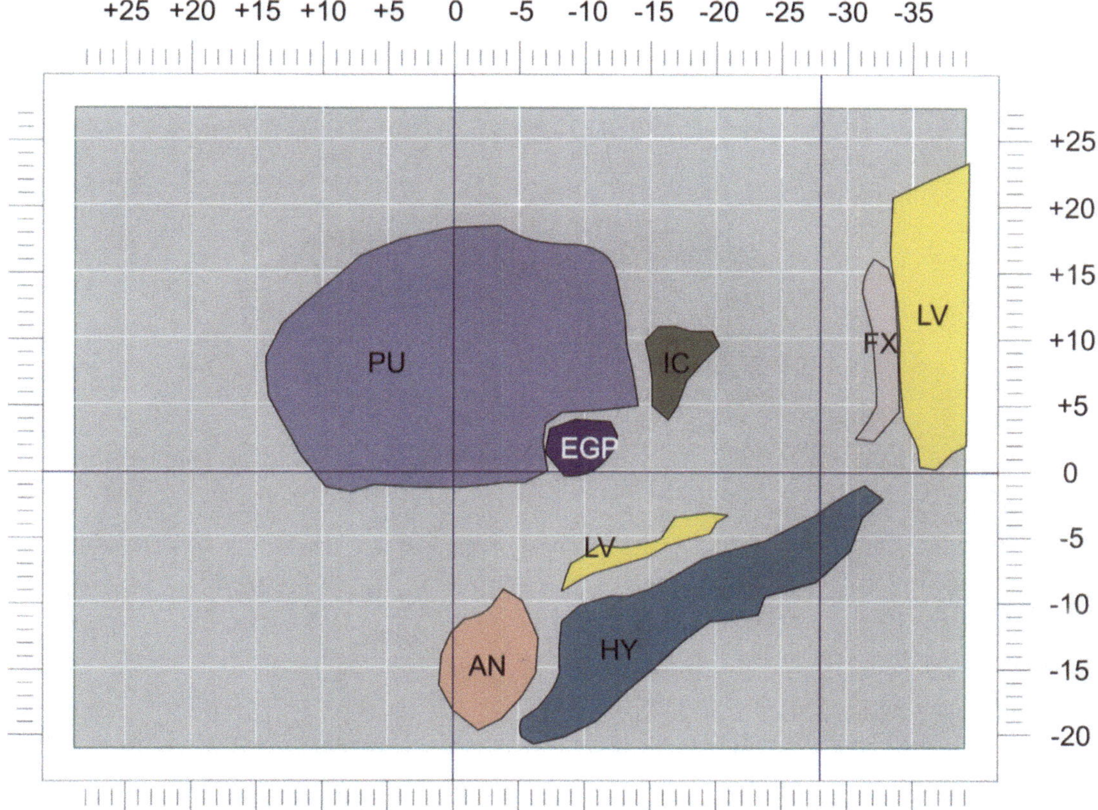


Sagittal 27 mm

# Plate 46a

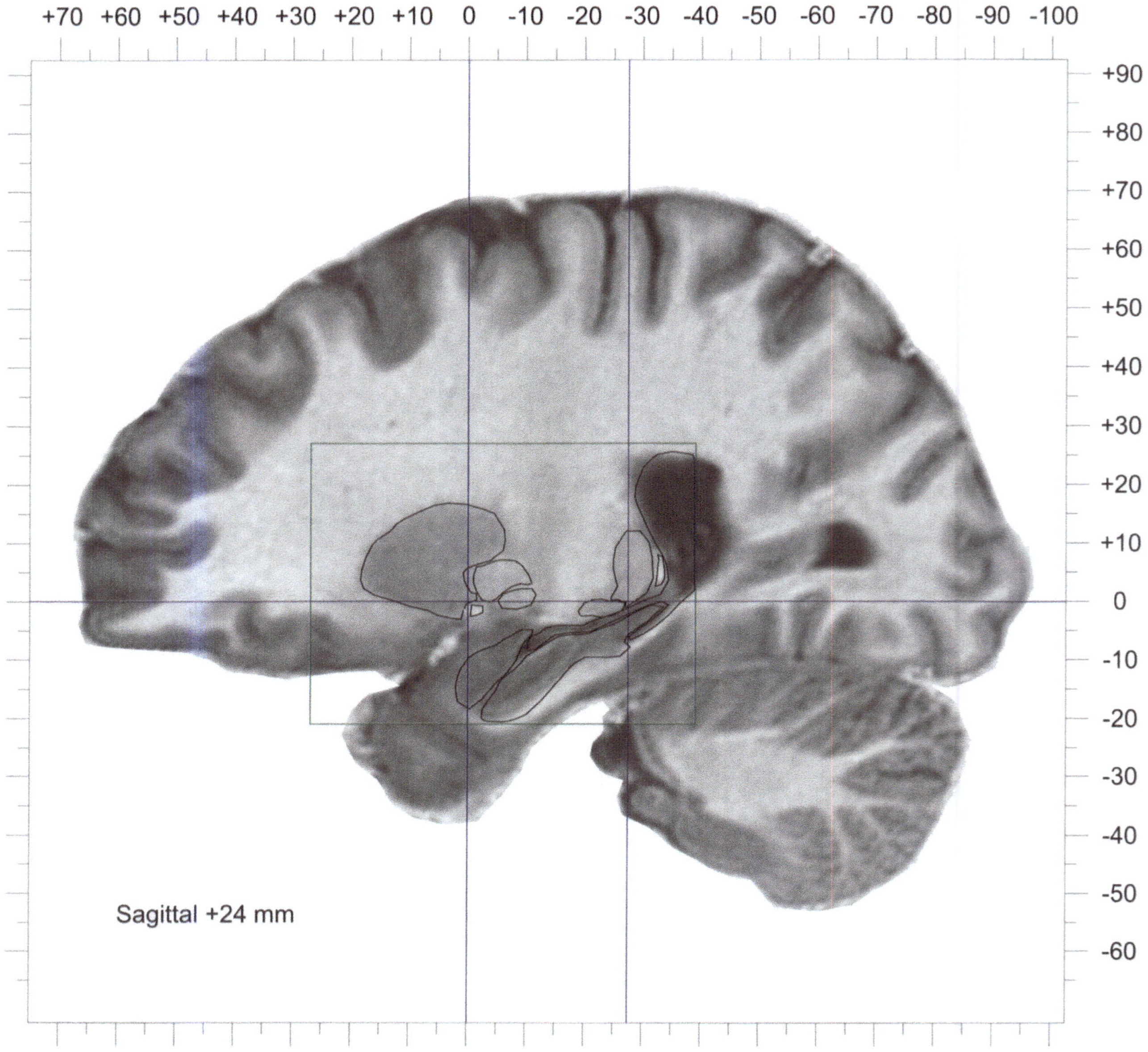

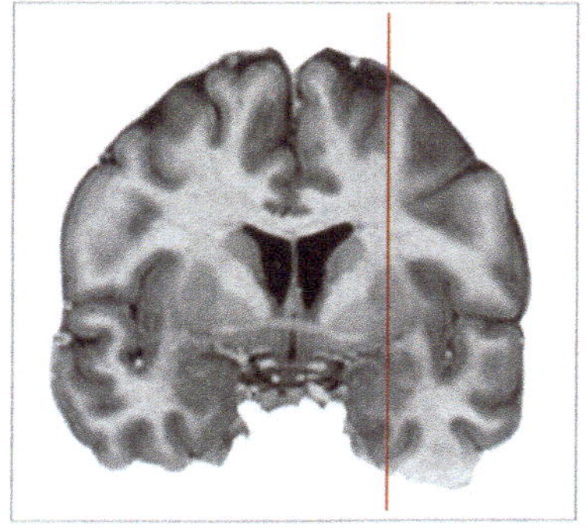

# Plate 46b

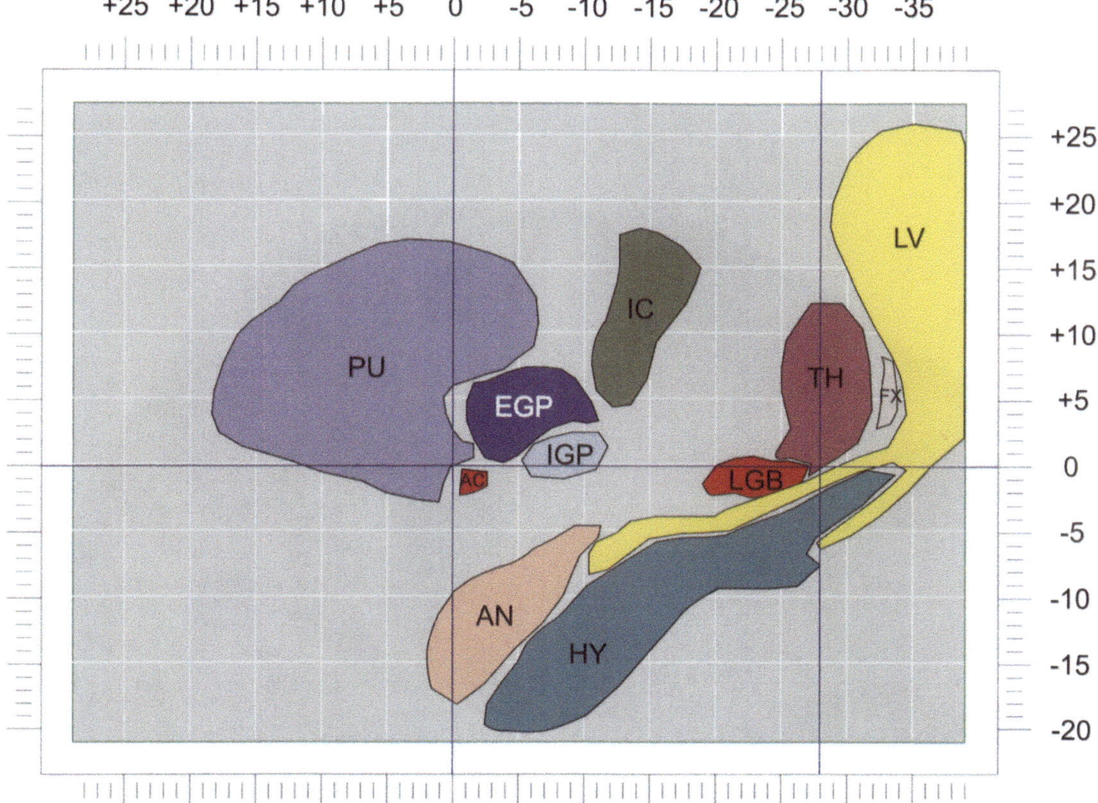


Sagittal 24 mm

# Plate 47a

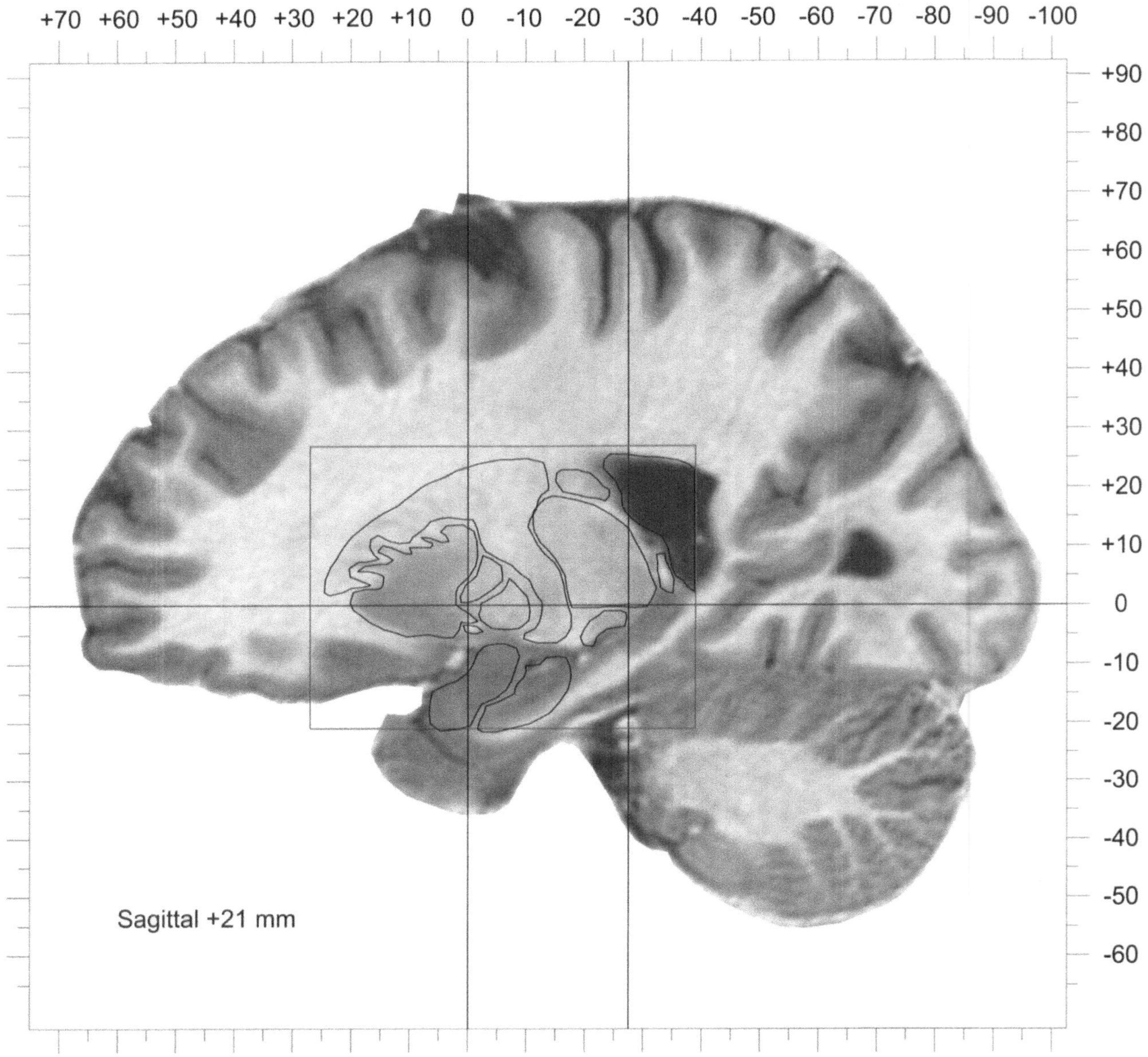

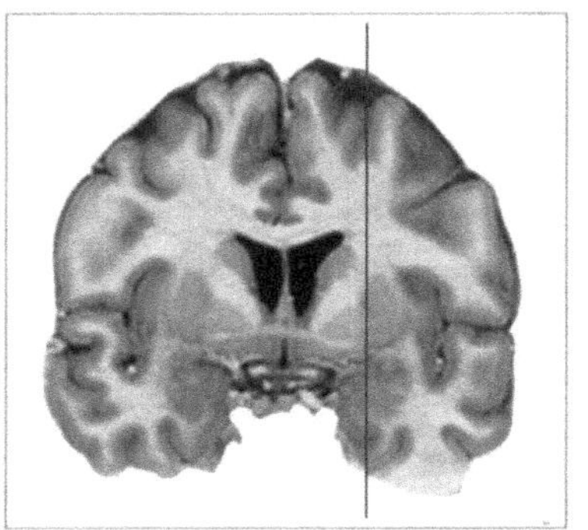

# Plate 47b

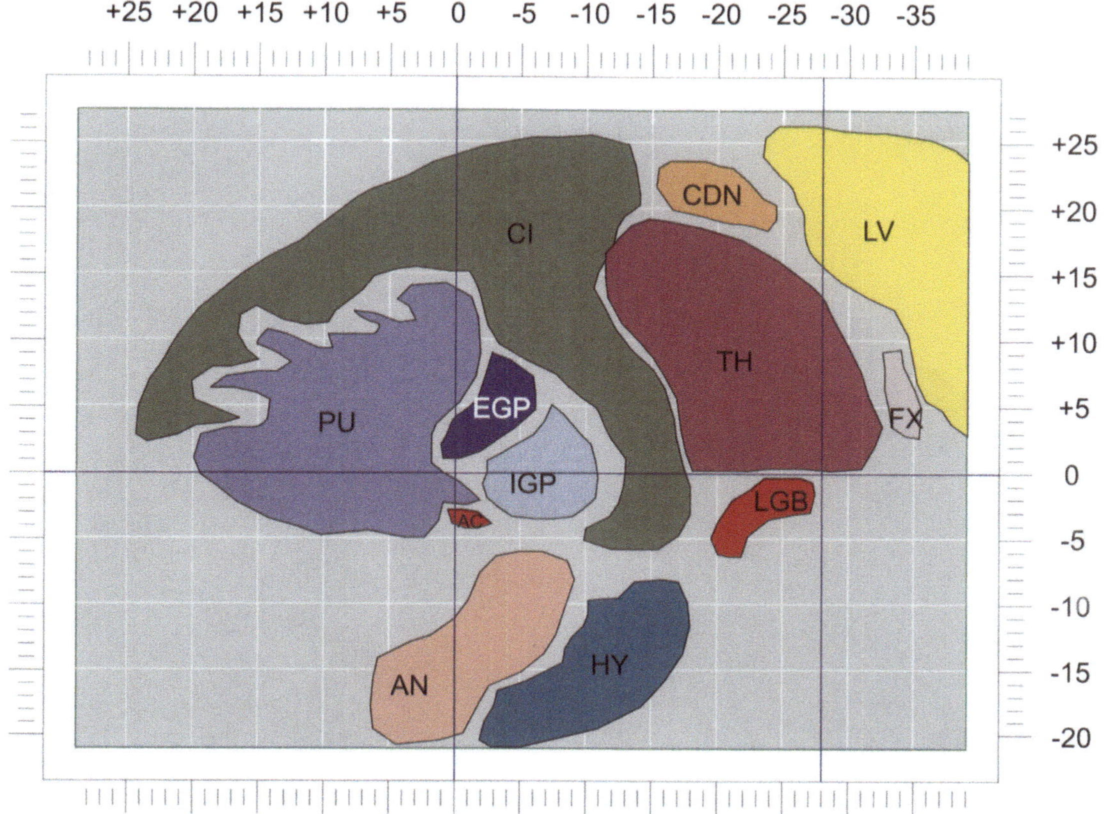



Sagittal 21 mm

## Plate 48a

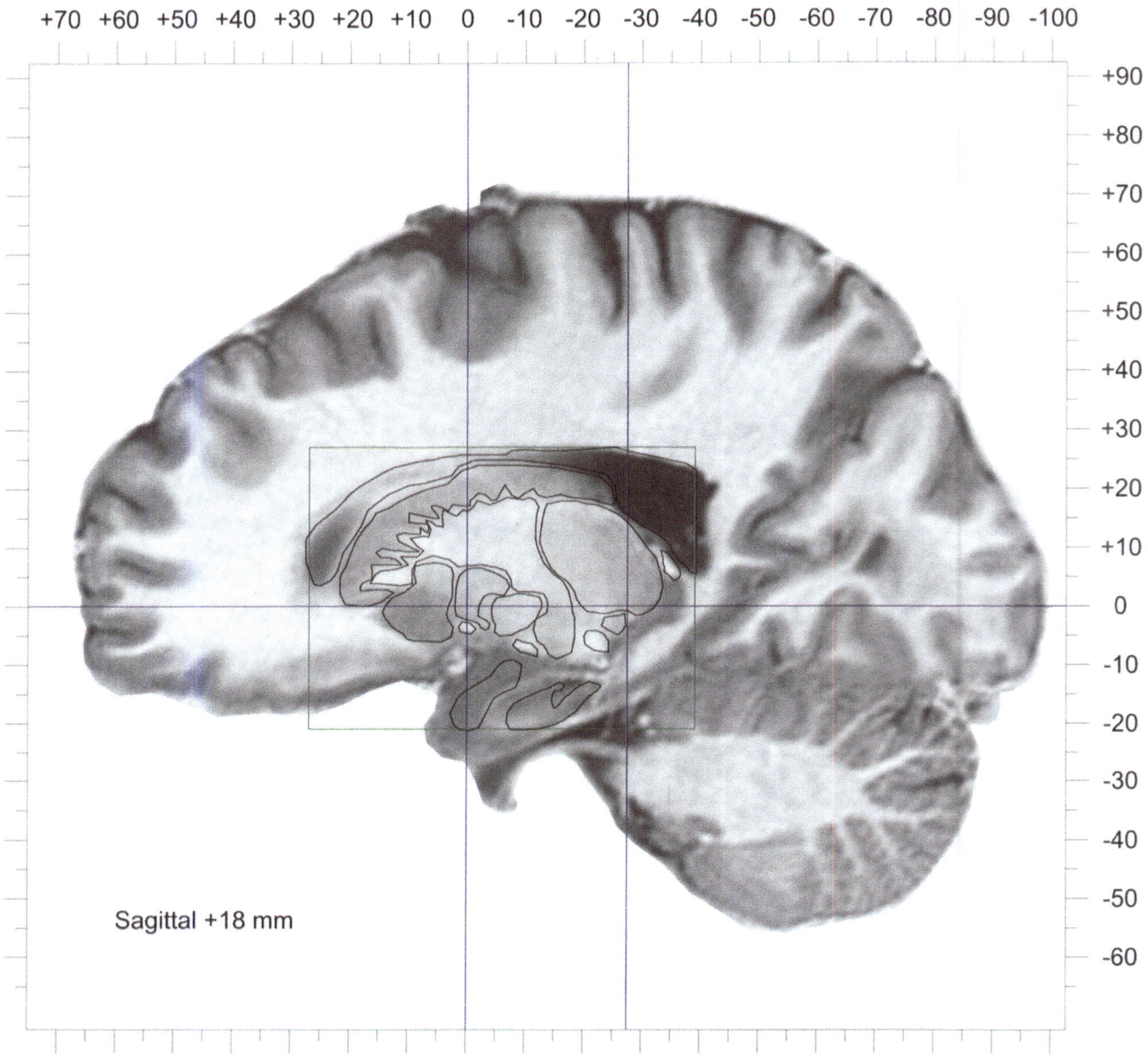

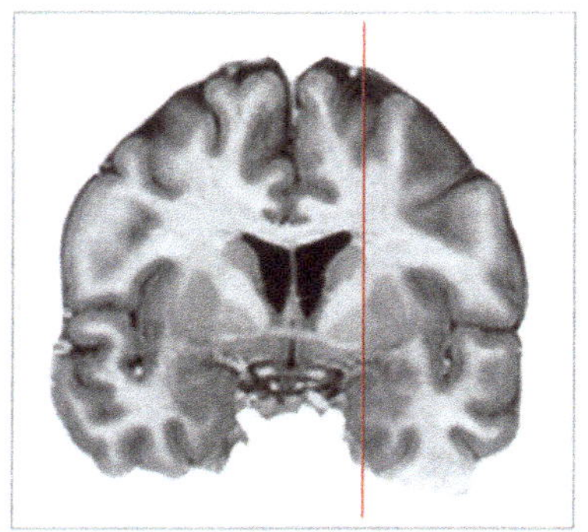

## Plate 48b

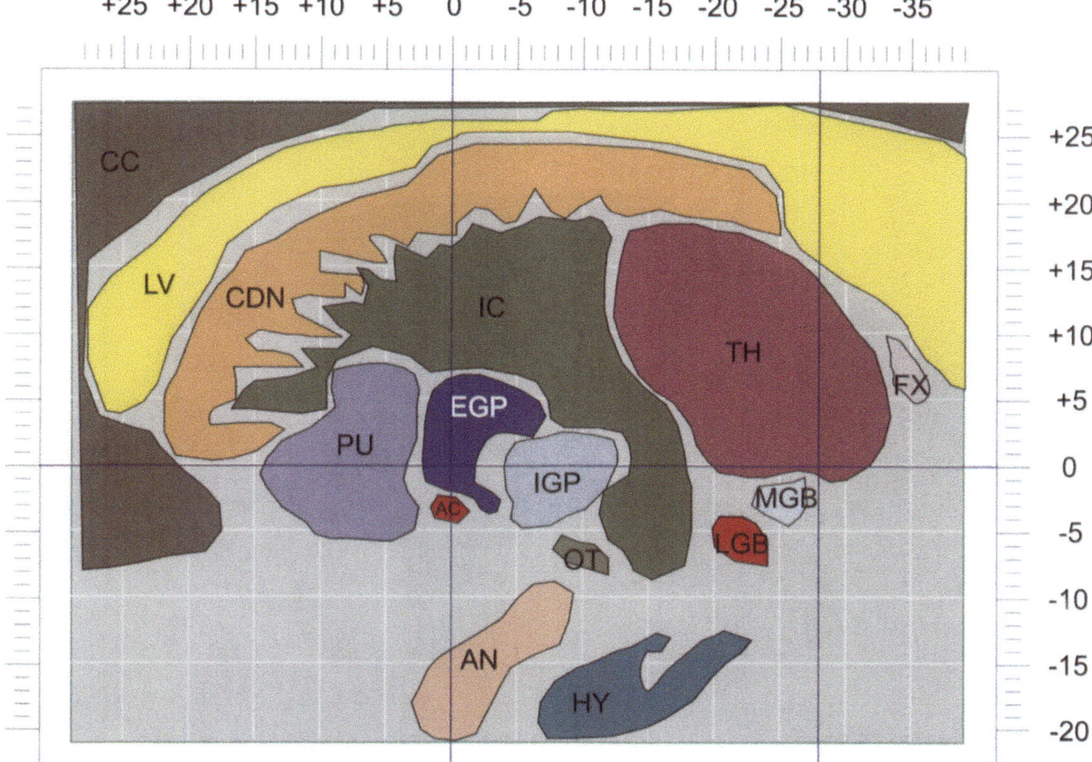



Sagittal 18 mm

## Plate 49a

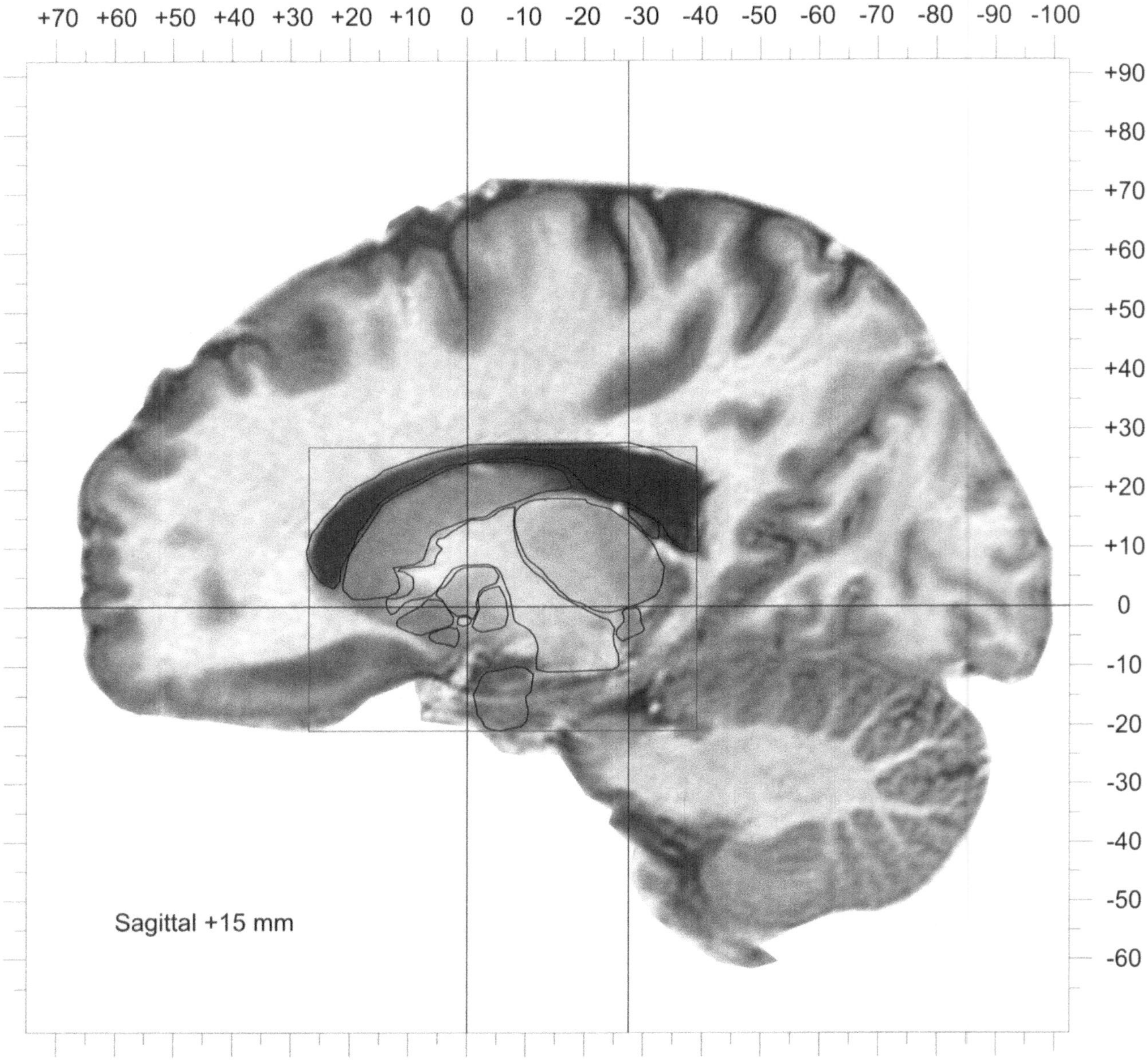

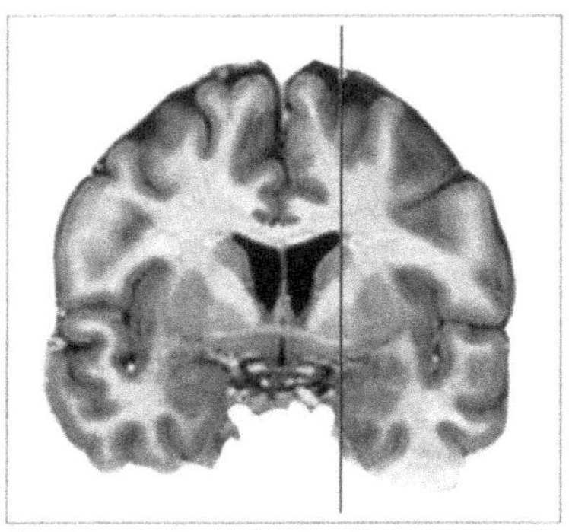

## Plate 49b

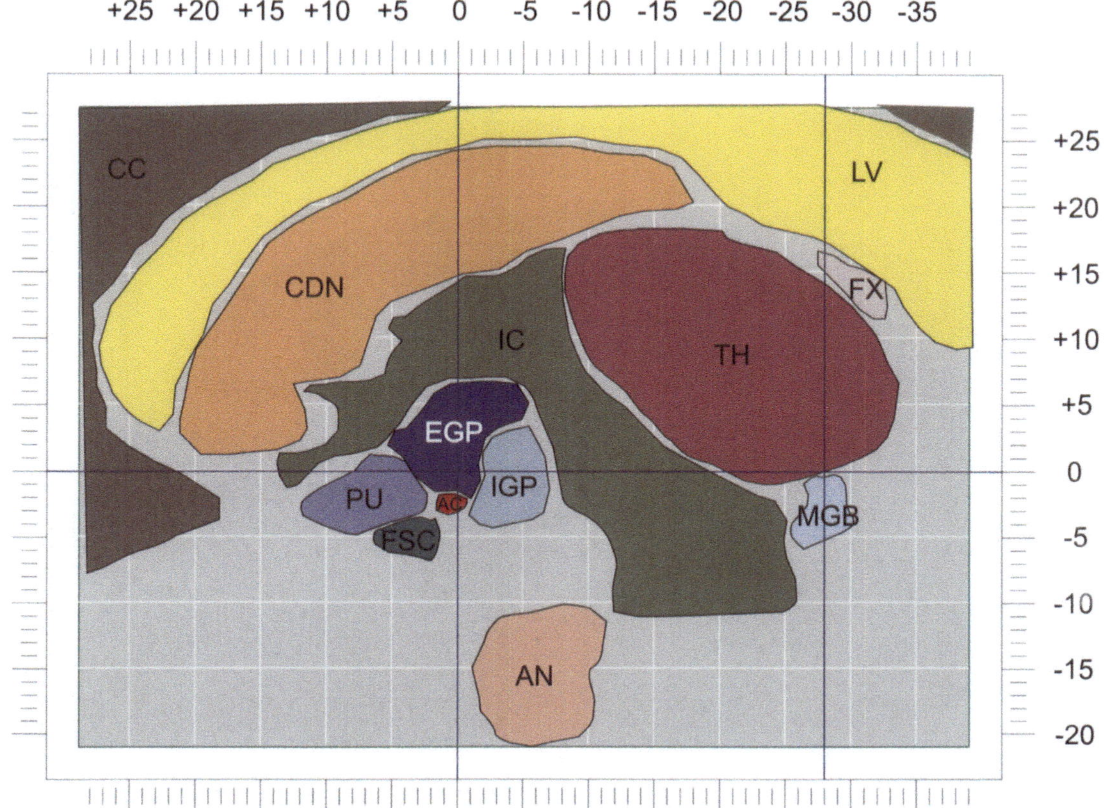


Sagittal 15 mm

## Plate 50a

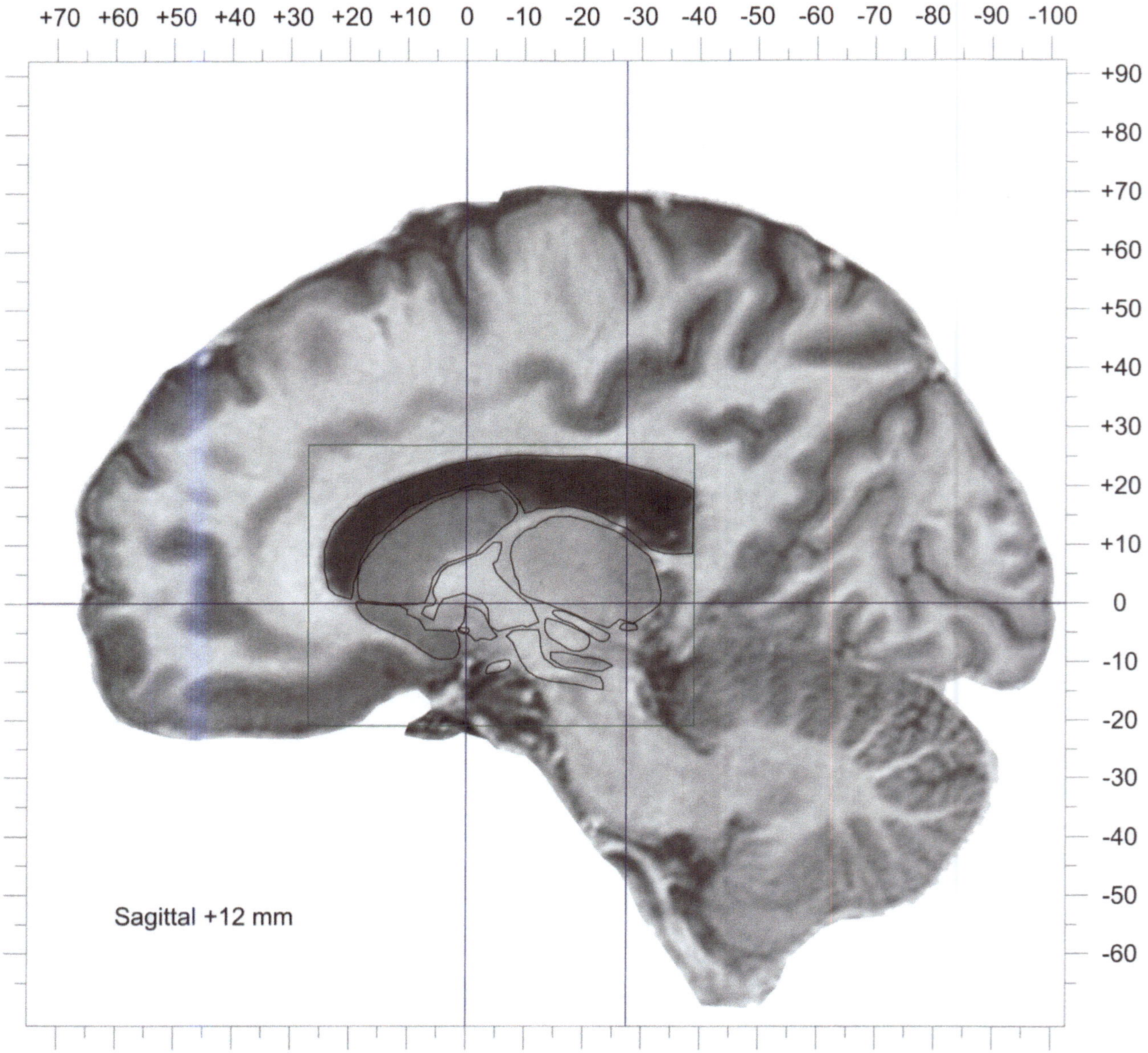

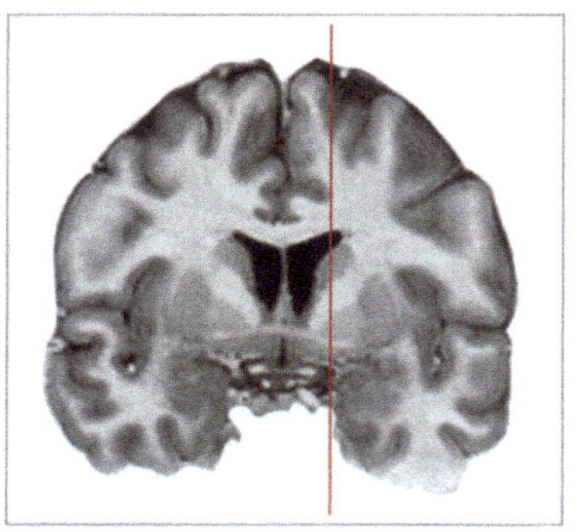

# Plate 50b

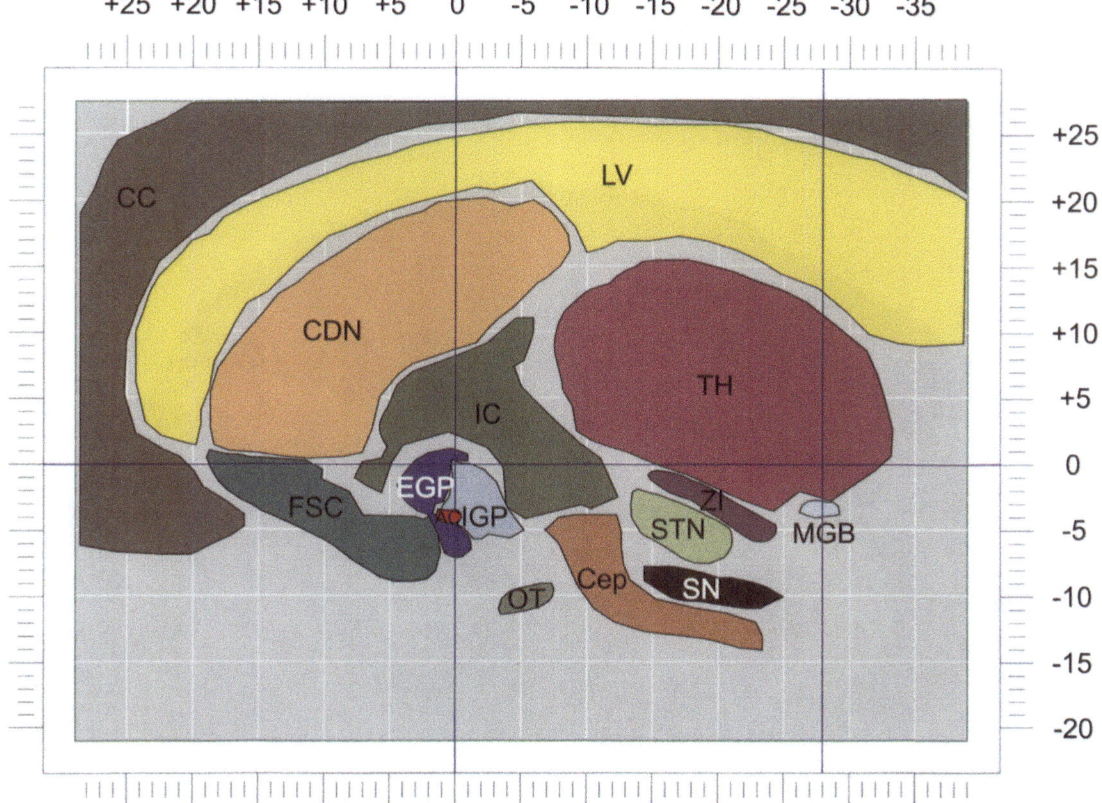


Sagittal 12 mm

# Plate 51a

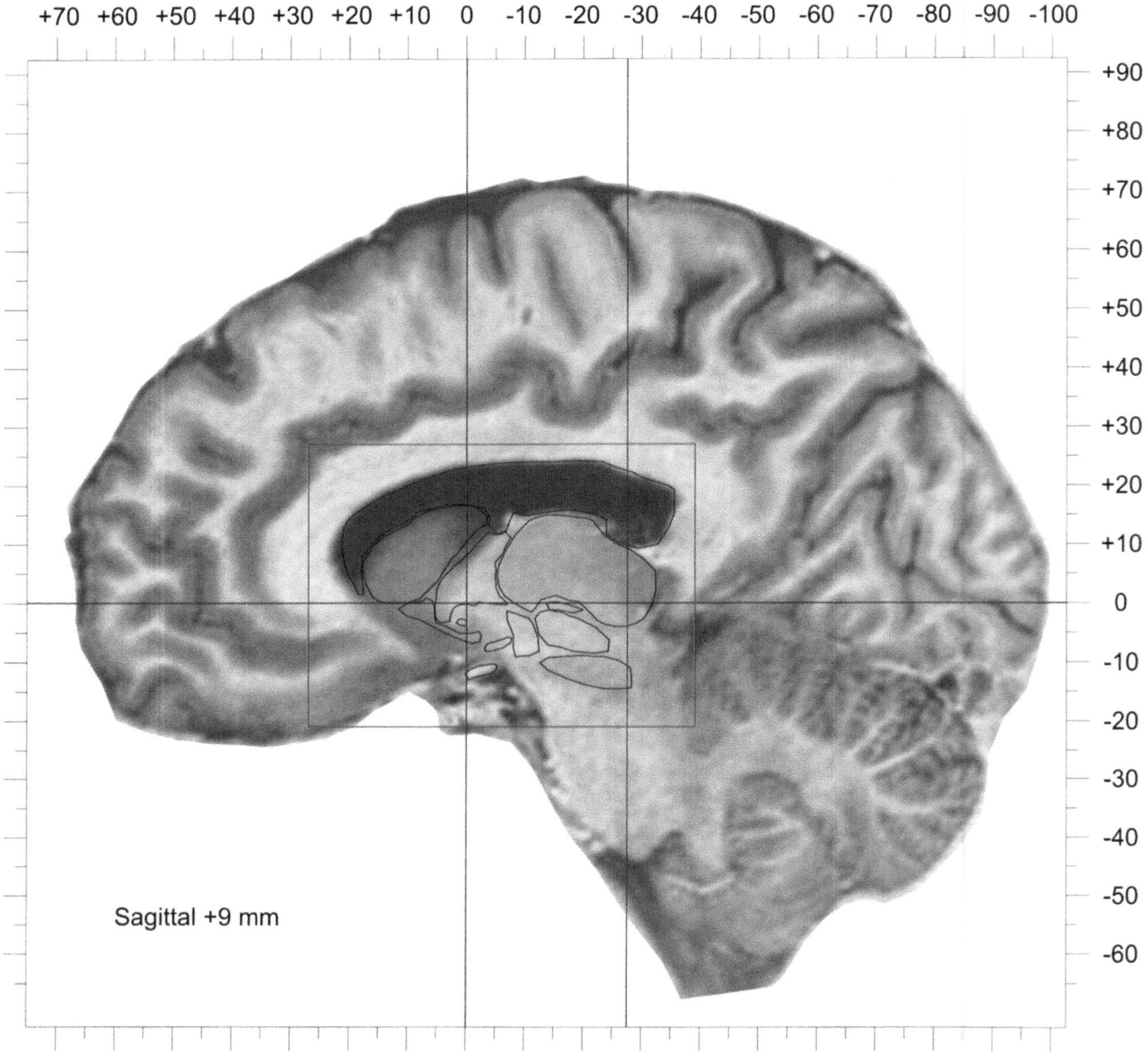

+70  +60  +50  +40  +30  +20  +10   0   -10  -20  -30  -40  -50  -60  -70  -80  -90  -100

+90
+80
+70
+60
+50
+40
+30
+20
+10
0
-10
-20
-30
-40
-50
-60

Sagittal +9 mm

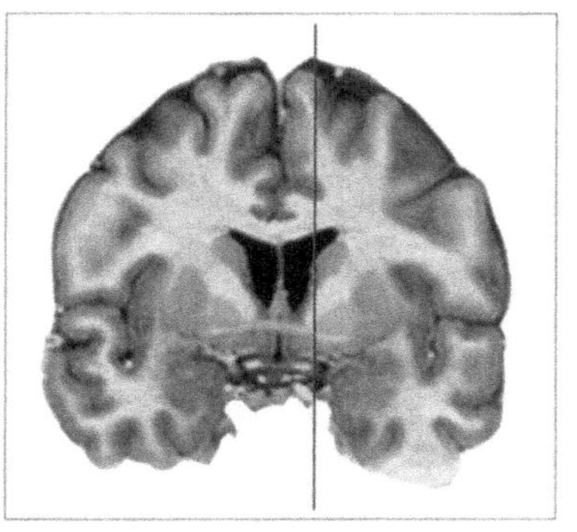

# Plate 51b

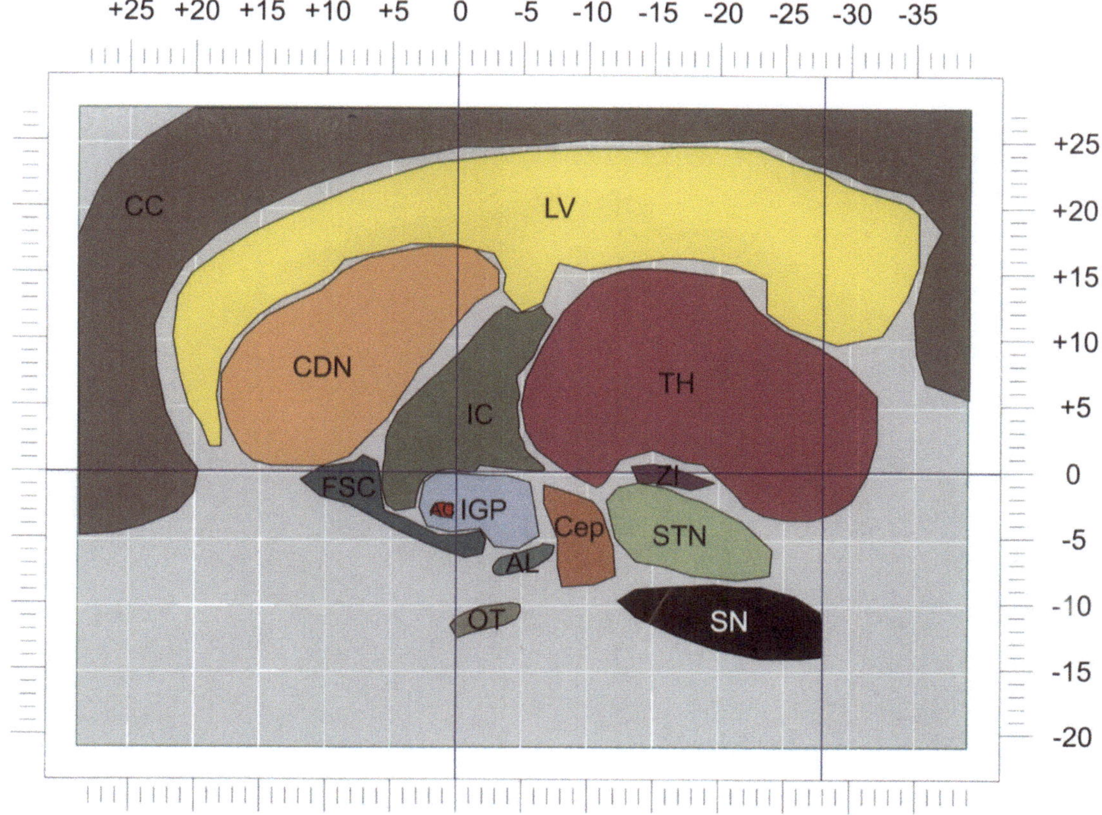


Sagittal 9 mm

## Plate 52a

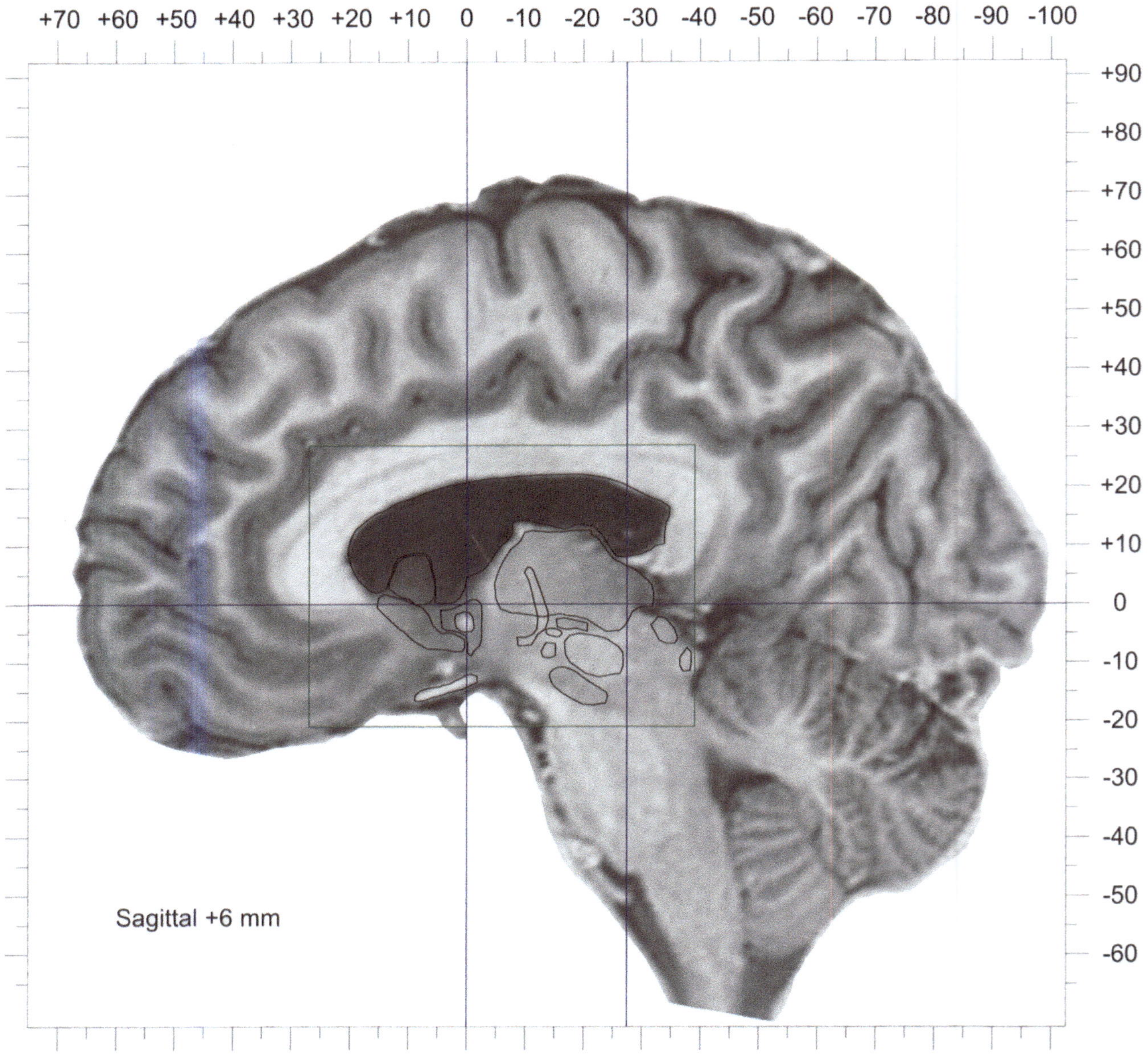

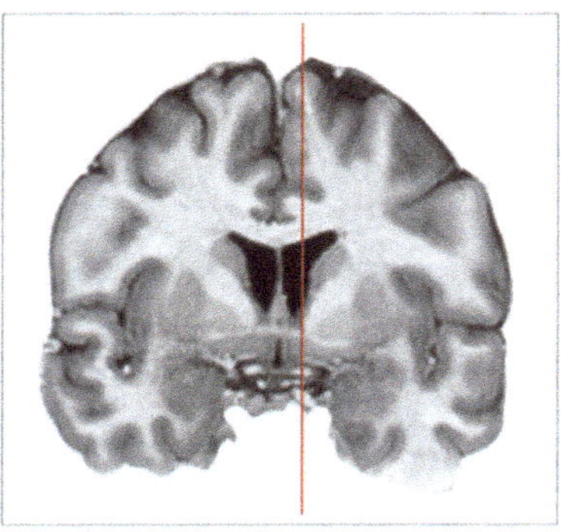

# Plate 52b

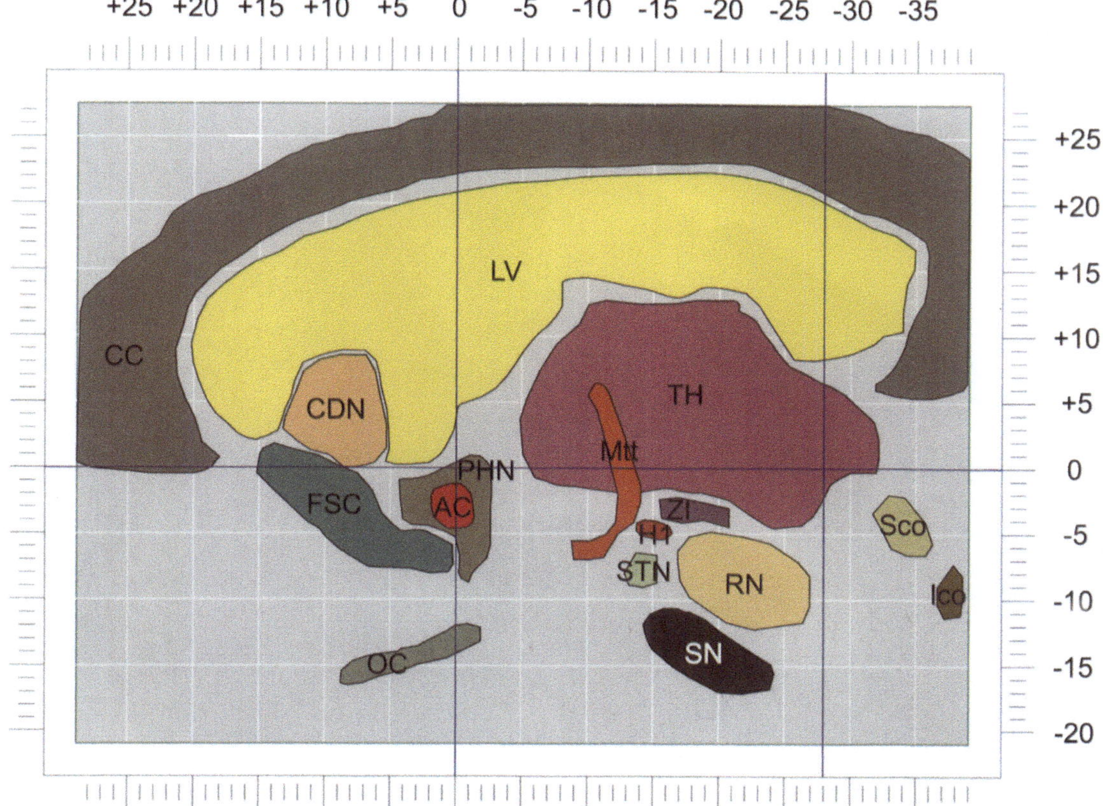


Sagittal 6 mm

# Plate 53a

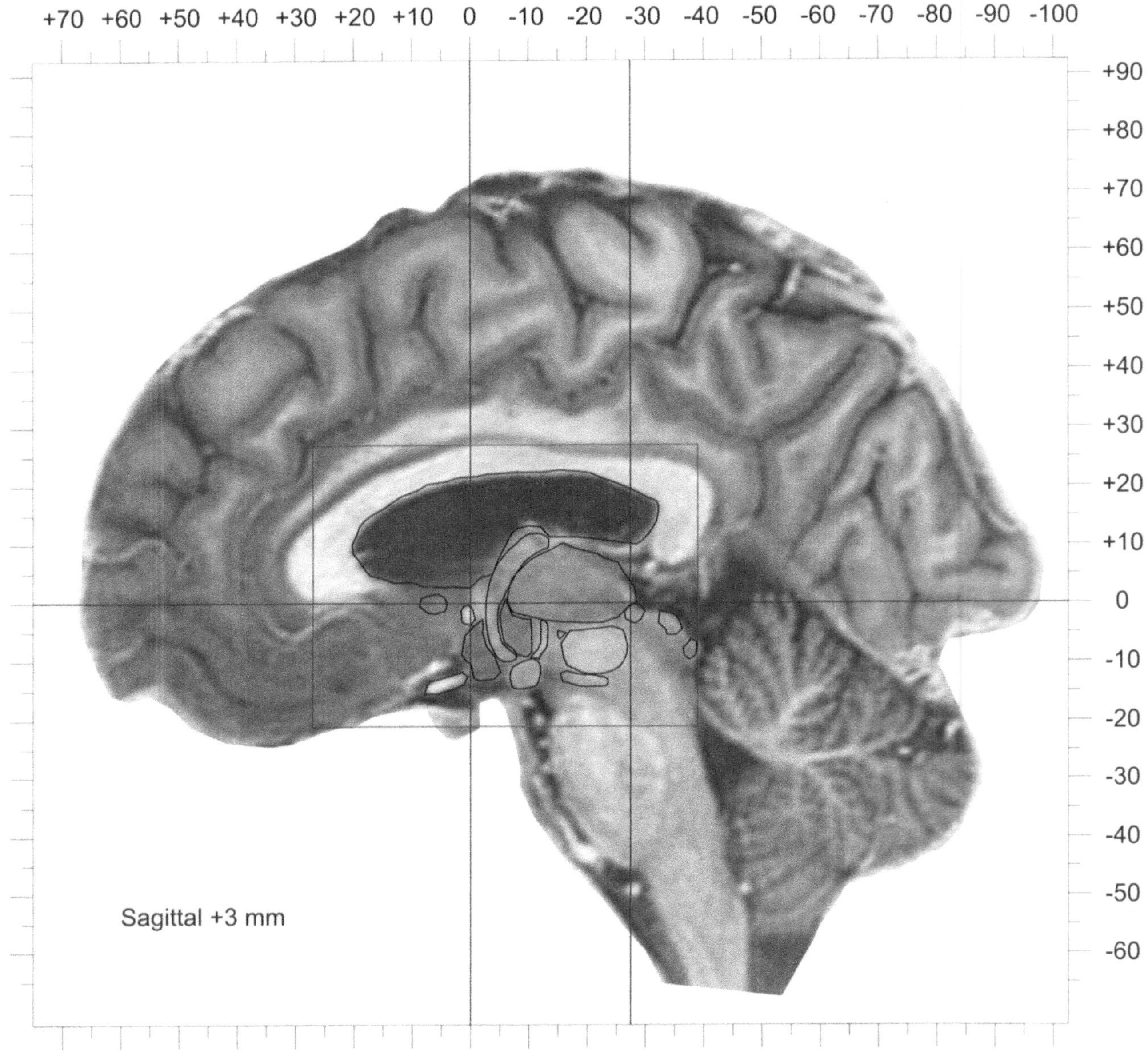

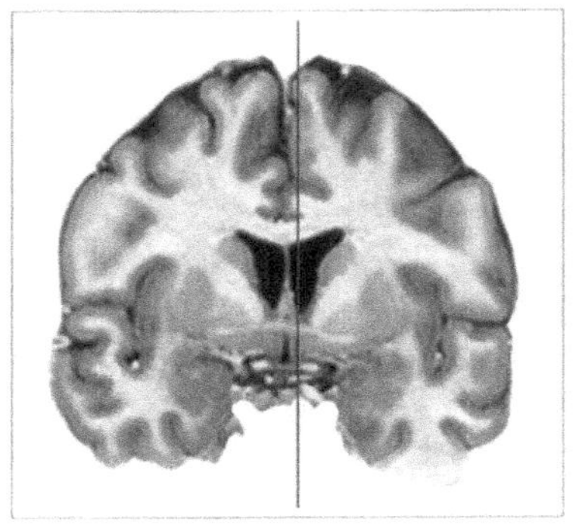

# Plate 53b

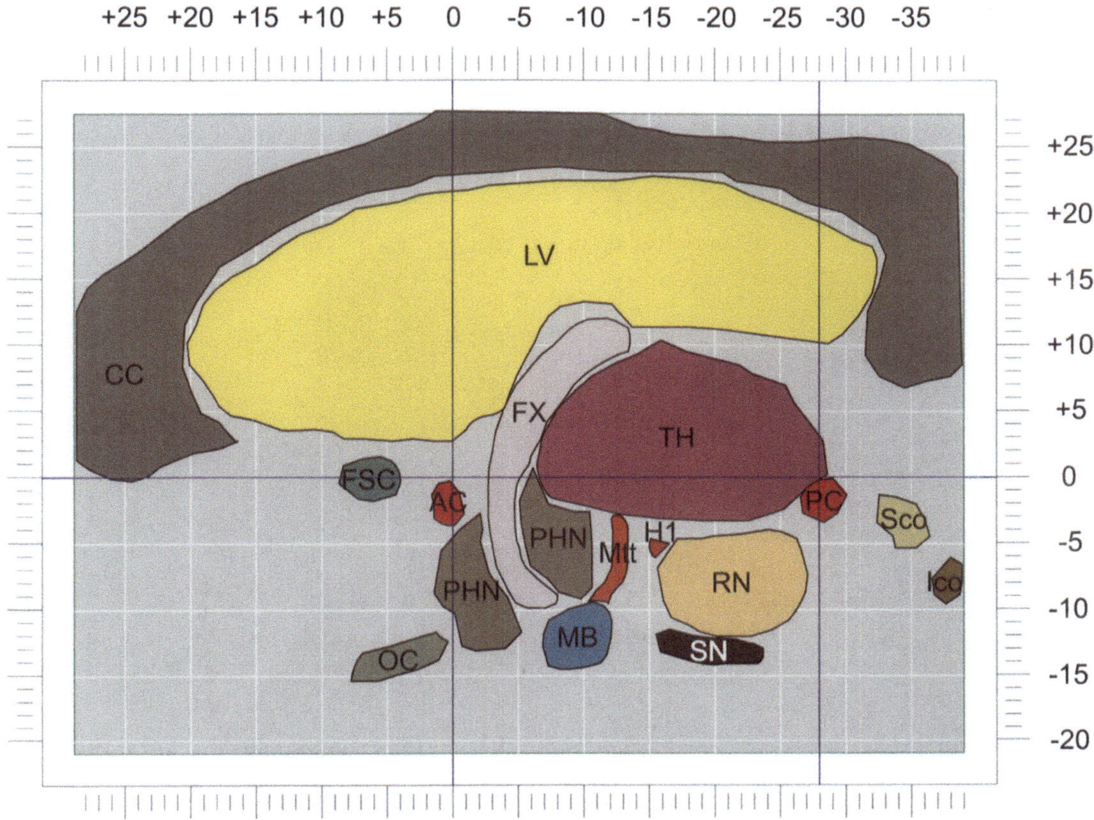


Sagittal 3 mm

# Plate 54a

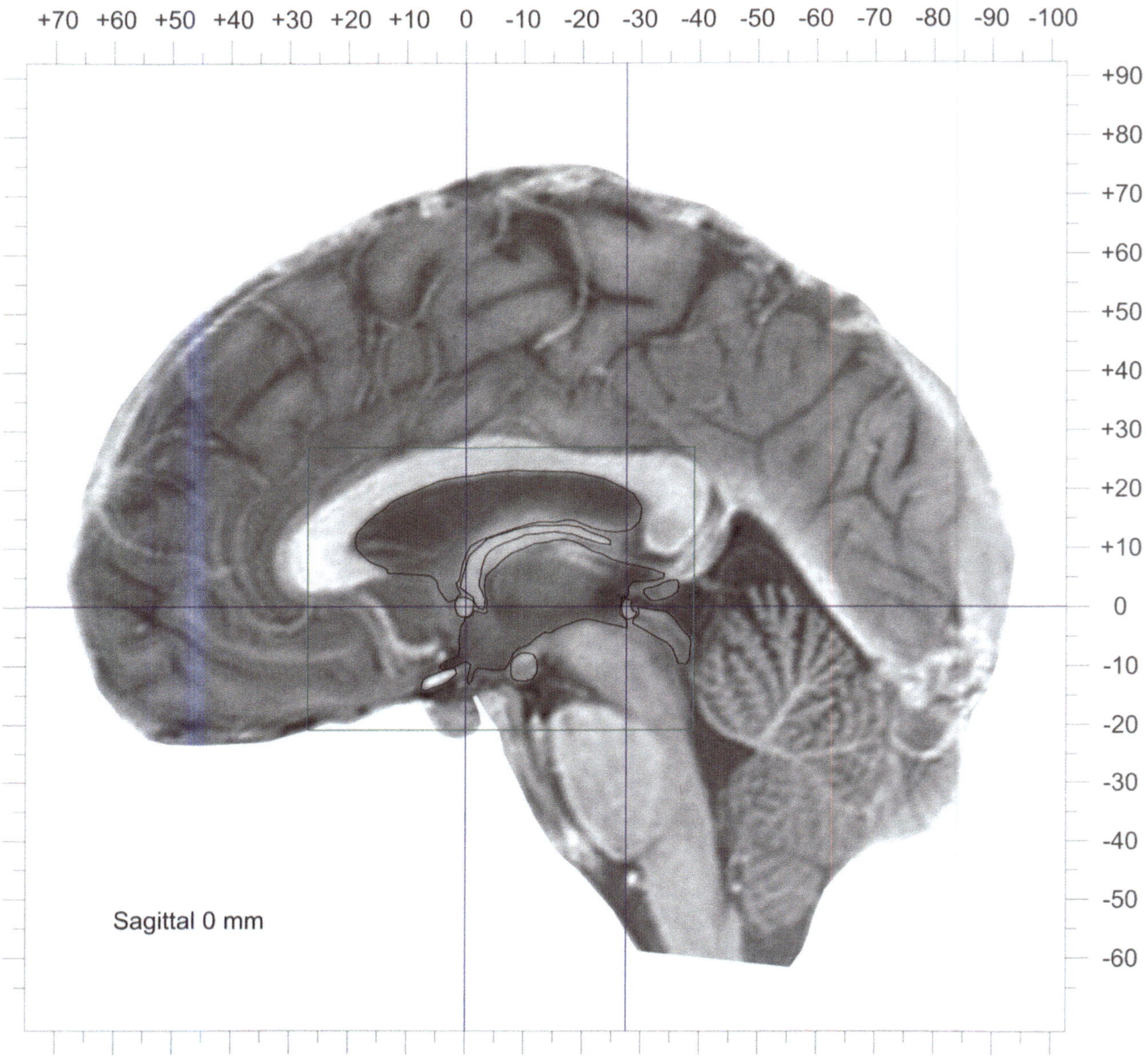

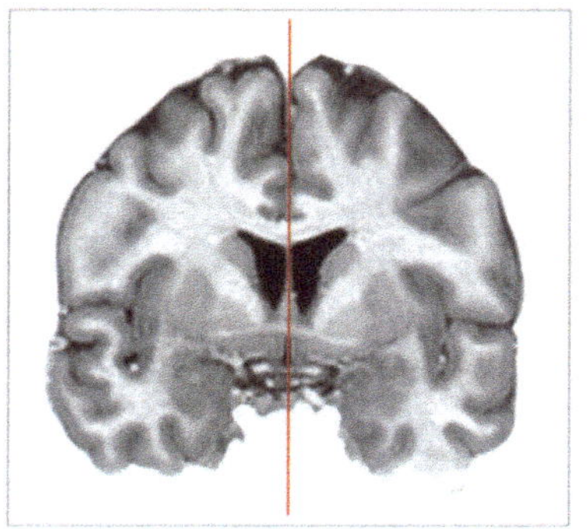


**Plate 54a**

## Plate 54b

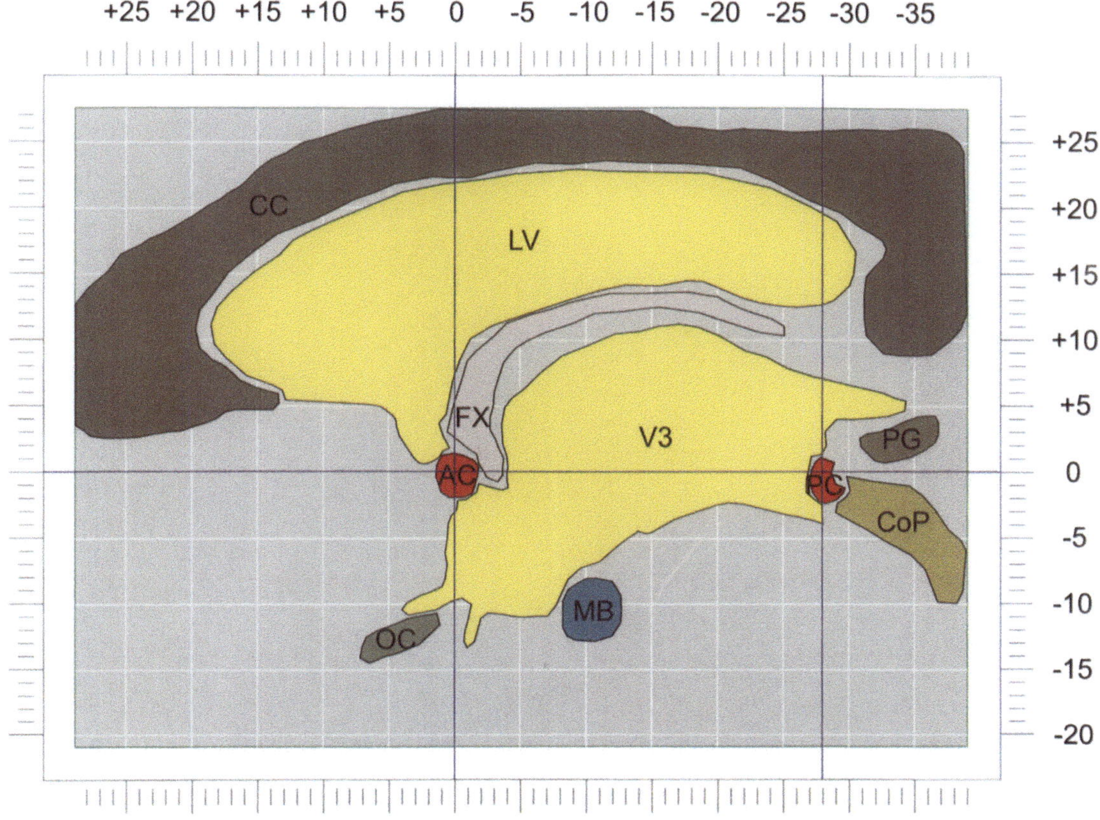


Sagittal 0 mm

# 3D Reconstructions

Combination of All Structures

Putamen, Globus Pallidus Medialis and Lateralis,
Ansa Lenticularis

Caudate Nucleus, Putamen,
Globus Pallidus Medialis and Lateralis, Ansa Lenticularis

The Thalamic Region

The Amygdala, Fornix and Periventricular Regions

# Abbreviation – Nomenclature – Color Codes

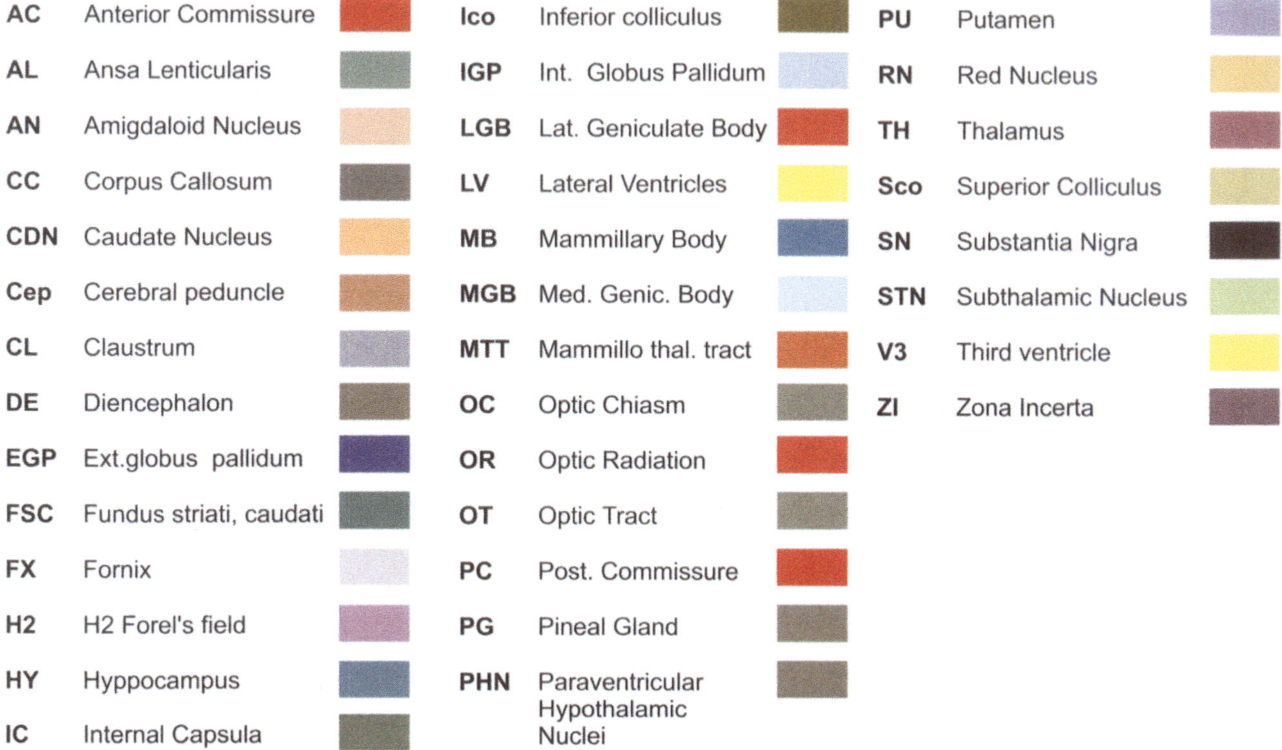

| | | | | | | | | |
|---|---|---|---|---|---|---|---|---|
| **AC** | Anterior Commissure | | **Ico** | Inferior colliculus | | **PU** | Putamen | |
| **AL** | Ansa Lenticularis | | **IGP** | Int. Globus Pallidum | | **RN** | Red Nucleus | |
| **AN** | Amigdaloid Nucleus | | **LGB** | Lat. Geniculate Body | | **TH** | Thalamus | |
| **CC** | Corpus Callosum | | **LV** | Lateral Ventricles | | **Sco** | Superior Colliculus | |
| **CDN** | Caudate Nucleus | | **MB** | Mammillary Body | | **SN** | Substantia Nigra | |
| **Cep** | Cerebral peduncle | | **MGB** | Med. Genic. Body | | **STN** | Subthalamic Nucleus | |
| **CL** | Claustrum | | **MTT** | Mammillo thal. tract | | **V3** | Third ventricle | |
| **DE** | Diencephalon | | **OC** | Optic Chiasm | | **ZI** | Zona Incerta | |
| **EGP** | Ext.globus pallidum | | **OR** | Optic Radiation | | | | |
| **FSC** | Fundus striati, caudati | | **OT** | Optic Tract | | | | |
| **FX** | Fornix | | **PC** | Post. Commissure | | | | |
| **H2** | H2 Forel's field | | **PG** | Pineal Gland | | | | |
| **HY** | Hyppocampus | | **PHN** | Paraventricular Hypothalamic Nuclei | | | | |
| **IC** | Internal Capsula | | | | | | | |

## Combination of All Structures

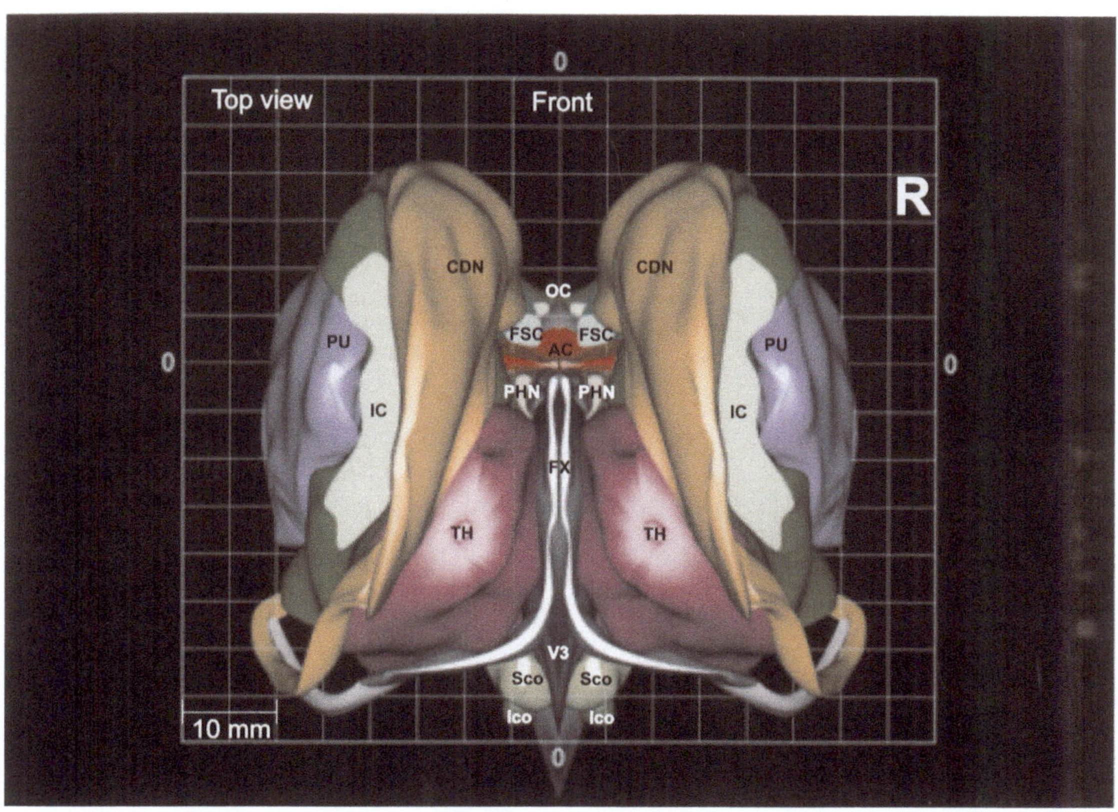


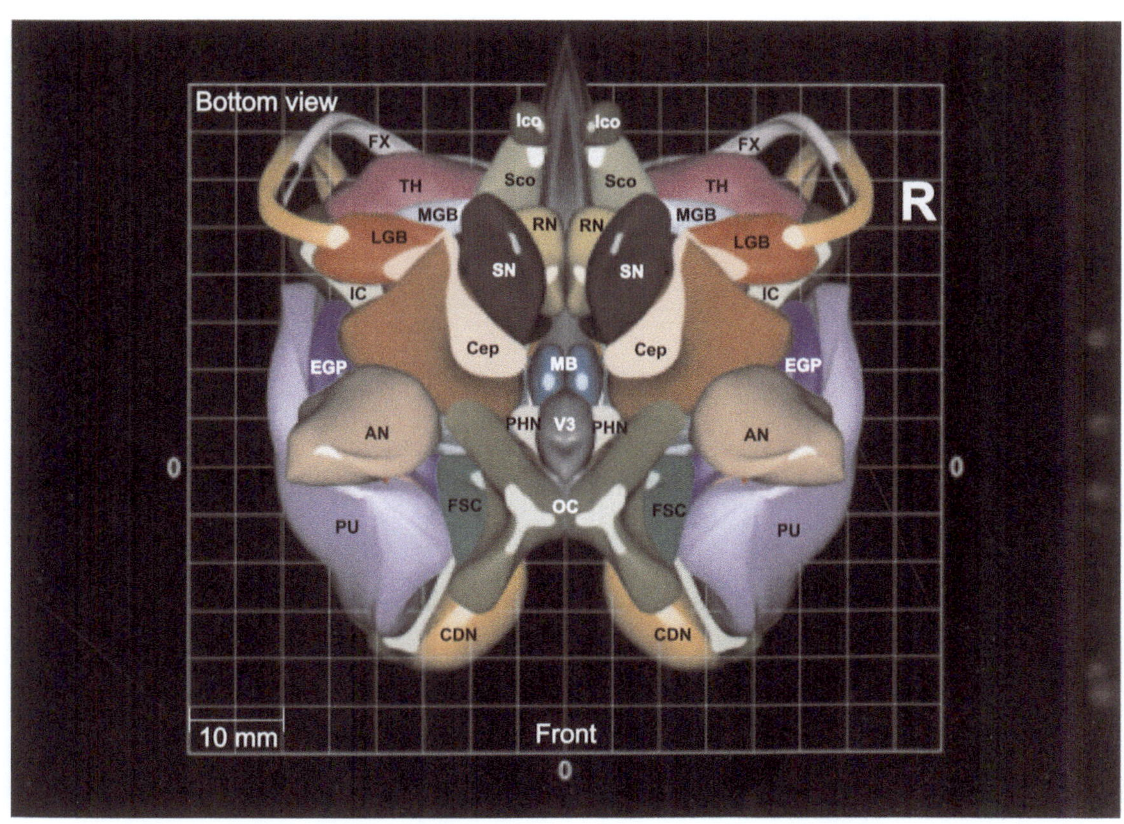

## Combination of All Structures *(continued)*

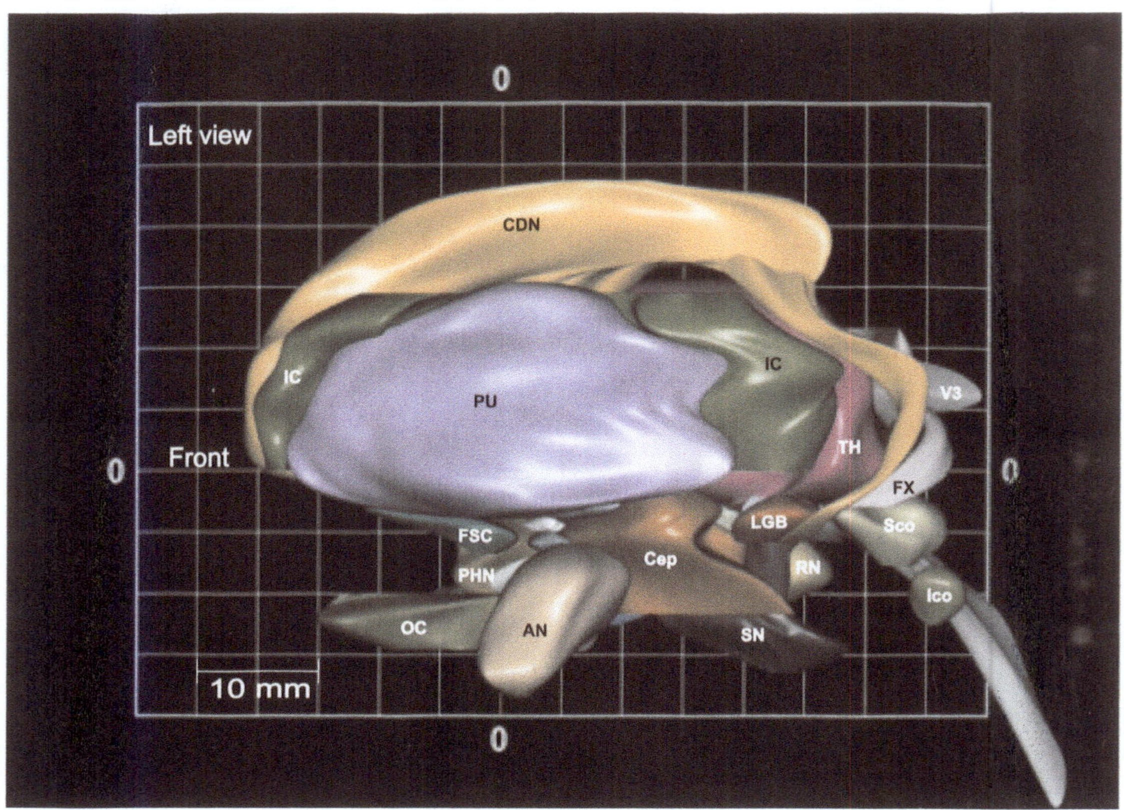


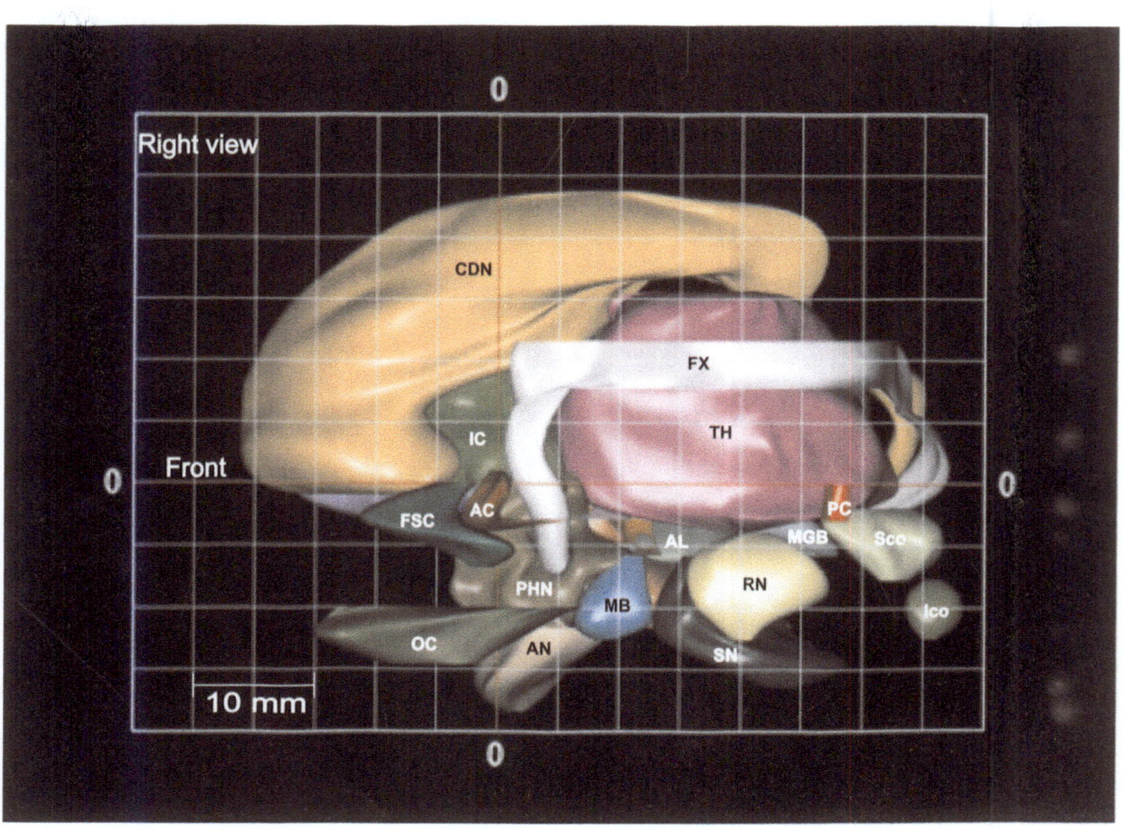

## Combination of All Structures *(continued)*

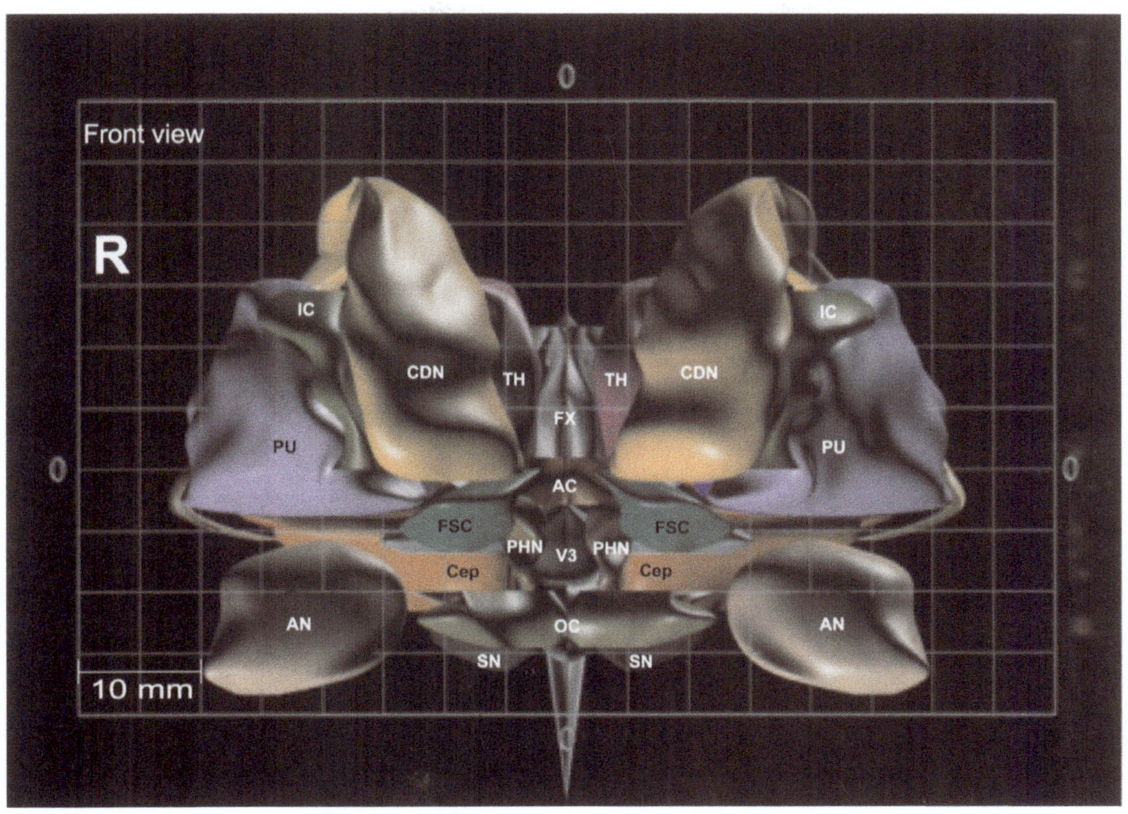


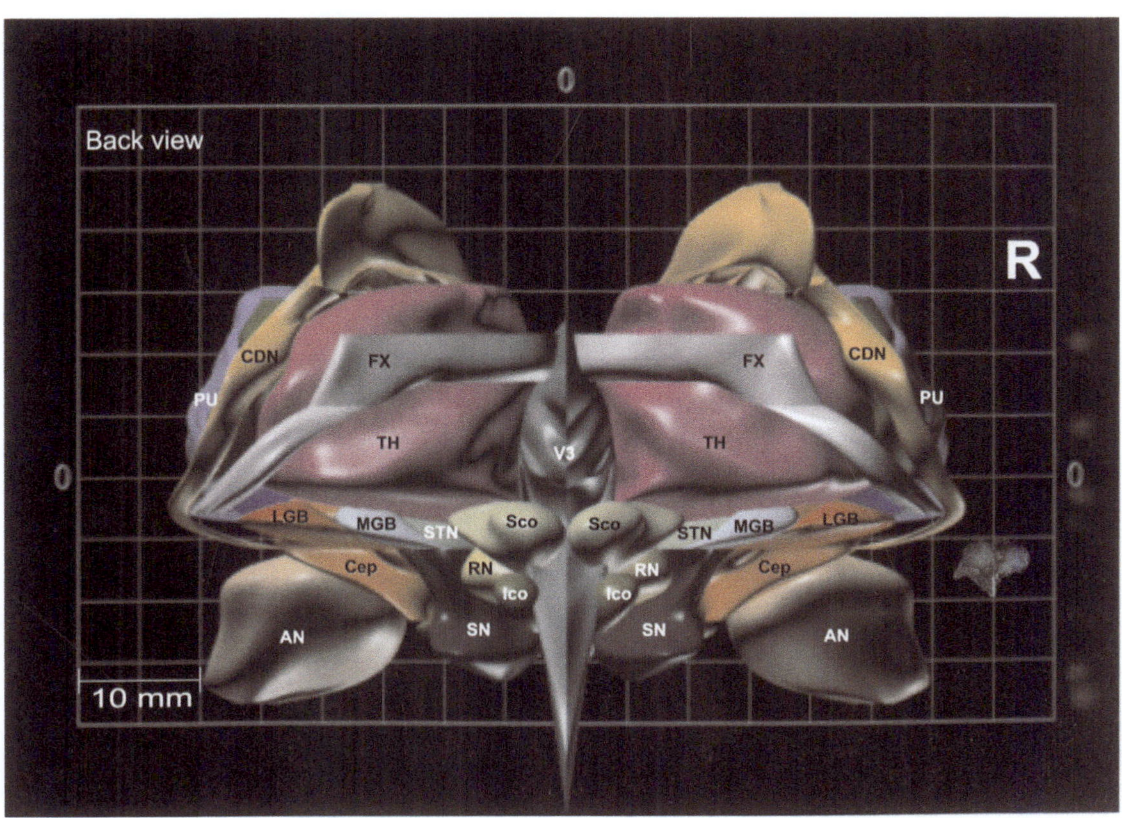

## Putamen, Globus Pallidus Medialis and Lateralis, Ansa Lenticularis

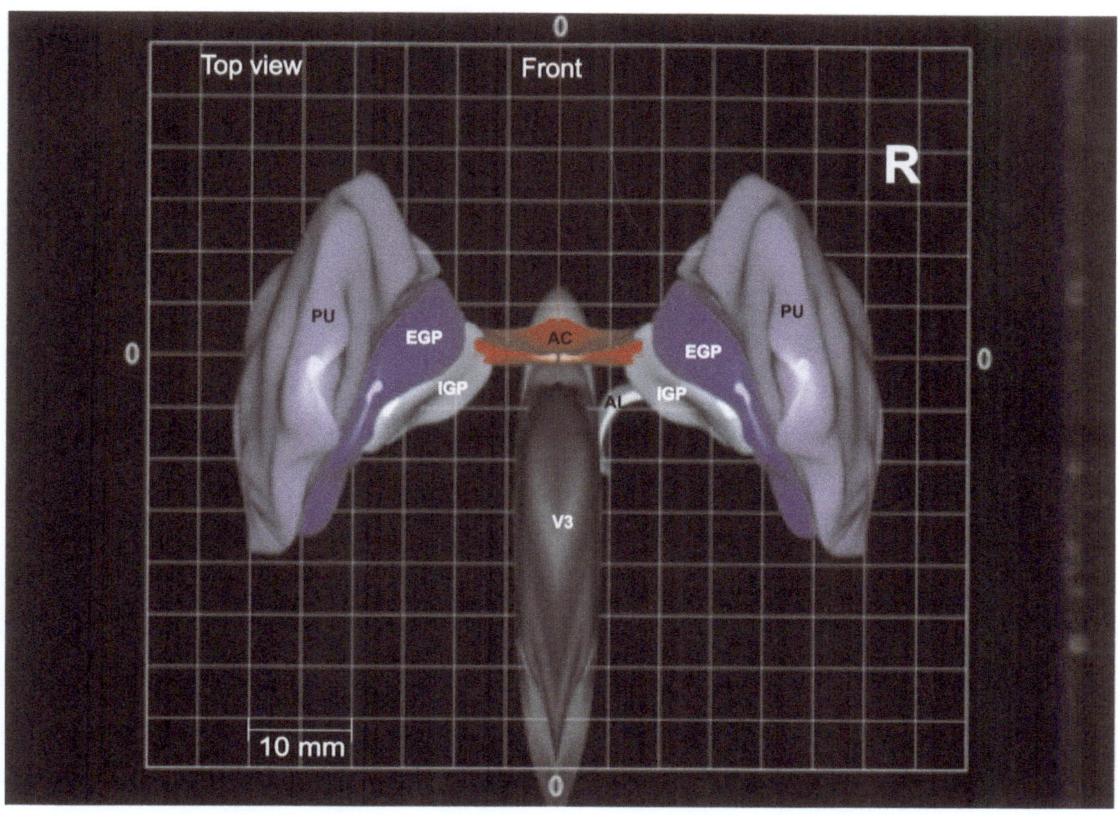


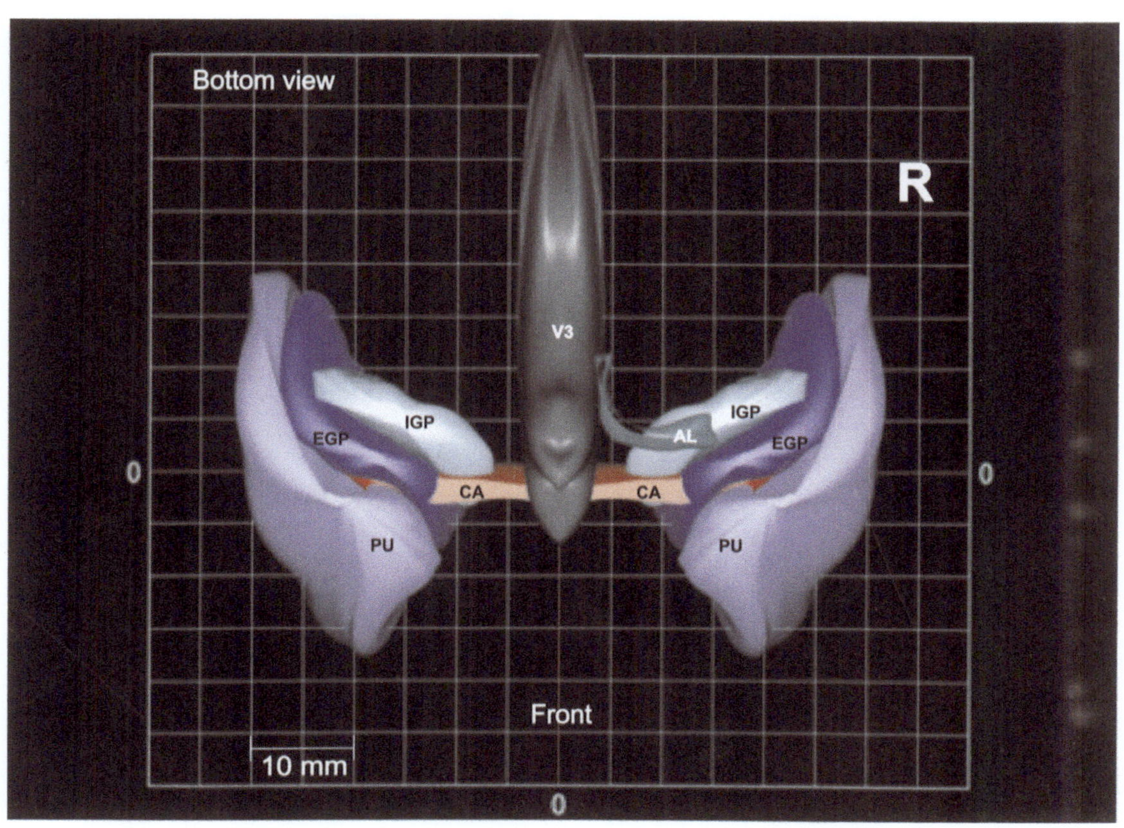

## Putamen, Globus Pallidus Medialis and Lateralis, Ansa Lenticularis *(continued)*

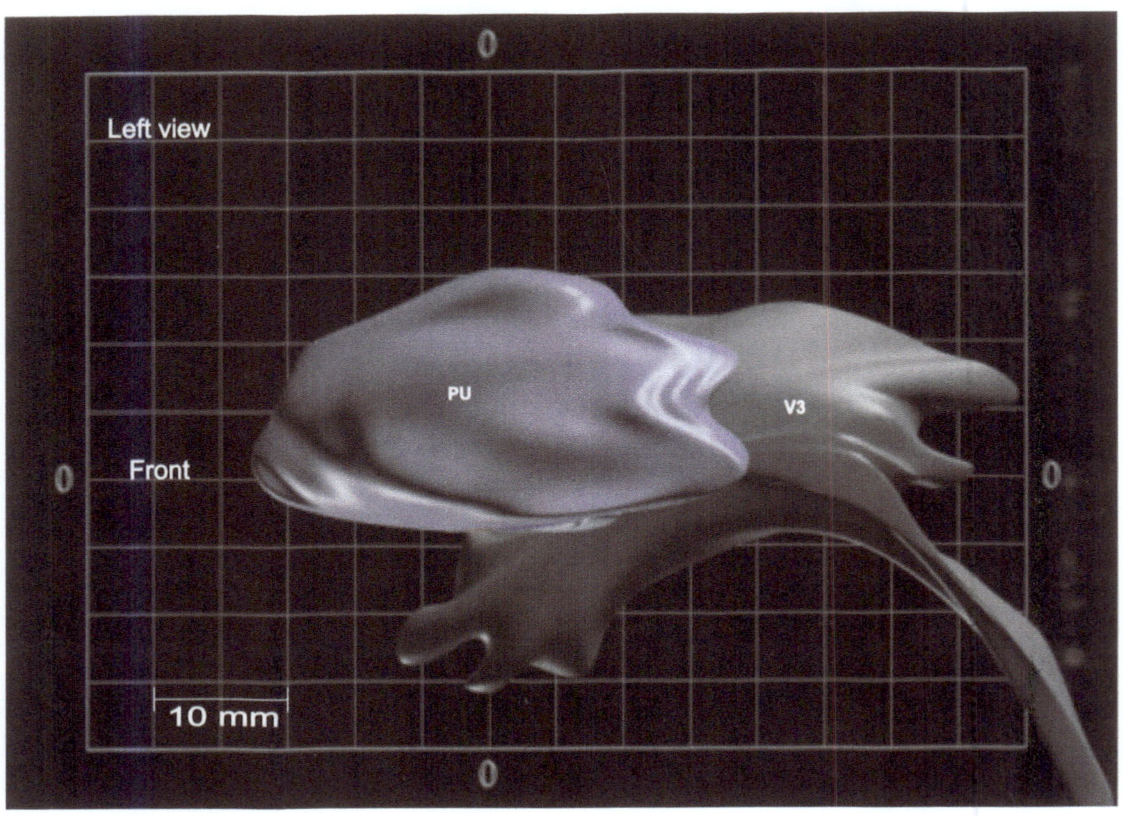


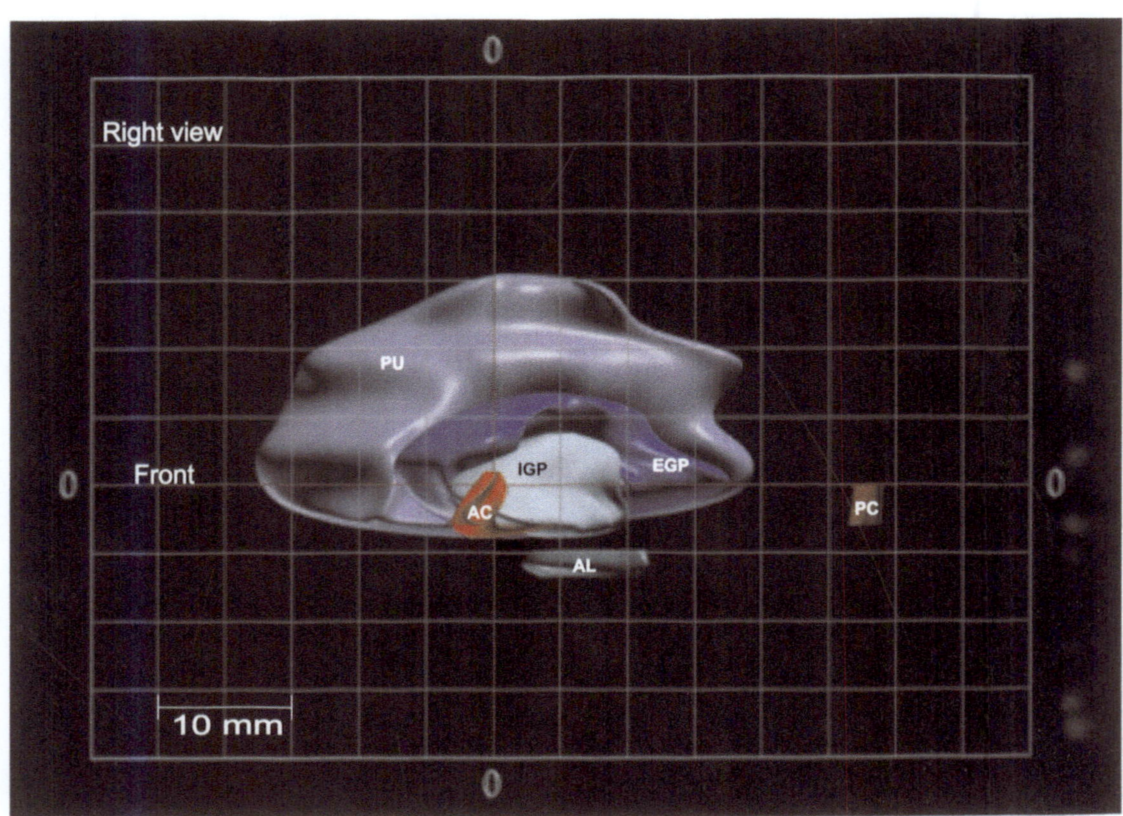

## Putamen, Globus Pallidus Medialis and Lateralis, Ansa Lenticularis *(continued)*

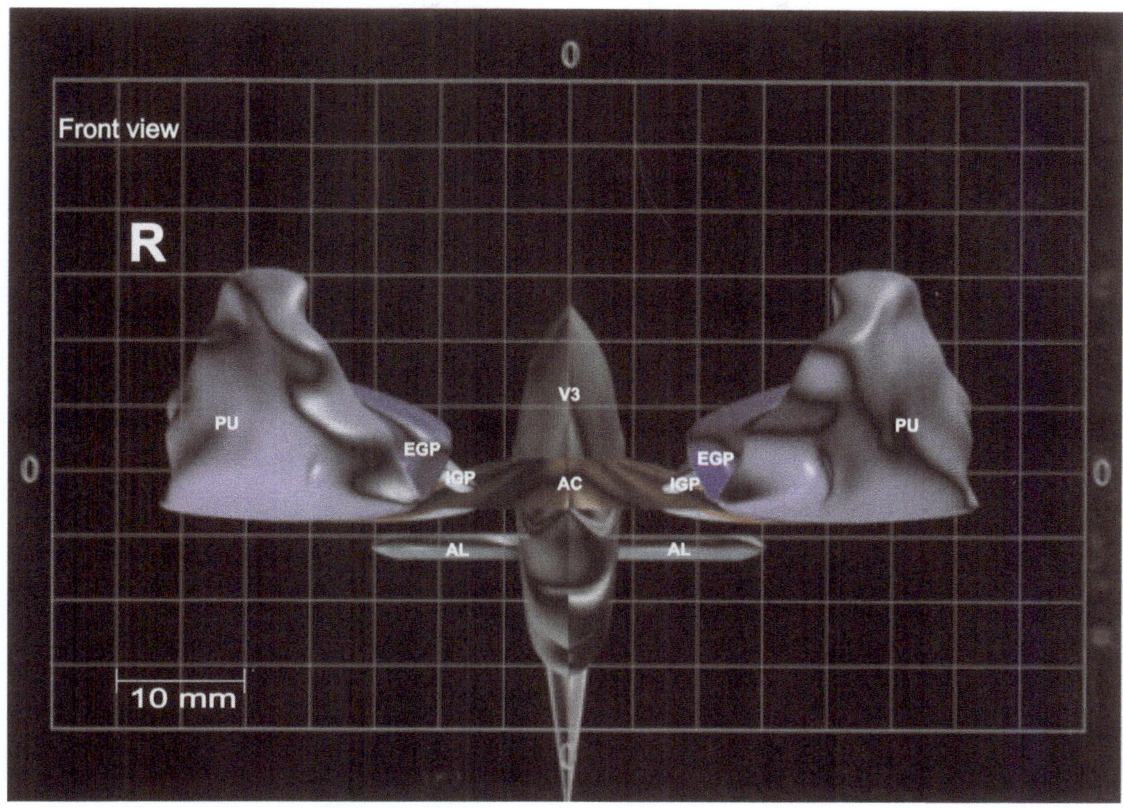


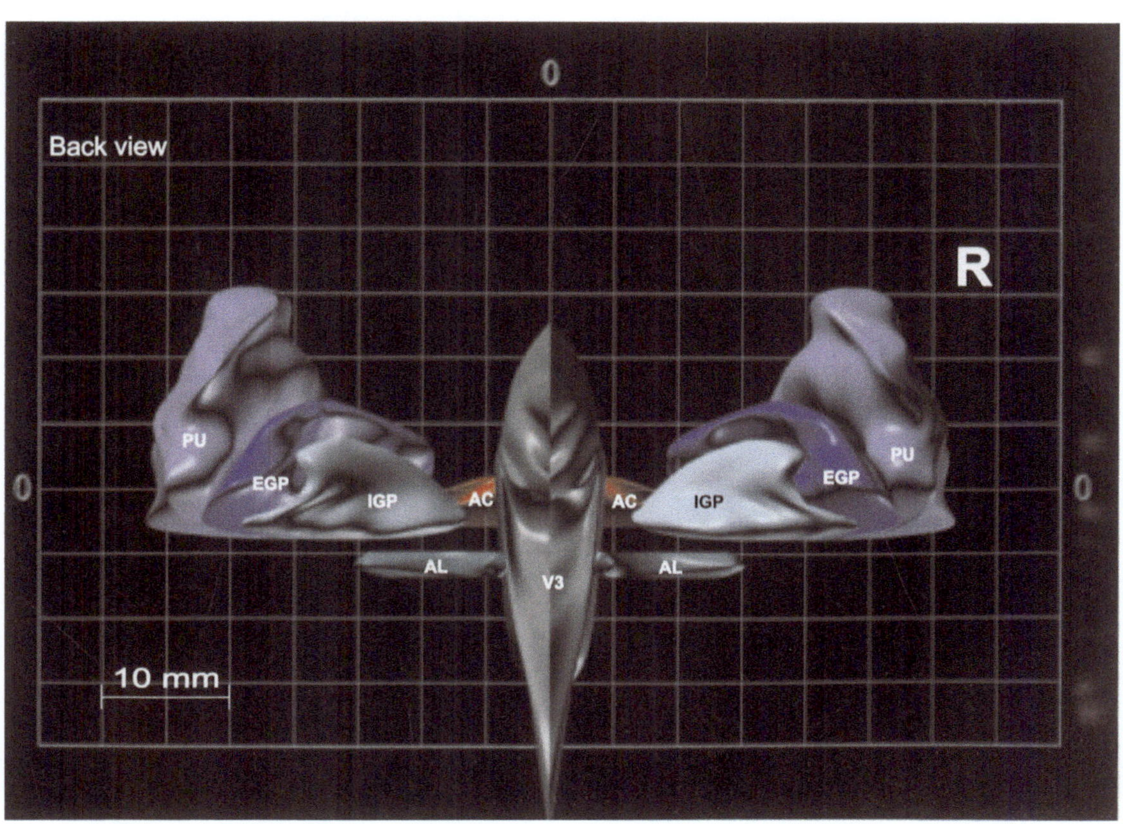

# Caudate Nucleus, Putamen, Globus Pallidus Medialis and Lateralis, Ansa Lenticularis

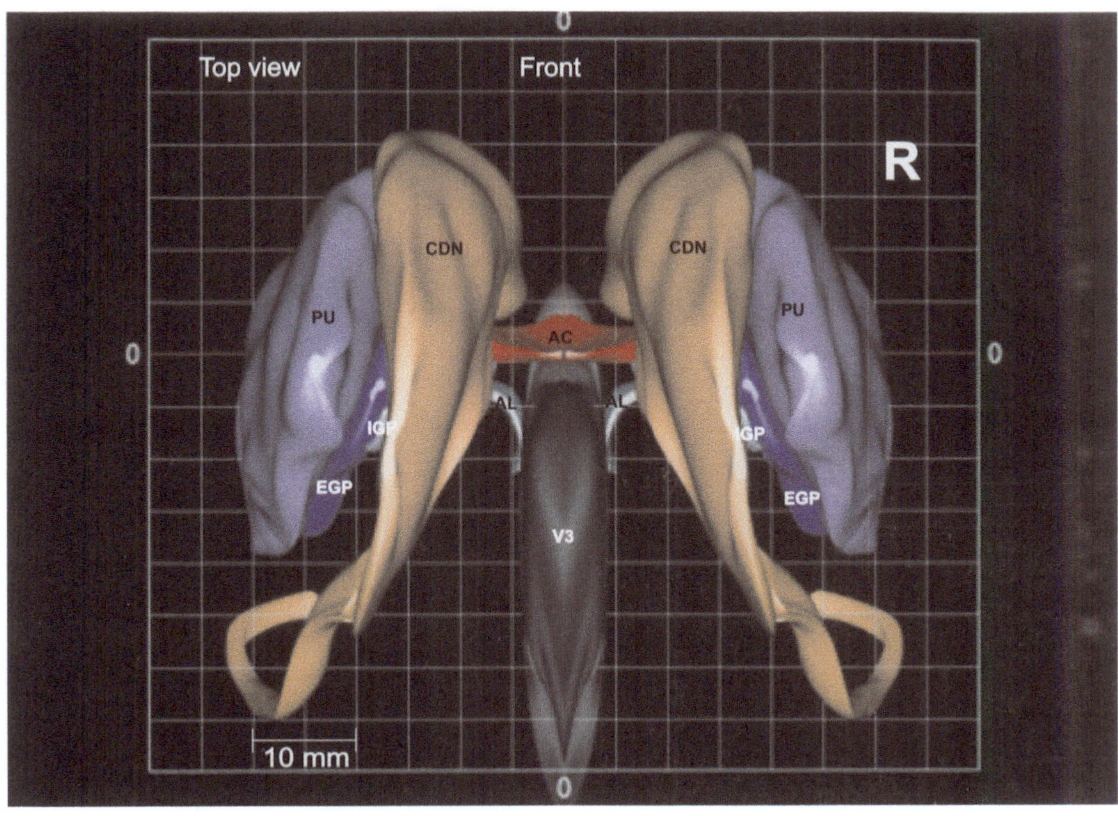


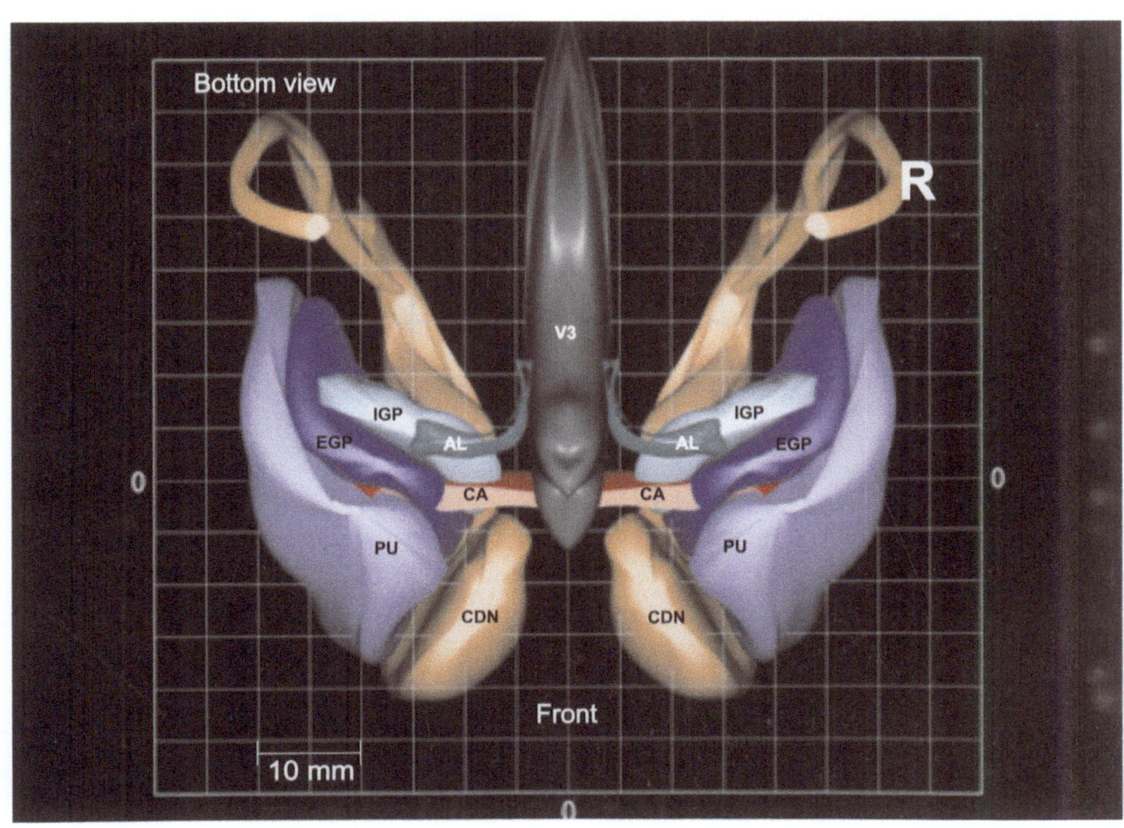

## Caudate Nucleus, Putamen, Globus Pallidus Medialis and Lateralis, Ansa Lenticularis *(continued)*

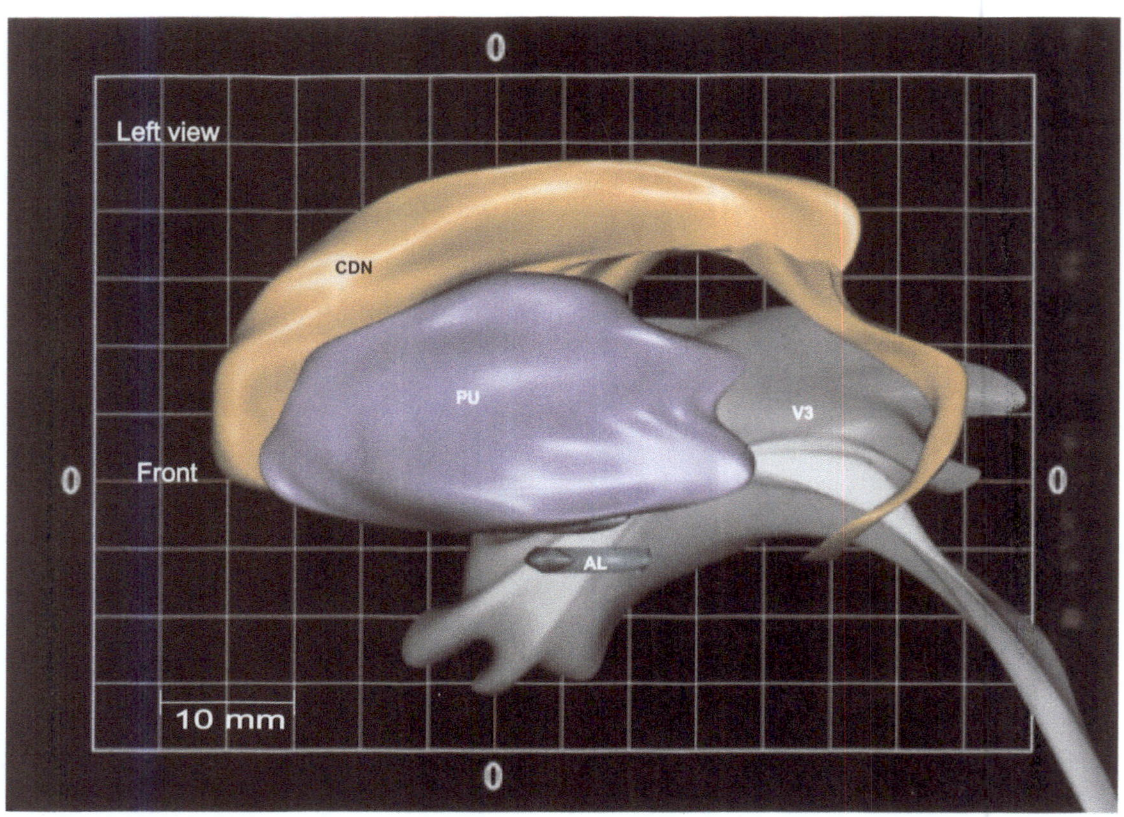


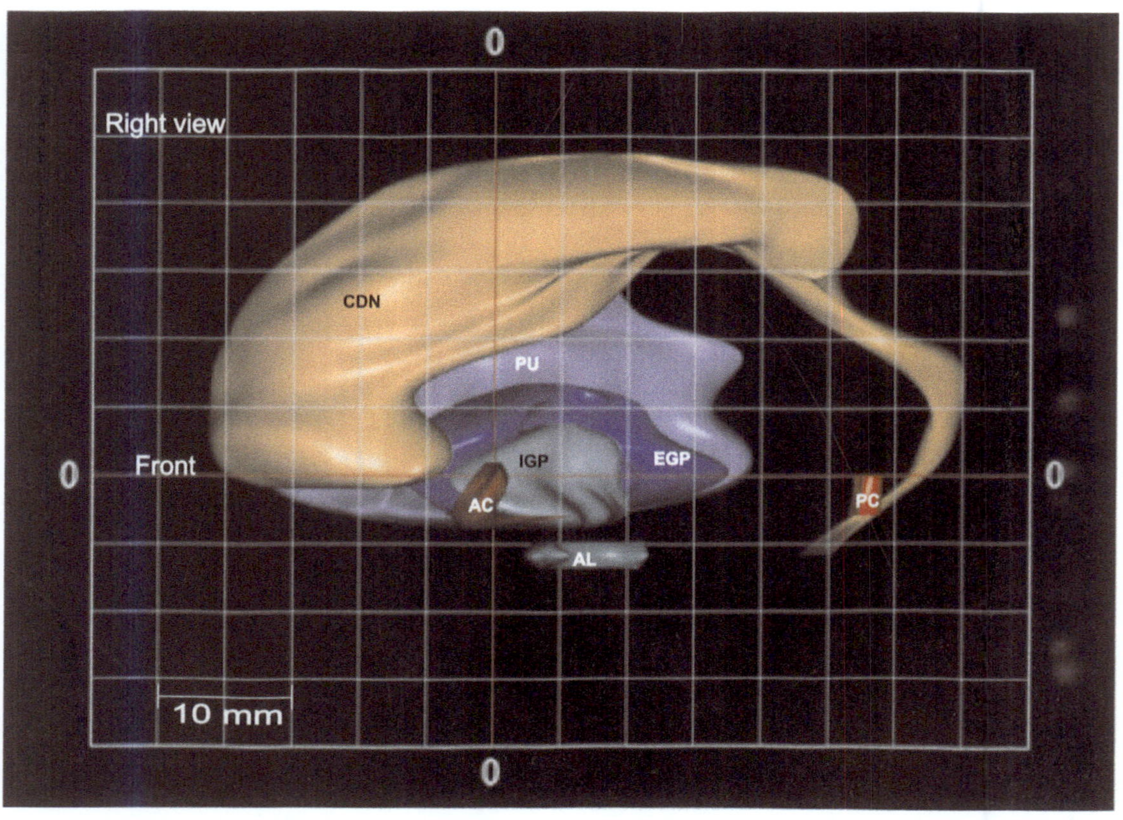

# Caudate Nucleus, Putamen, Globus Pallidus Medialis and Lateralis, Ansa Lenticularis *(continued)*

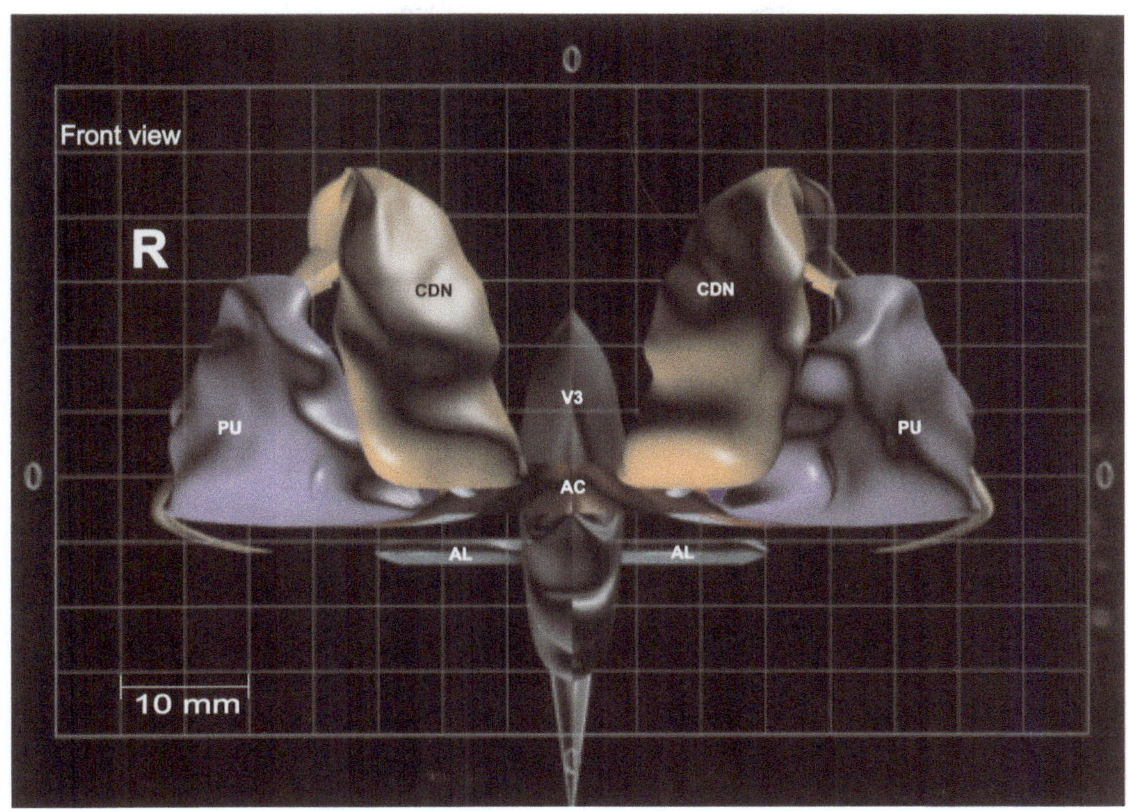


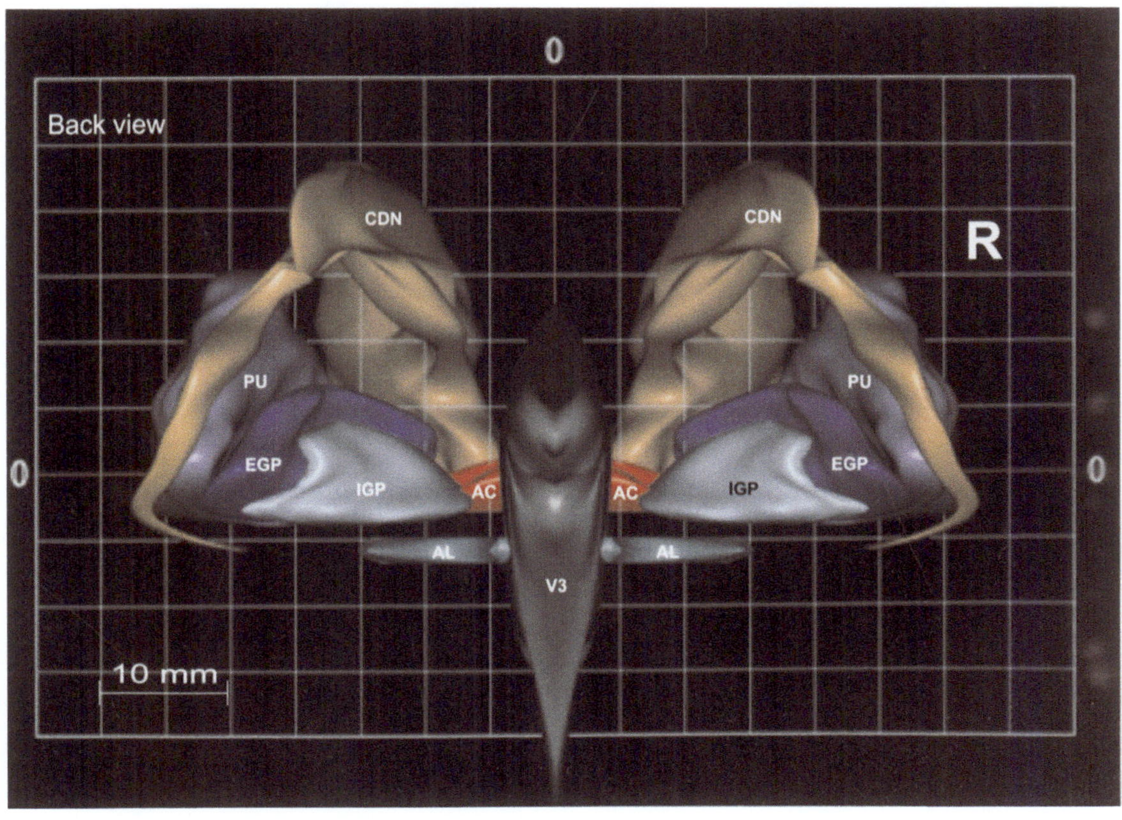

## The Thalamic Region

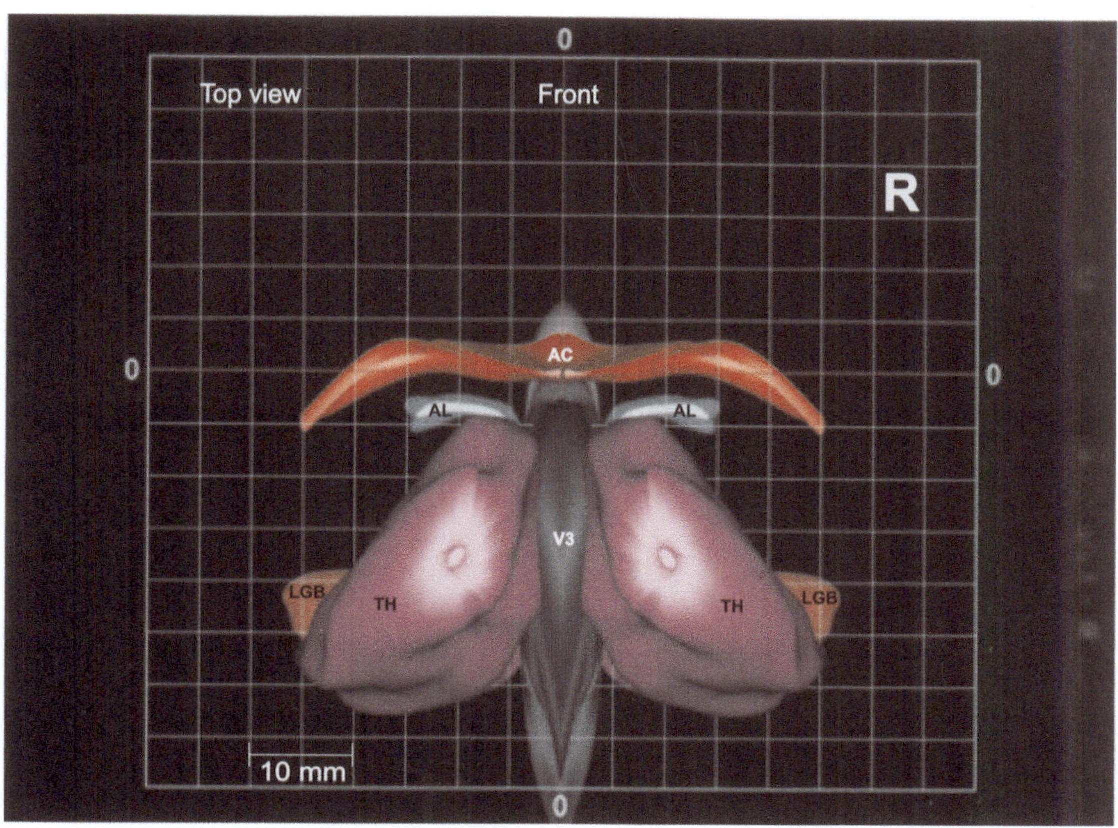


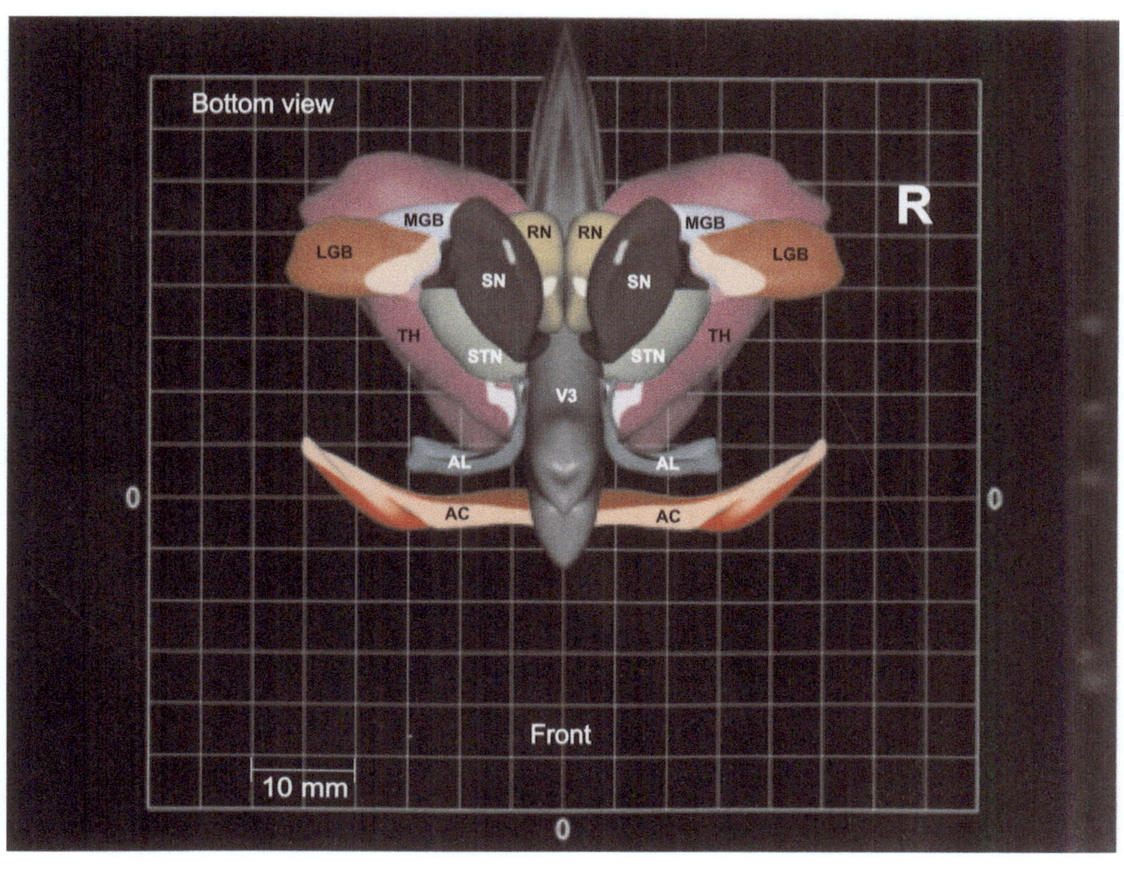

# The Thalamic Region *(continued)*

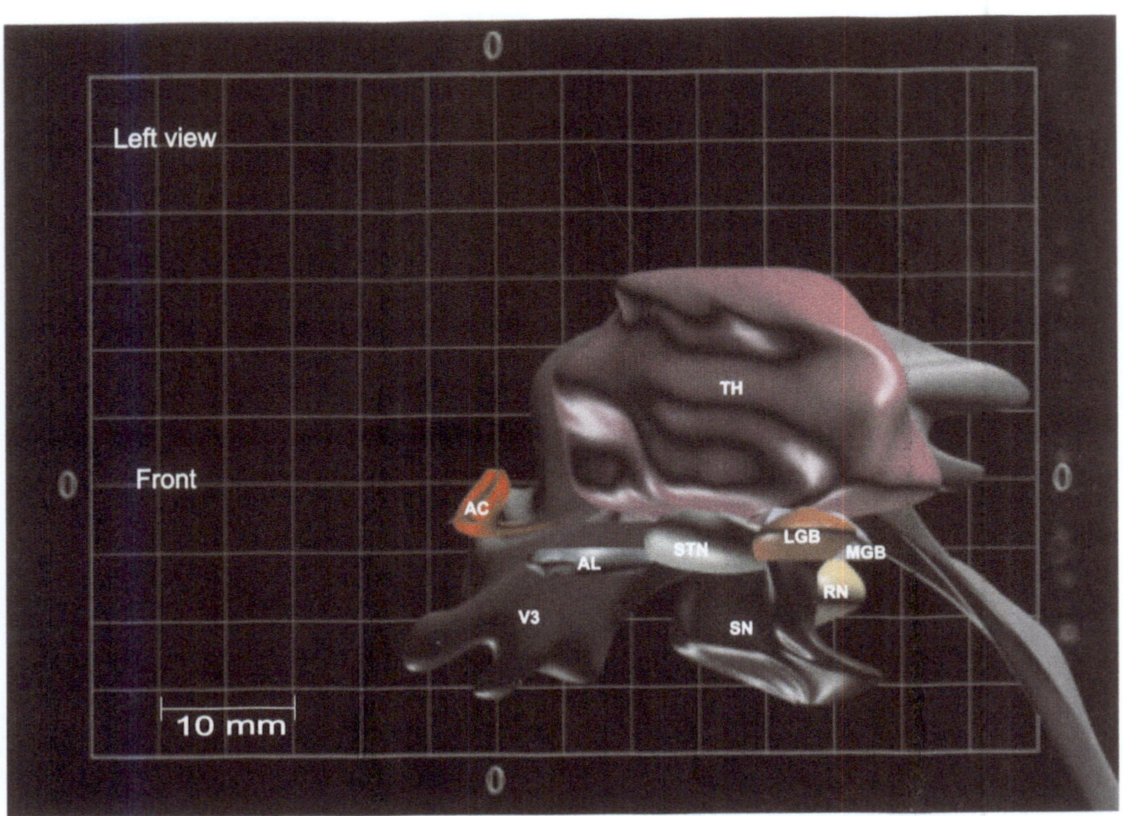


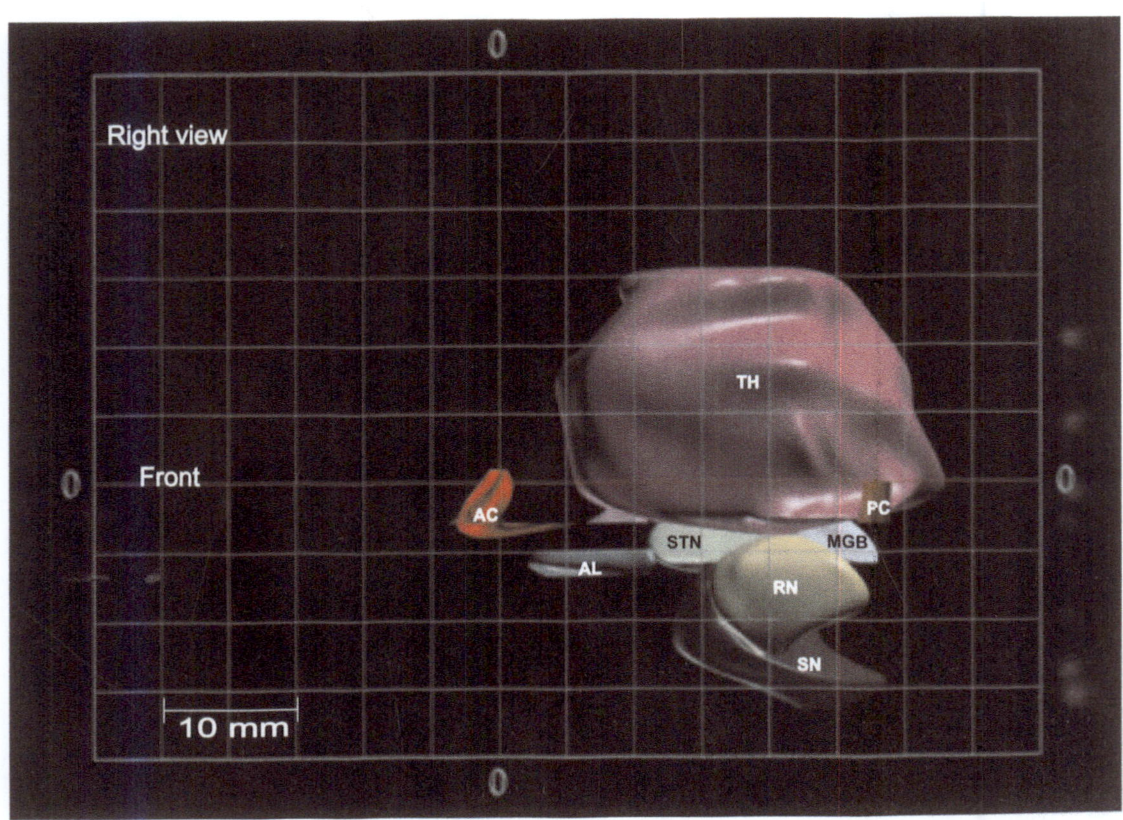

## The Thalamic Region *(continued)*

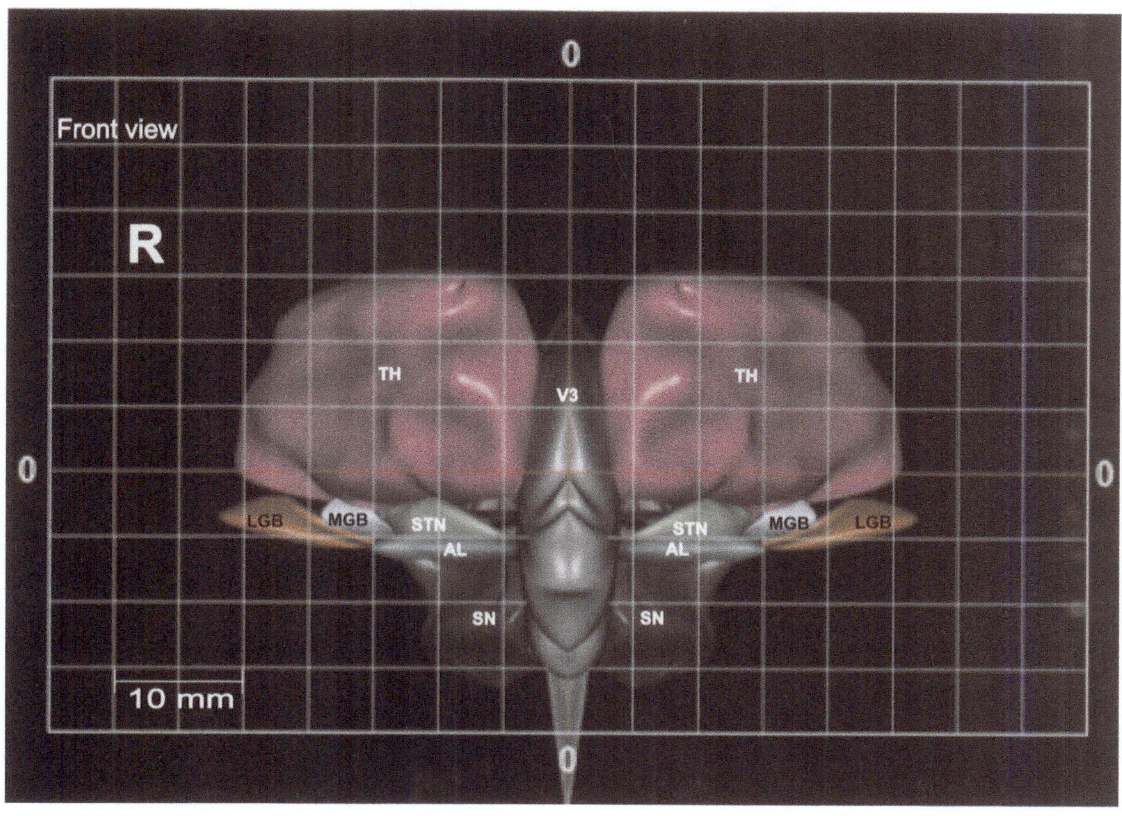


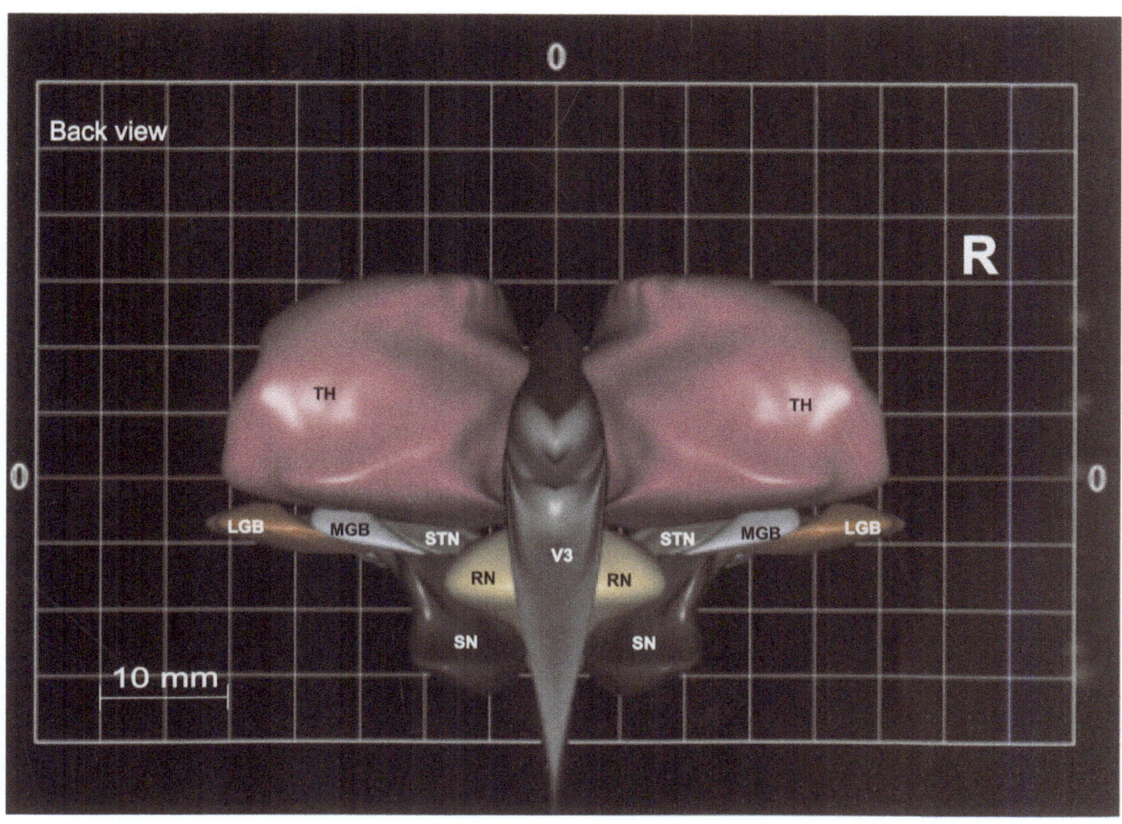

## The Amygdala, Fornix and Periventricular Regions

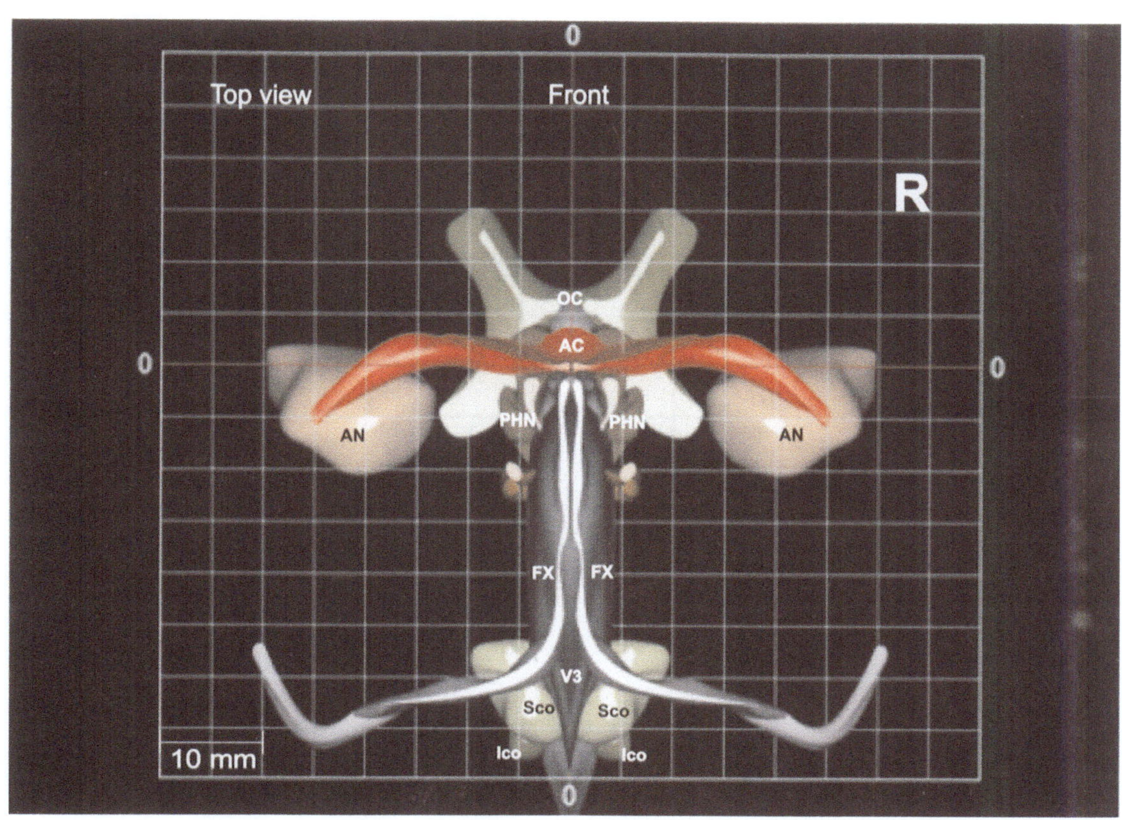


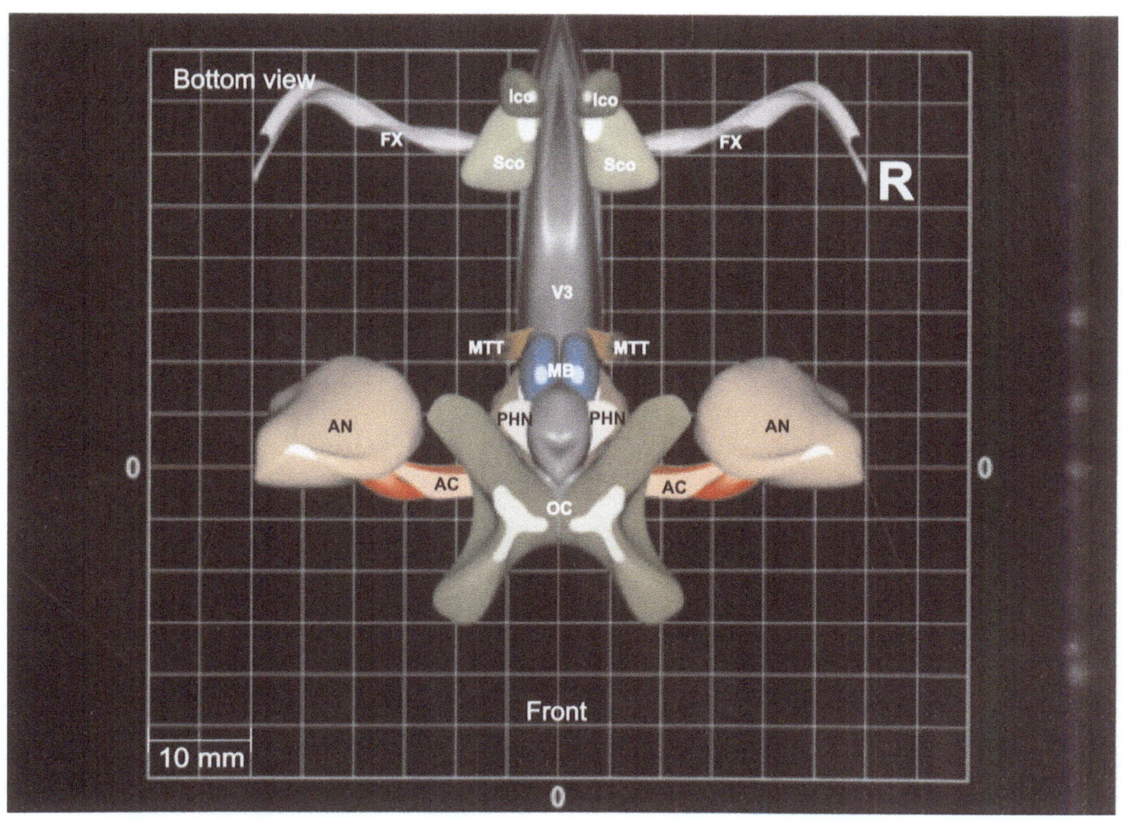

# The Amygdala, Fornix and Periventricular Regions *(continued)*

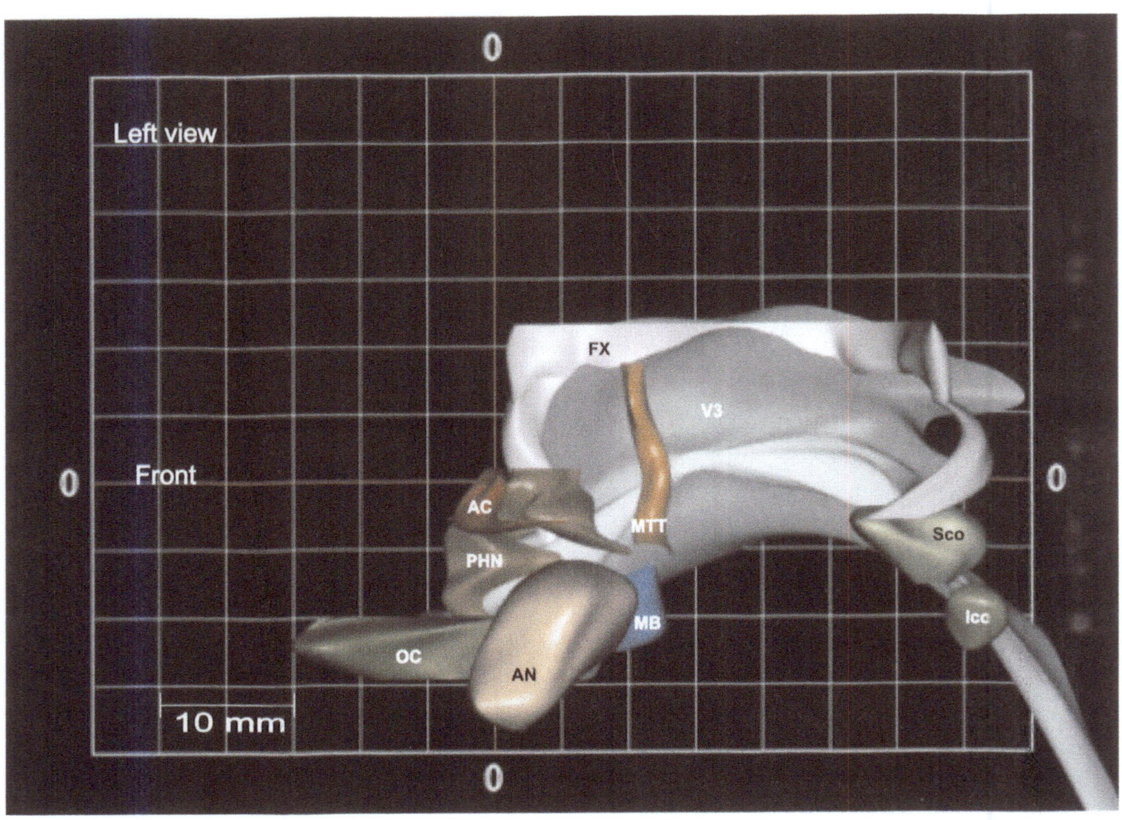


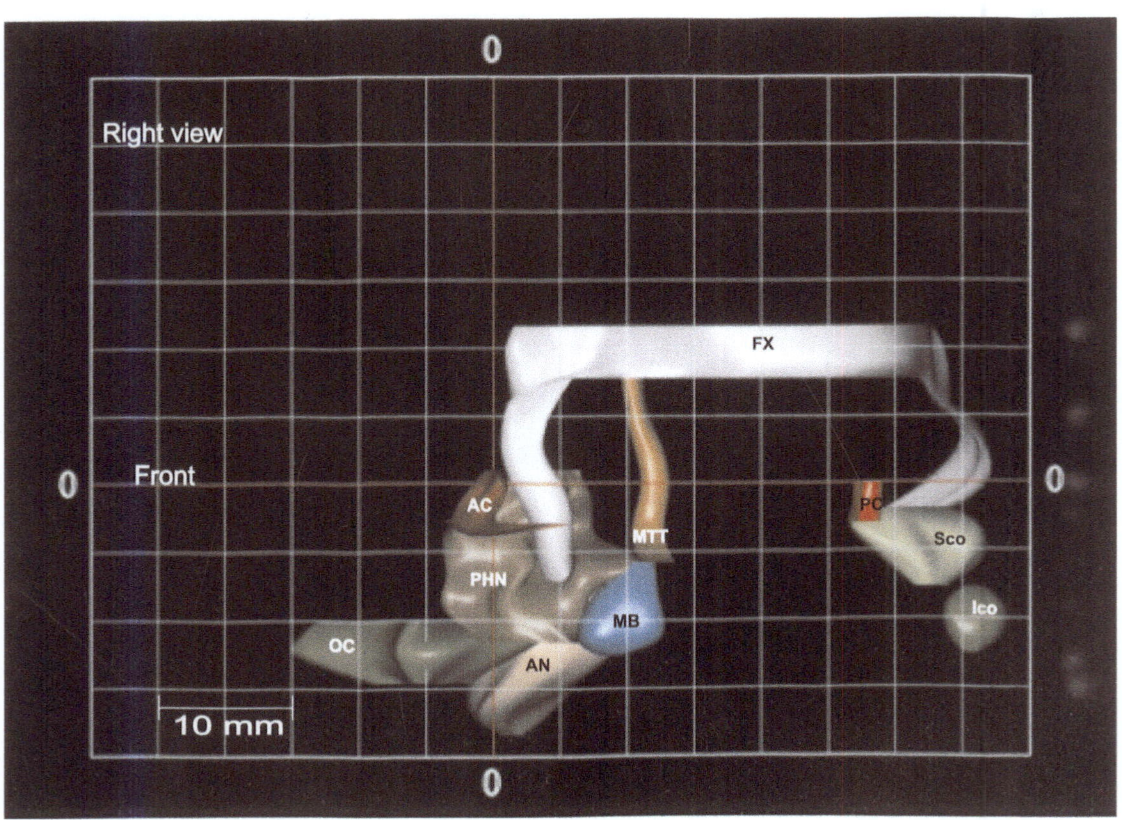

## The Amygdala, Fornix and Periventricular Regions *(continued)*

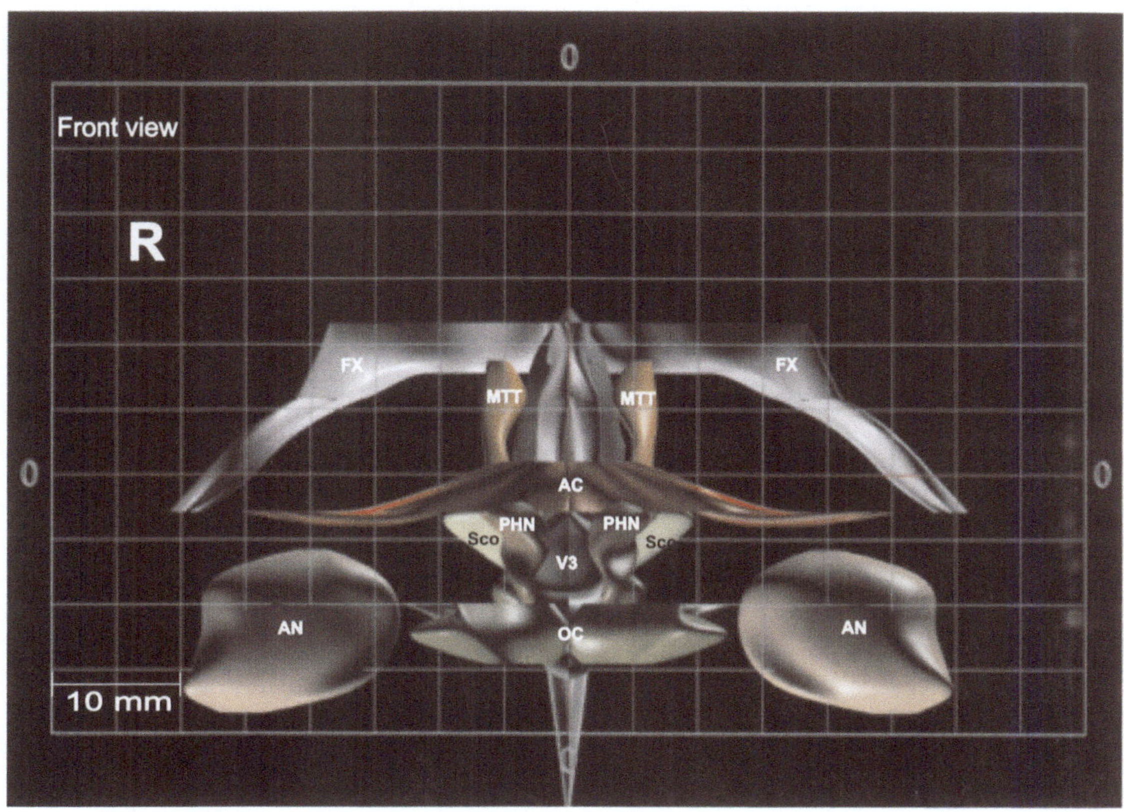


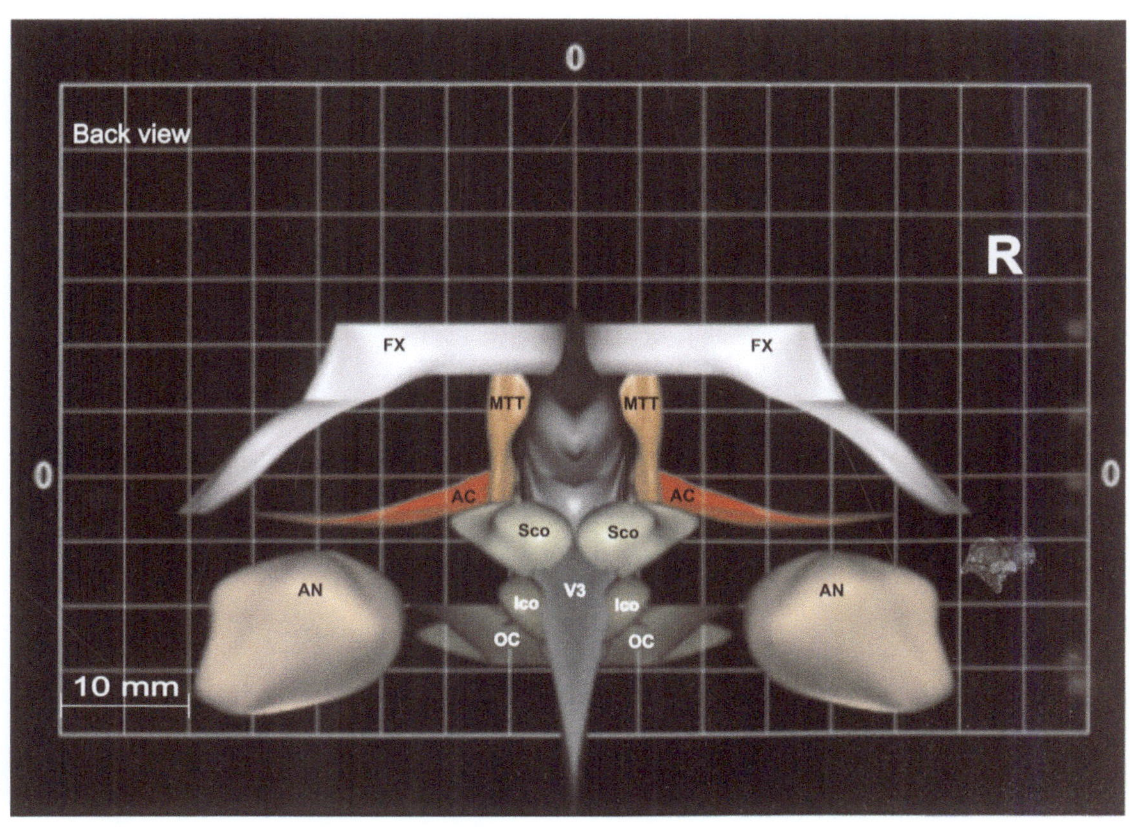

# Bibliography


Derosier C, Delegue G, Munier T, Pharaboz C, Cosnard G (1991) IRM: distorsion géométrique de l'image et stéréotaxie. J Radiol 72: 349–353

Dormont D, Zerah M, Cornu Ph, et al (1994) A technique of measuring the precision of a MR-guided stereotaxic installation using anatomical specimens. AJNR Am J Neuroradiol 15: 365–371

Duvernoy HM (1992) The human brain surfaces: three-dimensional sectional anatomy and MRI. Springer, Vienna

Evans AC, Dai W, Collins L, Neelin P, Marrett S (1991) Warping of a computerized 3-D atlas to match brain images: volumes for quantitative neuroanatomical and functional analysis in medical imaging. 5: Image processing. SPIE 1445: 236-244

Karavel Y, Cesaro P, N'Guyen JP (1985) Vues anatomiques commentées des noyaux gris centraux. Encycl Med Chir Neurologie 17001 H10. Masson, Paris

Kondziolka DE, Dempsey PF, Lunsford LD, et al (1992) Comparison between magnetic resonance imaging and computed tomography for stereotactic coordinate determination. Neurosurgery 30: 402–407

Kelly PJ (1991) Tumor stereotaxis. Saunders, Philadelphia

Kretschmann HJ, Weinrich W (1998) Neurofunctional systems. Thieme, Stuttgart

Lunsford LD (1988) Modern stereotactic neurosurgery. Martinus Nijhoff, Boston

Mai JK, Assheuer J, Paxinos G (1997) Atlas of the human brain. Academic Press, San Diego

Musolino A, Munari C, Betti O, et al (1987) Intérêt et technique du transfert des donnés tomodensitométriques dans les coordonnées stéréotaxique du système Talairach. Rev Electroencephalogr Neurophysiol Clin 17: 11-24

Ricciardi GK, Granata F, Tortorella G, Bramanti P, Longo M (1999) Ruolo della sequenza FIRMS nello studio delle anomalie della migrazione neuronale. Riv Ital Neuroradiol 12 (1): 73-76

Schaltenbrandt G, Wahren W (1977) Atlas for stereotaxy of the human brain, 2nd edn. Thieme, Stuttgart

Schaltenbrandt G, Walker AE (1982) Stereotaxy of the human brain. Thieme, Stuttgart

Szikla G, Bouvier G, Hori T, Petrov V (1977) Angiography of the human brain cortex. Springer, Berlin Heidelberg New York

Talairach J, Tournoux P (1988) Coplanar stereotaxic atlas of the human brain. Thieme, Stuttgart

Talairach J, Tournoux P (1993) Referentially oriented cerebral MRI anatomy. Thieme, Stuttgart

Talairach J, David M , Tournoux P, Corredor H, Ksasina T (1957) Atlas d'anatomie stéréotaxique des noyaux gris centraux. Masson, Paris

Talairach J, Szikla C, Tournoux P, et al (1967) Atlas d'anatomie stéréotaxique du télencéphale. Masson, Paris

Wolansky LJ, Evans A, et al (1996) Fast inversion recovery for myelin suppression (FIRMS). A new MRI pulse sequence for highlighting cerebral gray matter. Clin Imaging 20 (3): 164-170

Wolansky LJ, Chiang PK, et al (1997) Fast inversion recovery for myelin suppression (FIRMS). A new magnetic resonance pulse sequence. J Neuroimaging 7(3): 176-179

Wolansky LJ, Finden SG, Chen J, Hanna R, et al (1999) Optimization of gray/white matter contrast with fast inversion recovery for myelin suppression: a comparison of fast spin-echo and echo-planar MR imaging sequences. Am J Neuroradiol 20: 1653-1657